Moral Resilience

Moral Resilience

Transforming Moral Suffering in Healthcare

SECOND EDITION

Edited by

CYNDA HYLTON RUSHTON PHD, RN, FAAN

OXFORD
UNIVERSITY PRESS

OXFORD
UNIVERSITY PRESS

Oxford University Press is a department of the University of Oxford. It furthers the University's objective of excellence in research, scholarship, and education by publishing worldwide. Oxford is a registered trade mark of Oxford University Press in the UK and certain other countries.

Published in the United States of America by Oxford University Press
198 Madison Avenue, New York, NY 10016, United States of America.

Library of Congress Cataloging-in-Publication Data
Names: Rushton, Cynda H., author, editor.
Title: Moral resilience : transforming moral suffering in healthcare /
edited by Cynda Hylton Rushton.
Description: Second edition. | New York, NY : Oxford University Press, [2024] |
Includes bibliographical references and index. |
Identifiers: LCCN 2024013763 (print) | LCCN 2024013764 (ebook) |
ISBN 9780197667149 (paperback) | ISBN 9780197667163 (epub) |
ISBN 9780197667170 (digital)
Subjects: MESH: Ethics, Professional | Morals | Stress, Psychological |
Resilience, Psychological
Classification: LCC R724 (print) | LCC R724 (ebook) | NLM W 50 |
DDC 174.2—dc23/eng/20240507
LC record available at https://lccn.loc.gov/2024013763
LC ebook record available at https://lccn.loc.gov/2024013764

DOI: 10.1093/oso/9780197667149.001.0001

Printed by Marquis Book Printing, Canada

FSC www.fsc.org MIX Paper | Supporting responsible forestry FSC® C103567

Contents

Acknowledgments vii

Contributors ix

Introduction—CYNDA HYLTON RUSHTON 1

1. Moral Suffering: A Reality of Clinical Practice—CYNDA HYLTON RUSHTON 12

2. What Is Moral Distress? Understanding Context, Sources, and Consequences—ALISA CARSE, TESSY A. THOMAS, AND CYNDA HYLTON RUSHTON 29

3. Mapping the Path of Moral Adversity—CYNDA HYLTON RUSHTON 63

4. Integrity: The Anchor for Moral Resilience—CYNDA HYLTON RUSHTON 100

5. The Many Faces of Resilience—CYNDA HYLTON RUSHTON AND MEREDITH MEALER 133

6. Conceptualizing Moral Resilience—CYNDA HYLTON RUSHTON 162

7. Cultivating Essential Capacities for Moral Resilience—CYNDA HYLTON RUSHTON, ALFRED W. KASZNIAK, AND ROSHI JOAN S. HALIFAX 193

8. Strategies to Restore Integrity—CYNDA HYLTON RUSHTON 228

9. Building the Evidence Base for Moral Resilience—KATIE NELSON, KATHERINE (KATIE) BREWER, HEIDI HOLTZ, AND KATHERINE HEINZE 256

10. Designing Sustainable Systems for Ethical Practice—CYNDA HYLTON RUSHTON AND MONICA SHARMA 271

11. Creating a Culture of Moral Resilience and Ethical Practice—CYNDA HYLTON RUSHTON, MONICA SHARMA, KATHERINE (KATIE) BREWER, AND HEATHER FITZGERALD 309

Afterword: A Vision for the Future—CYNDA HYLTON RUSHTON 356

Index 361

Acknowledgments

No one ever travels alone—and this book is a testament to the synergy and creativity that arise when people with diverse perspectives come together around a shared purpose. I am deeply grateful to my co- authors— Alisa Carse, Roshi Joan S. Halifax, Al Kaszniak, and Monica Sharma. Together we have learned and shared generously in each other's work. I have been deeply inspired by each of you and your unique fingerprints are reflected throughout this book. This edition includes additional colleagues who have generated new insights and applications and extended our collective understanding of moral resilience and ethical practice. My deep gratitude to Heather Fitzgerald, Tessy A. Thomas, Meredith Mealer, Katie Nelson, Heidi Holtz, Katherine (Katie) Brewer, Katherine Heinze for your contributions and colleagueship.

Without the support of Patricia Davidson, former Dean of Johns Hopkins School of Nursing, and Ruth Faden, former Director of the Berman Institute of Bioethics, none of this work would have been possible. Both challenged and encouraged me to pursue documenting what has been learned so far about the concept of moral resilience. They diligently facilitated the opportunity to have the space and focused time to discover, explore, and write.

I am grateful for two fellowship opportunities that led to the inspiration for this book. A Contemplative Studies Fellowship from the Mind and Life Institute allowed me to work with Alisa Carse to refine the philosophical grounding of moral distress that contributed to the concept of moral resilience. The Brocher Foundation Residency Program in Geneva, Switzerland provided the opportunity for me to immerse myself in diverse scholarship and dialogue with other scholars to consider an alternative path for addressing moral suffering. It was during my tenure as a Visiting Scholar that I was inspired to write the proposal for this book. In addition, the opportunity to be a Visiting Scholar at the Upaya Institute in Santa Fe offered a unique opportunity to write in a container of contemplative practice beneath the vast New Mexican sky. The second edition was supported by a sabbatical from Johns Hopkins University that provided time in generative spaces around the world to pause, reflect, and create.

I am enormously grateful for the editorial expertise and advise of Judy Douglas, who was an unwavering partner in preparing the original manuscript for this book. Peter Young for his contribution to the preparation of the manuscript and Meredith Caldwell who stepped up when needed to provide valuable assistance during key periods of book preparation. Theresa Upshaw was instrumental in the management of the second edition. Our research team, including many of the co-authors, along with statistician Ginger Hansen and data analyst Danielle Boyce have contributed greatly to measurement of moral resilience and to our evolving program of research.

I am deeply grateful to the many colleagues, patients, and families who have influenced my career and my understanding of the concepts offered here. I am especially grateful for the clinicians who have shared their moral suffering with me in ways that have had a profound impact on my own journey. Without their honest engagement and willingness to be vulnerable amid their suffering, my own work would be incomplete. I am particularly grateful for my dear colleague, Lindsay Thompson, who has generously listened to and provided critical feedback throughout the writing process.

Finally, I am grateful for the support of my life partner, Weare Zwemer, and my daughters, Hilary and Callie, my most precious dimension of life. They are the light of possibility for the future.

Contributors

Katherine (Katie) Brewer, PhD, MSN, RN, is an assistant professor of nursing at Towson University in Towson, Maryland. Her research focuses on organizational determinants of clinician and healthcare worker well-being, including burnout and resilience. She specializes in the concept of institutional trust and betrayal in healthcare.

Alisa Carse, PhD, is an associate professor of philosophy, faculty affiliate of the Kennedy Institute of Bioethics, Georgetown University. Her teaching and research are centered in moral philosophy, social and political theory, moral psychology, and gender theory.

Heather Fitzgerald, DBe, MS, RN, is director of the Office of Professional Fulfillment and Resilience at Stanford Medicine Children's Health. She provides leadership, content expertise, and program development to promote resilience and well-being, deepen ethical competence, and mitigate moral distress. Her scope includes culture and ethical climate work to create the conditions for healthcare professionals to thrive in their work. Fitzgerald serves nationally on the American Nurses Association Ethics Advisory Board.

Joan S. Halifax, PhD (Roshi), is a Buddhist teacher, author, anthropologist, and social activist. She is the founder, abbot, and head teacher of Upaya Zen Center. She is the author of a number of books, including *Being With Dying: Cultivating Compassion & Fearlessness in the Face of Death; and Standing at the Edge: Finding Freedom Where Fear and Courage Meet.* She is the originator of Upaya's Being With Dying and G.R.A.C.E. programs.

Katherine Heinze, PhD, RN, is an assistant professor at the Christine E. Lynn College of Nursing at Florida Atlantic University. Her teaching and research are centered in Caring Science, moral resilience, and creating ethical systems of practice.

Heidi Holtz, PhD, RN, is an assistant professor of nursing, Barnes Jewish College of Nursing. She is a nurse scientist conducting research designed to promote a healthy work environment, support nurses' well-being, and improve patient outcomes by creating models for high-quality patient care in critical care settings.

Alfred W. Kaszniak, PhD, is a clinical neuroscientist, emeritus professor, and former head of the department of psychology at the University of Arizona, and a Zen Buddhist teacher. He is the author, co-author, or editor of seven books, including the three-volume *Toward a Science of Consciousness*, and over 160 journal articles and scholarly book chapters.

Meredith Mealer, PMHNP, PhD, is an associate professor of medicine at the University of Colorado Anschutz Medical Campus in the Department of Physical Medicine and Rehabilitation. She works clinically as a psychiatric mental health nurse practitioner and her research focuses on depression, anxiety, PTSD, burnout syndrome, and resilience. As a nurse scientist, she has conducted research focusing on resilience, mental health, and healthy workplaces.

Katie Nelson, PhD, RN, is a nurse scientist, clinician, and educator passionate about healthcare access and provision for socially marginalized populations disproportionately burdened by serious illness. Dr. Nelson received her PhD from the Johns Hopkins University School of Nursing and currently works as an assistant scientist in the Johns Hopkins Center for Indigenous Health in the Johns Hopkins Bloomberg School of Public Health.

Cynda Hylton Rushton, MSN, PhD, RN, FAAN, is the Anne and George L. Bunting Professor of Clinical Ethics in the Johns Hopkins Berman Institute of Bioethics and the School of Nursing, with a joint appointment in the School of Medicine's Department of Pediatrics. A founding member of the Berman Institute of Bioethics, Dr. Rushton co-chairs the Johns Hopkins Hospital's Ethics Committee and Consultation Service. She is a Fellow of the American Academy of Nursing, a Hasting's Center Fellow and author of over 250 journal articles and scholarly book chapters. She is co-creator of the Rushton Moral Resilience Scale-16 (RMRS-16) and leads Maryland's R^3:Resilient Nurses Initiative.

Monica Sharma, MD trained as a physician and epidemiologist, worked for the United Nations for twenty-three years, directing programs for whole systems transformation and leadership development worldwide.

Currently, she works with the United Nations, universities, management institutions, governments, non-governmental organizations, business, media, and other organizations. She created a unique response based on extensive application—a conscious full-spectrum model—and generated equitable and sustainable results related to several Sustainable Development Goals, worldwide. She is the author of the award-winning book *Radical Transformational Leadership*.

Tessy A. Thomas, DO, MBE, is an assistant professor of pediatrics and bioethics at Geisinger Commonwealth School of Medicine and Geisinger Medical Center in Pennsylvania. Clinically, she is a pediatric critical care physician. Her teaching and research interests are centered on moral distress, professional integrity, professionalism, and professional identity formation of healthcare professionals.

Introduction

Cynda Hylton Rushton

MY PERSONAL AND professional journey with suffering began when I was a nursing assistant, witnessing the incredible resilience of young children with cystic fibrosis as they struggled with the intensive treatment regimen, the frequent and prolonged setbacks, hospitalizations, and their slow and untimely dying process. Alongside them were parents, sometimes dealing with more than one affected child, doing their best to meet the demands of their child's illness and treatment while balancing myriad competing obligations, confusion, uncertainty, and grief. After I graduated from nursing school, I began my career as a graduate nurse in the pediatric intensive care unit, at a time when technological advances were escalating but there were many diseases and injuries still not amenable to cure or rehabilitation. Suffering was a constant companion alongside miraculous and unpredicted recoveries. Later, I helped care for an infant who was neurologically devastated following accidental asphyxiation. For almost two years, my fellow nurses and I went through the motions of caring for her body while trying to make sense of a situation riddled with dissonance and conflicting emotions. When her parents' request that life-sustaining treatments be ended, allowing her to die, was rejected, we practiced in a climate of moral outrage and fear. When she died from sepsis, we experienced profound relief. In a culture of "power on," I had no words to articulate the impact of my own suffering. This was the job; there was no time for sadness or despair. Ethics committees or staff support systems were non-existent; we were expected to take care of it ourselves and not let visible evidence of our distress accompany us to work.

Cynda Hylton Rushton, *Introduction* In: *Moral Resilience*. Second Edition. Edited by: Cynda Hylton Rushton, Oxford University Press. © Oxford University Press 2024. DOI: 10.1093/oso/9780197667149.003.0001

In the mid-1980s, I practiced at a children's hospital where I cared for very premature neonates and infants suffering from congenital malformations, children experiencing trauma or cancer treatment. Ethical questions about the boundaries of innovative therapies to extend life and their consequences on the infants and their families were a daily conundrum. When a series of "Baby Doe" cases fueled a national debate on this issue, I was invited to represent the nursing perspective in the hospital's newly created interdisciplinary infant care review committee.[1]

Later, at another children's hospital, I became involved in one of the first institutionally based clinical ethics programs in the nation. There I worked with a physician and a philosopher to implement an ethics consultation process, develop policies, and stimulate interdisciplinary dialogue through routine ethics rounds. I became engaged in a wide range of ethics issues and began to work as a clinical ethics consultant and educator, translating complex ethical concepts into clinical practice within an interdisciplinary model. In my newly created role as nursing liaison, I learned from other nurses and clinicians that the moral suffering they experienced was often a response to their sense of moral failing and threats or violations to their integrity.[1,2,3,4]

These ongoing encounters led me to write about professional caregiver suffering. It was influenced by my conversations over several years with Warren T. Reich, who had written one of the seminal articles on suffering, together with my personal experiences as a nurse and ethicist. Reich defined suffering as "an anguish experienced as a threat to our composure, our integrity, the fulfillment of our intentions, and more deeply as a frustration to the concrete meaning that we have found in our personal experience. It is the anguish over the injury or threat to the injury to the self and thus the meaning of the self that is at the core of suffering."[5(p85)] I seized upon this definition to expand my understanding of the clinical realities facing nurses and other healthcare professionals. For me, it became a vehicle that allowed me to articulate positive and negative responses to suffering and to explore the relationships between concepts related to moral suffering, including conscience violations and moral distress. Participating in clinical ethics education and consultation, together with ongoing conceptual and theoretical exploration, naturally led to an exploration of the meaning of integrity. Given Reich's definition of suffering, the threat to one's wholeness is a particular kind of suffering that engages the moral aspects of our lives.[5] I began to examine the contours of integrity and conscience in clinical practice[3,4].

Beginning in the late 1990s, my clinical interests and clinical ethics consultation practice led me to focus on the ethical issues embedded in palliative and end-of-life care. As co-chair of the Johns Hopkins Hospital Ethics Committee and Consultation Service since 1999, I found that many consultations involved to some extent moral suffering and distress. My exploration of the nature of suffering within this context expanded to include different worldviews that yielded a deeper understanding of compassion, empathy, and the nature of suffering itself. As part of a Kornfeld Fellowship in ethics and palliative and end-of-life care, I participated in a novel interdisciplinary program, *Being With Dying: Compassionate Care of the Dying,* that introduced me to previously unexplored methods to address the inevitable suffering that arises at the end of life. I found that the Buddhist notions of suffering and compassion resonated with my clinical experiences and offered a new lens with which to engage, rather than reject, the suffering that patients, families, and clinicians were experiencing. More and more I grew to understand what His Holiness the Dalai Lama meant when he wrote, "It is our suffering that is the most basic element that we share with others, the factor that unifies us with all living creatures."[6]

I spent the next year developing a mindfulness practice with training in Mindfulness-Based Stress Reduction (MBSR)[7] and exploring how experiential programs such as the Healer's Art could be applied to the care of dying people.[8] As I explored how clinicians experienced suffering and moral distress, the interconnections came into sharper focus, clarifying how best to cultivate individual skills and create more holistic and healing practice environments.[9]

My interest in the moral aspects of suffering led to examining the concept of moral distress through the lens of contemplative practice and an evolving vision of ethics as embodied, lived, and embedded in all aspects of our interconnected existence rather than a more narrowly defined view of ethics as limited to moments of conflict, confusion, or dilemmas alone. As I joined the faculty of the *Being With Dying* program[10] and developed my own meditation practice and insights along my personal journey, I began to realize the importance of training the mind to reduce reactivity and confusion, to focus on what really mattered, and to cultivate the conditions that supported compassionate, ethical practice.[11] These skills, cultivated over more than two decades, have informed my approach to clinical ethics and the elements so often missing in typical bioethics discourse, in particular the absence of somatic grounding within the practice of clinical ethics and the need for specific skills and practices to enable integrity and ethical practice. Likewise, a shift in thinking occurred: our suffering was not something to hide or be suppressed.[12] It must be skillfully worked so that we can transform it to fuel a future of integrity and compassion rather than allow it to disable our basic human goodness and moral community. Rather than seeing our suffering as weakness, we can view it as a raw material that is needed to build strength and resilience that we can leverage to sustain our integrity, caring practices, clinical expertise, and well-being so that our patients and their loved ones receive quality, safe, and compassionate care.

Leveraging the growing body of neuroscience research related to our work in the *Being With Dying* program,[10,11] I partnered with Dr. Al Kazniack and Dr. Joan Halifax, Roshi to apply the neuroscientific research and contemplative practice to develop a framework for understanding and responding to morally distressing situations.[12,13] This led to new insights for designing interventions to support clinicians so they can be with the inevitable situations of moral distress by employing new tools, practices, and mindsets. These were refined and used within the *Being With Dying* professional training and in continuing education offerings locally and nationally. Later, they were incorporated into the design of the Mindful Ethical Practice and Resilience Academy, a program designed to cultivate mindfulness, ethical competence, and resilience in nurses.[14,15]

During this time, I was fortunate to receive a Mind and Life Institute Contemplative Science Fellowship to explore the how strategies for moral distress might be enhanced with contemplative practices. Dr. Alisa Carse, a moral philosopher, and I embarked on a philosophical journey to deepen our understanding of the concept and to develop an alternative paradigm for understanding it. As a doctoral student taking bioethics courses at Georgetown University, Dr. Carse, along with Warren Reich, introduced me to an emerging and contemporary perspective of an ethic of care as a means for understanding moral and ethical complexities from a new vantage point. It was a rich area of exploration that resonated with my clinical experience and instincts about the territory of clinical ethics. We share a longstanding line of inquiry into various dimensions of moral psychology and its application to the challenges that arise in various contexts, including clinical practice. Dr. Carse was already steeped in philosophical inquiry into vulnerability, shame, regret, and the importance of pro-social skills such as empathy.[17,18] These insights were instrumental in shifting our understanding of the phenomena involved.[19,20,21]

Simultaneously, I was examining how the evolving concept of organizational ethics aligned with efforts to address individual moral suffering. It led me to consider the broader context of organizational ethics and the implications for integrity.[4,22] Creating an environment that allows caregivers to practice with integrity is no simple task. Strategies to promote the integrity of the person being cared for, their family, the healthcare professional, the institution, and the community require multi-pronged efforts.[4,22,23] Understanding the suffering of another demands that we enter into that individual's experience and engage in the dynamic process of learning to be with it, understand it, and potentially give meaning to it. Only through a commitment to a shared vision that embodies robust values of respect, compassion, and justice can clinicians and healthcare institutions successfully impact the experience of suffering and its effect on the quality of patient care. After years of focusing on the hospital context, I met and began to collaborate with Dr. Monica Sharma, former director of Leadership and Capacity Building at the United Nations, who developed a highly effective and sustainable approach to systems transformation and leadership. We worked together for three years as consultants to support the launch of the University of Virginia's Compassionate Care Initiative using the Conscious Full Spectrum model.[24,25] This spurred interest in examining the contours of an enabling environment that supported integrity and ethical practice and continued practice in using the methods in various contexts. In parallel to this, I began collaborating with colleagues at the Johns Hopkins Hospital to design interventions aimed at bolstering a healthy workplace. Several years later we developed a three-part series, Toward a Culture of Ethical Practice in Healthcare (TCEP), that engaged teams from healthcare institutions across the country to apply the model to their own environments.

As the years unfolded, I became increasingly concerned about the lack of meaningful strategies to change the reality of the moral suffering of clinicians, particularly moral distress. Innovative and passionate leaders had embarked on a broad range of strategies, yet the data continued to mount indicating that the prevalence of moral distress was escalating and expanding to other members of the clinical team. I spent the better part of two years examining the burgeoning scholarship on the sources and consequences of moral distress on clinicians and the relative dearth of solutions to the individual- and system-level contributions to the problem. While a visiting scholar at the Brocher Institute in Geneva, Switzerland, in 2015, I had the space and time to step back from the work and to explore two critical questions: What is the alternative to moral distress and suffering? What would help us shift our thinking in a way that might produce alternative solutions? In this process, a few authors suggested the term *moral resilience* as a promising direction. The concept, although not well developed, resonated as a concept worth pursuing. That began the next phase of my conceptual, theoretical, and empirical research[26].

The first edition of this book was the culmination of over three years of conceptual research and synthesis of empirical evidence. Since 2018, the concept has evolved,[27,28,29] a measure of moral resilience has been developed and tested,[30,31] and a program of research has been launched.[29,32,33,34,35,36,37] Concurrently, the issues of burnout and the contribution to it of moral suffering were gaining national attention. I was honored to be part of the National Academies committee that produced the report: Taking Action Against Clinician Burnout: A Systems Approach to Professional Wellbeing.[38] The report outlined the complex interplay of individual and systemic factors that combine to create the conditions for workplace burnout. Since then, a variety of national organizations have aligned to focus support for research, education, policy, and practice innovations. Importantly, the COVID-19 pandemic focused attention again on these long-standing fissures in the healthcare system that have contributed to moral suffering and degraded well-being. These systemic factors have been exacerbated by the crush of the pandemic and have left a deep and painful moral residue and an alarming exodus of trained clinicians from their jobs and the profession. These realities are fuel for designing comprehensive, multi-faceted interventions that restore the integrity and well-being of clinicians and help to dismantle the systemic patterns that have undermined it. There is renewed urgency for foundational paradigm shifts and new models of designing and implementing change. Our hope is that our scholarship and vision will offer fuel for those courageous innovators who will lead us into the future.

The Contours of This Book

What is included in this book is truly a work in progress. While progress has been made, much more conceptual, empirical, and practical work needs to be done. This edition represents the collaboration of wise and generous colleagues who have substantially informed the direction of my scholarship and thinking in a hybrid edited text that explicitly honors their seminal contributions. It is one pathway for approaching the complex and interconnected realities of clinicians who are exposed daily to moral adversity. It is a humble offering of what we have gleaned so far from a synthesis of literature, experience, and ongoing contemplative practice. We have extensively reviewed the literature within specific contexts, and there are likely areas deserving of more exploration and applied perspectives outside of traditional healthcare contexts. We invite others to work with us to expand our understandings and to embrace new ways of approaching the persistent and recalcitrant problem of moral suffering and burnout in the health professions.

In the first two chapters, we explore the nature and consequences of moral suffering, a concept that is ripe for further refinement and exploration as a broader container for the many forms of moral suffering that arise in clinical practice. This broader lens offers an opportunity to explore the contours of the anguish and despair that clinicians carry with them and to consider what might be needed to transform their experience in ways that would reduce their distress and potentially propel them toward new understanding and meaning of themselves and others. Next, we examine the extensive and excellent scholarship focused on moral distress as a particular type of suffering. The literature is summarized and a call for a new paradigm is offered. In Chapter 3 we turn to synthesizing several conceptual views to create a conceptual map that suggests a pathway for examining their interrelationship, beginning with moral adversity as the instigator of moral stress, which unrelieved can lead to various forms of moral suffering, including moral distress and moral injury. We explore collateral responses of moral apathy, moral outrage, moral disengagement, and moral decline. The concepts of moral resilience and moral repair are introduced.

In Chapter 4, the concept of integrity as the core of moral resilience is examined through the lens of personal, professional, and relational integrity and the role of conscience in detecting situations that imperil our integrity. We elaborate on the various situations and circumstances that imperil integrity in clinical practice. With this as the foundation, we explore the concept of moral resilience in Chapter 5 by first exploring the extensive scholarship on the broader concept of resilience in the context of biology, psychology, and social ecology, and as applied to clinicians. Building on these threads, in Chapter 6 we define and articulate the concept of moral resilience with particular emphasis on the context of clinical practice.

In Chapters 7 and 8, we turn to specific strategies for cultivating various individual capacities for moral resilience. These include strategies to foster self-awareness and self-regulation, reflection and insight, ethical competence, self-stewardship, and transformational learning. Alongside these foundational capacities and skills, attention is needed to restore integrity by developing specific methods for moral repair.

Chapter 9 explores the evolution of measuring moral resilience using the Rushton Moral Resilience Scale (RMRS).[31] This scale is the only validated measure of moral resilience to date, and the chapter highlights the development of the scale and results from various studies.[29] Future directions for measurement of moral resilience are examined.

In Chapters 10 and 11 we shift to exploring the interface between individual moral resilience and a culture of ethical practice. Using the Conscious Full Spectrum Response (CFSR), we apply the concepts to create a template for moral resilience and ethical practice. This template offers a promising direction for leveraging individual moral resilience capacities to design systemic solutions to the sources of moral suffering that are results-oriented and sustainable. The Conscious Full Spectrum Response has been used worldwide and applied to diverse contexts to address recalcitrant systemic problems.

This book is offered as a catalyst for ongoing refinement and empirical exploration. We look forward to learning of the constructive and innovative ways our work will inform future breakthroughs. The goal is to support clinicians to transform their moral suffering with the capacities of moral resilience so that they can serve the people they are dedicated to with greater compassion, wisdom, and ease. Our research has demonstrated that moral resilience offers clinicians a protective resource that can be amplified. We also have evidence that the combination of empowered moral resilience and increased organizational effectiveness has the greatest potential to reduce the detrimental effects of moral adversity and suffering.[29,34,36] This cannot occur without fundamental shifts within our healthcare organizations and society. The solutions to the current reality so beleaguered by the weight of moral suffering will require new mindsets and paradigms and innovative methods to make and sustain progress. The needs are urgent, and we must take the long view in designing solutions that leverage both individual and system strategies—one without the other will be insufficient. Our hope is that clinicians and healthcare leaders will commit to bold steps to address the systemic patterns that undermine clinician integrity by being part of an emerging learning community where innovation and trust thrives. Readers are invited to explore this context with a generous and open heart and leverage the possibilities for healing our healthcare system and ourselves. Together we can transform ourselves and align our efforts in ways we cannot currently imagine creating a new paradigm for healthcare and healing the wounds of moral suffering.

References

1. Rushton C. Caregiver suffering: finding meaning when integrity is threatened. In Haddad A, Pinch W, editors, Nursing and health care ethics: a legacy and a vision. Washington, DC: American Nurses Publishing; 2009, 293–306.
2. Rushton CH. Caregiver suffering in critical care nursing. Heart Lung. 1992; 21:303–306.
3. Rushton CH. The baby K case: ethical challenges of preserving professional integrity. Pediatr Nurs. 1995;21:367–372.
4. Rushton CH, Scanlon C. When values conflict with obligations: safeguards or nurses. Pediatr Nurs. 1995;21:260–261, 268.
5. Reich WT. Speaking of suffering: a moral account of compassion. Soundings. 1989;72:83–108. Available at http://www.jstor.org/stable/41178467
6. Lama D (HH), Cutler H. Art of happiness. London: Hodder-Stoughton; 1998.
7. Kabat-Zinn J. Full catastrophe living: using the wisdom of your body and mind to face stress, pain and illness. New York: Delacourt Press; 2005.
8. Remen RN. The healer's art [Internet]. n.d. [cited August 12, 2023] Available at www.rachelremen.com/learn/medical-education-work/the-healers-art/.
9. Rushton CH, Reder E, Hall B, Comello K, Sellers DE, Hutton N. Interdisciplinary interventions to improve pediatric palliative care and reduce health care professional suffering. J Palliat Med. 2006;9:922–933.
10. Halifax J, Dossey B, Rushton C. Compassionate care of the dying: an integral approach. Sante Fe, NM: Prajna Mountain Publishers; 2006.
11. Rushton CH, Sellers DE, Heller KS, Spring B, Dossey BM, Halifax J. Impact of a contemplative end-of-life training program: being with dying. Palliat Support Care. 2009;7:405–414.
12. Rushton CH. Caregiver Suffering In Carter BS, Levetown M, editors. Palliative care for infants, children & adolescents: a practical handbook. Baltimore, MD: Johns Hopkins University Press; 2004: 220–243.
13. Rushton CH, Kaszniak AW, Halifax JS. A framework for understanding moral distress among palliative care clinicians. J Palliat Med. 2013;16:1074–1079.
14. Rushton CH, Kaszniak AW, Halifax JS. Addressing moral distress: application of a framework to palliative care practice. J Palliat Med. 2013;16:1080–1088.
15. Rushton C, Swoboda S, Reller N, Skrupski K, Prizzi M, Young P, Hanson G. Mindful ethical practice and resilience academy: equipping nurses to address ethical challenges, Amer J Crit Care. 2021;30(1): e1–e11.
16. Rushton C, Swoboda S, Reimer T, Boyce D, Hansen, G. The Mindful Ethical Practice & Resilience Academy (MEPRA): Sustainability of impact. Amer J Crit Care. 2023;32(3):184–194.

17. Carse A. Vulnerability, agency and human flourishing. In Taylor CR, Dell'Oro R, editors. Health and human flourishing: religion, medicine, and moral anthropology. Washington, DC: Georgetown University Press; 2006, 33–52.
18. Carse A. The moral contours of empathy. Ethical Theory Moral Pract. 2005;8:169–195.
19. Carse A. Moral distress and moral disempowerment. Narrat Inq Bioeth. 2013;3(2):147–151.
20. Rushton, CH, Carse, A. Towards a new narrative of moral distress: realizing the potential of resilience. J Clin Ethics, 2016;27:214–218.
21. Carse A, Rushton CH. Harnessing the promise of moral distress: a call for re-orientation. J Clin Ethics. 2017;28:15–29.
22. Rushton, CH., Brooks-Brunn, JA. Environments that support ethical practice. New Horizons. 1997;5:20–29.
23. Rushton CH. Creating a culture of ethical practice in health care delivery systems. Hastings Cent Rep. 2016;46(S1):S28–S31.
24. Sharma M. Radical transformational leadership: strategic action for change agents. San Francisco, CA: North Atlantic Books; 2017.
25. Fontaine DK, Rushton CH, Sharma M. Cultivating compassion and empathy. In Plews-Ogan M, Beyt G, editors. Wisdom leadership in academic health science centers: leading positive change. London: Radcliffe Publishing; 2014, 92–110.
26. Young P, Rushton C. Concept analysis Moral Resilience, Nursing Outlook. 2017;65(5): 579–587.
27. Rushton CH, Schoonover-Shoffner K, Kennedy MS. A collaborative state of the science initiative: transforming moral distress into moral resilience in nursing. Amer J Nurs. 2017; 117(S2): S2–S6.
28. Rushton CH. Cultivating moral resilience. Amer J Nurs. 2017; 117(2-S1): S11–S15.
29. Rushton, C. Transforming moral suffering by cultivating moral resilience and ethical practice. Amer J Crit Care. 2023;32 (4): 238–248.
30. Holtz H, Heinze K, Rushton C. Inter-professionals' definitions of moral resilience. J Clin Nurs. 2017;27(3-4):e488–e494.
31. Heinze KE, Hanson G, Holtz H, Swoboda SM, & Rushton CH. Measuring health care interprofessionals' moral resilience: validation of the Rushton Moral Resilience Scale. J Pall Med. 2021;24(6): 865–872.
32. Antonsdottir I, Rushton CH, Nelson KE, Heinze KE, Swoboda SM, & Hanson GC. Burnout and moral resilience in interdisciplinary healthcare professionals. J Clin Nurs. 2021;00: 1–13
33. Thomas TA, Davis FD, Kumar S, Thammasitboon S, & Rushton CH. COVID-19 and moral distress: a pediatric critical care survey. Amer J Crit Care. 2021; e1–e19.

34. Rushton CH, Thomas T, Antonsdottir I, Nelson K, Boyce D, Vioral A, Swavley D, Ley C, Hanson G. Moral injury, ethical concerns and moral resilience in health care workers during COVID-19 pandemic. Jour Pall Med. 2021; 25(5):712–719.
35. Swavely D, Weissinger G, Holtz H, Aldi T, Alderfer M, Lynn L, Rushton C. The impact of traumatic stress, resilience, and threats to core values on nurses during a pandemic. J Nurs Admin. 2022;52(10): 525–535.
36. Rushton C, Nelson K, Antonsdottir I, Hanson G, Boyce D. Perceived organizational effectiveness, moral injury, and moral resilience among nurses during the COVID-19 pandemic: Secondary analysis. Nurs Manag. 2022;53(7):12–22.
37. Rushton, C. Transforming moral suffering by cultivating moral resilience and ethical practice. American Journal of Critical Care. 2023; 32 (4): 238–248.
38. National Academies of Sciences, Engineering, and Medicine. Taking action against clinician burnout: a systems approach to professional well-being. Washington, DC: The National Academies Press; 2019.

1

Moral Suffering

A REALITY OF CLINICAL PRACTICE

Cynda Hylton Rushton

SUFFERING IS AN inherent dimension of being human. None of us is immune to its consequences; all of us experience some adversity that gives rise to various forms and intensities of suffering throughout our lives. *The way suffering is experienced is dependent upon context, capabilities, and resources. There is no uniform experience of suffering; it is experienced personally and uniquely and impacts one's whole being. Clinicians have been engaged in an intimate relationship with suffering since there have been disease, treatment, and death. Its incidence and intensity have increased with the growth of technology, complexity of care, organizational and societal demands, and diversity of moral viewpoints. Clinicians regularly confront the pain and suffering of the treatments they prescribe and administer in the attempt to ameliorate or palliate disease, injury, or symptoms. They witness the attempts of the people they serve as they struggle to navigate often-unfathomable challenges and sometimes defy predictions of disability, quality of life, or death. They see firsthand the indignities of treatment and disease that erode a person's moral agency, self-image, and confidence and,

* Portions of this chapter are from *Nursing and Health Care Ethics: A Legacy and A Vision* (p. 360), by A. Haddad and W. Pinch, 2008, Silver Spring, MD: American Nurses Association. Copyright 2008 by the American Nurses Association. Adapted with permission.

Cynda Hylton Rushton, *Moral Suffering* In: *Moral Resilience*. Second Edition. Edited by: Cynda Hylton Rushton, Oxford University Press. © Oxford University Press 2024. DOI: 10.1093/oso/9780197667149.003.0002

more subtly, the sense of meaning and hope. All the while they also bear witness to the depletion of financial resources and the stress of those who desperately hope for their loved one's recovery or continued life. Increasingly these forms of suffering are intensified because of systemic societal, political, and organizational constraints and disparities. And they witness the strength of people's life force, determination, and resilience as they transcend their physical, emotional, or spiritual suffering to overcome adversity and become whole again after devastating circumstances.

Suffering can arise intermittently or be sustained over long periods along a spectrum of intensity and consequences. It can involve feelings such as unsettledness, irritation, anxiety, frustration, or disappointment over situations or experiences that provoke confusion or uncertainty or do not turn out as we had hoped. More intense feelings such as desperation, sadness, agony, or anguish also arise when our aspirations, goals, values, and commitments are imperiled in some profound way. Suffering leaves an indelible imprint on the psyche of the person experiencing it. We are hardwired, it seems, to remember our suffering; we integrate its details into both conscious and unconscious parts of our psyches, our bodies, and our minds. When a suffering experience is unprocessed or unresolved and remains outside conscious awareness, the response to it may reappear when similar experiences of suffering occur or appear in unrelated situations as inappropriate or disproportionate responses.

The experience of suffering often leaves the person feeling exposed and vulnerable. At its root is the sense of having no control over one's destiny, "of submitting to or being forced to endure some particular set of circumstances."[1(p28)] This view of suffering as a passive process tends to leave the person feeling victimized and powerless; it is often reinforced by a view of suffering as an inevitable part of certain experiences, diseases, or roles. Some clinicians, for example, view the suffering they experience on behalf of the people they serve as an expected aspect of their profession and therefore reject their own suffering as a legitimate moral claim. Others believe that suffering has redemptive value and "builds character," while still others hold that it does not build character, but rather reveals it.[1] Regardless of the meaning assigned to the experience of suffering, both positive and negative consequences are possible. Suffering may offer the motivation to grow, learn, re-order one's priorities, and transcend its despair and anguish or it may lead to a fragmented, tormented way of being that is alienated from what matters most and leaves the person in a perpetual and unrelenting experience of misery and despair. According to Hauerwas, "[Suffering] may reveal us as better or worse than we thought ourselves to be. Suffering can just as easily destroy us as it can make us more resolute."[2(p26)]

Clinicians who are dedicated to serving others suffer in myriad ways. Although the source and consequences of their suffering may be unacknowledged, honored, or addressed, the residue can persist. When asked to reflect on situations in their clinical practice that have stayed with them, clinicians can recount the events surrounding a situation that caused them suffering many years later, with more vivid detail than they can give for an event occurring only a few days previously.[3] Their version of suffering can be related to failing to prevent or causing harm to self or others; witnessing acts of interpersonal violence ranging from disregard for the opinions of others to blatant bullying or misuse of power or authority; or pervasive injustices of our social and economic systems that contribute to disease, disability, or death.[4] They also suffer when they witness or participate in decisions or activities that cause senseless or unnecessary suffering to others. These and other examples are part of everyday clinical practice. Suffering is an inescapable aspect of clinical practice and embedded in it is a deep moral thread. Although some specialties and settings seem to carry a greater intensity than others, it is present in some form in all aspects of clinical care. Many clinicians have never had the opportunity to acknowledge, name, or release the grip of their own suffering or the suffering of those they are dedicated to care for. There is a reticence to share their suffering with others fearing that doing so will render them weak, ineffective, or incapable of managing the fallout. This "conspiracy of silence" extends to unspoken professional norms that seemingly prohibit clinicians from sharing their concerns about their actions with the people they serve to protect them from the confusion or to share in their struggles to be with the dissonance created by their competing moral obligations and responsibilities. These realities are exacerbated by the systems and structures of healthcare organizations that contribute to them. New evidence suggests that discordant values between clinicians and their organizations contribute to decreased compassion and job satisfaction and increased absenteeism, burnout, and contemplation of early retirement.[5] While there is no prescriptive way to suffer or respond to it, there is a moral art in doing so.

The Moral Dimensions of Suffering

Broadly understood, suffering is the anguish in response to real or perceived threats to our intentions, commitments, personal/professional identity, meaning in life, and sense of wholeness as a person.[6] Within the moral domain, it involves various forms of moral investment or commitment that are threatened or imperiled. Specifically, it is the anguish experienced in response to various forms of moral adversity including moral harms, wrongs or failures, or unrelieved moral stress. It is an embodied state of awareness that begins with the perception of somatic sensations or symptoms before the individual becomes cognitively aware of the source of it.[7,8,9] Moral suffering can be triggered by witnessing, participating in, or directly precipitating situations that produce a wide range of negative moral outcomes, such as observing a clinician speak to a patient who has recently immigrated to America in a condescending or disrespectful manner; participating in treatment plans that prolong an inevitable death; handling the bodies of unconscious patients in harsh, uncaring ways; or observing members of our team demean or dismiss our moral concerns or those of others. It can also arise when one fails to uphold an important moral value or standard or in some other way falls short from a moral point of view; in these situations, the response commonly includes the activation of conscience signifying a threat to one's integrity. Clinicians who work in situations where pressures for efficiency, throughput, or inadequate staffing are prominent may acutely or chronically experience moral suffering in response to the dissonance between their professional values and their organizational mandates. Most fundamentally at stake are one's moral values and commitments that can be ignored, challenged, or violated, leading to a loss of self-esteem, self-confidence, or moral wholeness. It can also be precipitated in response to moral betrayal and unresolved moral dissonance that can lead to various forms of moral alienation, fatigue, or indifference.

Moral suffering has its roots in our concern for others and our intention to bring about beneficial outcomes, to relieve the pain and suffering of others, or to rectify an injustice. Suffering for and with another person ignites our innate capacities for compassion. We are intrinsically oriented toward compassion in response to suffering. Caring for others signifies a moral concern for them as persons and for their well-being and a commitment to act on their behalf to reduce or relieve their suffering. It involves being able to be present to their suffering, attune to it, and leverage moral investment, emotional engagement, and wise discernment to act on behalf of another. It connotes a strong sense of responsibility to attend to and respond to the holistic needs of another and, in the case of healthcare professionals, to provide individualized care and services to those in their care. These moral sentiments are reflected in the foundational documents of the medical, nursing, and social work professions and the intentions arising from the calling to serve others.[10,11,12]

Clinicians witness the suffering that accompanies illness or injury—the indignities and the damage to the patient's self-image, the depletion of financial and human resources, the stress of families who desperately hope for their loved one's recovery and the anxiety born of the sense of powerlessness in a situation beyond their control. Clinicians suffer because they understand and identify with the sufferings of the patient and family. Nurses, in particular, experience this suffering in an intimate way. In their roles, they have the most sustained proximity to the patient and they directly carry out the treatment plan. They witness the impact of their ministrations on the patient and family and sometimes struggle to make sense of interventions they may view as harmful or senseless.

The threat to one's wholeness is a particular kind of suffering that engages the moral aspects of our lives; integrity is a central feature of moral suffering. Clinicians struggle to find the place of integrity in their relationships so that they do not suffer for and with others to the point of their own detriment or the detriment of their patients. As they fulfill their obligations and expectations as professionals, they may encounter threats to their ideal of their profession and professional goals, their self-image, moral character, and personal or professional identity. Suffering, loss, and fear are intrinsic and inevitable dimensions of caring for patients and their families. Many clinicians have reported being ill prepared to address suffering with their patients, much less their own. Claiming their own suffering with its inherent threats to integrity may be why professionals caring for patients may feel threatened if they "get too close" and allow themselves to experience grief or love. As Barnard[13] noted, they may fear that this level of intimacy will threaten their ability to continue to function in their professional roles. These threads of the culture of clinical care contribute to the isolation, lack of acknowledgment, fear, and deficiency in meaningful and sustainable solutions.

Moral suffering is distinguished from other types of physical or somatic suffering reflective of disease or injury. While moral suffering can lead to a compromise or disintegration of a person's health, in this context it is likely a consequence of the moral suffering rather than the cause of it. Admittedly, there may be interplay between these dimensions, but for our purposes we focus more on consequences of moral suffering. An extreme form has been called "soul pain," a sense of alienation from one's deepest values and convictions. It can result in an emotional response primarily motivated by fear and an all-pervading sense of emptiness, hopelessness, meaninglessness, or numbness.[14] Embedded in these processes is a sense of loss of moral agency, identity, held beliefs or assumptions, unmet goals or expectations, and loss of relationships. In response to these losses, we experience grief and its own particular type of suffering connected to the moral aspects of our essence, purpose, values, and commitments.

Clinicians may also judge themselves harshly if the outcomes they pursue do not occur, if they are treated with disrespect or punished by other healthcare professionals or the institution where they practice, or if they fail to act because they lack skills or the fortitude to persist in the face of resistance. Their attempts to resolve the dissonance arising from conflicting or incommensurate goals, values, or treatment options can lead to a growing sense of deficiency and failure. The encroachment on their basic values—their understanding of life, death, disability, and relationships—may compromise how they perceive the meaning of their work and the satisfaction they derive from it.[4] According to Reich,[6] disruptions in integrity may appear as changes in clinicians' autonomy, moral well-being, character, or self-esteem, and unintentionally manifest in the care they provide and intensify their suffering.

Real or perceived, powerlessness—the inability to cause or prevent change—contributes to caregiver suffering and undermines moral agency. A clinician's perceived inability to minimize or eliminate tragic outcomes brings on feelings of powerlessness and helplessness. These feeling are magnified when clinicians feel that they have no control over their practice, no input into the treatment plan, or no recourse in carrying out a plan they find morally objectionable, such as providing disproportionately burdensome treatments to dying patients. These experiences are often intensified when there are institutional, community, or societal barriers to enacting what clinicians believe to be the ethical response. If other members of the healthcare team or the institution where they practice do not legitimize their moral concerns, their moral agency is threatened, their values supplanted, and their capacities for compassion and resilience imperiled.[15] These outcomes have been starkly illustrated during the COVID-19 pandemic.[16,17,18]

In clinical environments, primacy is often placed on expertise and mastery, on "heroic" intervention and competence. Stakes are high, pressures and expectations can be great, and disappointments and frustrations are often intense. When a sense of personal deficiency, frustration, or failure is in the mix, it can lead to attempts to divert attention from one's own suffering and to focus on the failings of others—for example, blaming the patient, or family, vilifying the surgeon for his aggressive efforts to sustain life despite overwhelming complications, or blaming "the system" for one's inability to bring about the outcome one regards as optimal for one's patient. It is important to acknowledge the broader constraints and pressures affecting what one can do, to recognize the challenges of navigating morally complex circumstances with integrity. It is also the case that others' failings or the failings of the "system" are oftentimes central to one's own moral agency and integrity.[4] But displacing responsibility and blame onto others can also risk reinforcing a sense of helplessness, a perception of oneself as a mere pawn in the system. Too often both individual and collective narratives are created that reflect these themes and become ingrained in the clinical culture itself. Shared frustration and despair can be contagious, deflecting attention away from the actual root causes of the moral suffering and the responsibility of everyone for creating the conditions for the adversity and the corollary responsibility to be engaged in solutions to address them. In such situations, one may cease to see avenues that are open and within reach and expend disproportionate energy railing against "the system" without demonstrable impact. A significant source of moral suffering involves the experience of imperiled integrity that remains unrelieved. Threats, challenges, or violations of integrity occur when our intentions, behavior, and actions are incongruent with our own values, character, conscience, and commitment to do what is best—all things considered. Dissonance is a common feature of clinical work. It involves how we experience and respond to inconsistencies in our thoughts, behaviors, and actions.[19] It can be particularly distressing when it diminishes or disregards the value of human life, a common source of moral distress.[20] Exceptions and contradictions in the application of moral norms and rules are expected—for example, the doctrine of double effect or the withdrawal of life-sustaining therapies as generally accepted exceptions to a moral prohibition against killing—in clinical practice, yet there are social rules and processes that exist, in part, to resolve moral dissonance.[21,23] For example, when decisions are made that define the boundaries of end of life care and produce dissonance for members of the healthcare team, procedural safeguards that involve consultation with others, such as palliative care or ethics consultants, may be required.[22,23a,23] Increasingly, clinicians are faced with incommensurate moral choices that reflect the breakdown of systemic values of respect for the dignity of every person and inequities in access and outcomes of healthcare interventions. These sustained moral conflicts and dilemmas were pronounced during the COVID-19 pandemic.[18,24,25,26,27]

When moral dissonance is unresolved, it generally involves a choice that must be made between competing or incommensurate moral claims, commitments, or responsibilities. In such instances, the usual decision-making processes, sanctioned exceptions to general rules, or processes of remediation or reconciliation are either unavailable or inadequate to define acceptable behavior in ways that are seen to uphold fundamental moral values and norms.[23,23a] When dissonance cannot be adequately resolved, we are at risk of rationalizing our actions with justifications that "get us off the hook," trivializing the inconsistency, using denial, or seeking distraction as a means to reduce our distress.[20(p6)] It can result in what Cribb calls "ethical laziness," doing what is required and moving on, or "ethical arrogance."[28(p123)] ignoring the rules or standards and doing what one believes to be the more justified response. Such dissonance also arises between professional and organizational priorities and values that leave clinicians in the position of implementing the decisions of organizational leadership without input or engagement in the decision itself. In this case, clinicians struggle to find a place of integrity between what they believe to be true about their roles and the reality of what they are mandated to do by their organization or external forces. They find themselves traversing the territory between resistance, resignation, and acceptance without complacency.

Protracted moral dissonance can be psychologically unsustainable, leading to moral suffering, especially when it threatens the norms that uphold human dignity and worth that form the social fabric of moral solidarity and trust, especially in health care.[29,30] When integrity is imperiled, fundamental concerns about moral identity and responsibility become prominent. These themes were intensified during the COVID-19 pandemic and bring into greater focus the cost of erosion of moral and professional identity on the workforce.[31,32] Moral suffering also involves an appraisal and interpretive process to make sense out of one's experiences and assess and assign them a valence as threat or opportunity. While appraising moral suffering suggests continued movement, some clinicians become stymied in an ongoing and relentless cycle of moral suffering, including moral distress, moral injury, or moral apathy, outrage or disengagement that persistently fragments their sense of wholeness and well-being.

Moral suffering tends to activate negative, self-directed emotions such as guilt, shame, anger, and regret in response to one's involvement, direct or indirect, in moral compromises. People with strongly internalized values generally experience anxiety, guilt, or distress when they have some moral culpability for compromises or wrongdoing, especially when such acts have violated a shared moral code. Moral suffering can also ensue as a response to actions of others that constrain the exercise of one's moral agency, such as when a physician commits the other members of the healthcare team to a plan of care they had no input into designing but are required to implement, or when organizational leaders make policy decisions that thwart safe, quality patient care, violating foundational ethical precepts.

Moral suffering—and at its most intense, moral injury or moral outrage—can be triggered by threats, such as retaliation by superiors when moral concerns are voiced, or by moral loss or disappointment when one is unable to fulfill one's ideal of professional identity because of individual, collective, or systemic obstacles. Such obstacles may reflect the rules of professional behavior that must be followed and whose consequences and ethical values may themselves reflect ethically suspect or outright violations of what is needed or what one considers morally and ethically correct.[33]

Understanding these threats is the key to understanding suffering, particularly moral suffering. Underlying them all is a threat to the individual's integrity, an internal state of wholeness in all dimensions of a person's being—physical, emotional, behavioral, and spiritual. Integrity relies on the balance and harmony of the various dimensions of human existence. Since we are whole beings, suffering occurs at the level of the whole being.[34] Threats to bodily integrity, for instance, can become evident as disease, injury, or illness. For clinicians, the occurrence of physical symptoms, particularly those unresponsive to usual treatments including muscle tension, headaches, and the like, may be a manifestation of their own suffering within their professional roles. Likewise, psychological integrity may be undermined by a disintegration of the self by psychopathology or threats to personhood or identity. The self-image of clinicians can be undermined by various threats, from unrealistic expectations, suppressed feelings that mute the authentic self, and maladaptive coping to dysfunctional relationships and ineffective communication. Because spiritual integrity involves an integration of moral character, adherence to moral norms, and coherent and consistent behavior within a set of principles or commitments, it too is vulnerable to disruptions. For clinicians, treatment decisions or organizational mandates may threaten their understanding of justified and unjustified burdens, obscure or extinguish the meaning of their work, or even lead to a crisis of faith.

Threats to the integrity of healthcare professionals may alienate them from their values and convictions and cause them to neglect what matters most—in many cases, their sense of being a "good" physician, nurse, social worker, or other professional. When clinicians act in a way they believe is contrary to their values and commitments, their loss of integrity results in moral suffering. Physicians, nurses, social workers, chaplains, and others may struggle to determine whether they did all they could to help a patient or whether they missed any signs or symptoms that could have altered the outcome, were inaccurate in diagnosis, or did not fulfill their professional obligations or moral code. Their sense of what is required in their role is often framed by their expectations and desire to alleviate or improve the patient's condition. During the COVID pandemic, clinicians struggled with providing treatment in ways that were contrary to their usual practice patterns because of overwhelming numbers of people needing treatments, scarcity of human or material resources, or government or organizational mandates.[33,35,36,37] They may believe that if they "try hard enough" or are "smart enough," they can accomplish the outcomes they desire. When death is the outcome, their self-image may be altered, their integrity compromised because the outcome is incongruent with the ideals of their profession to relieve suffering, to benefit those they serve as best they can, and to provide care that is fair and dignified.[16] Alongside these concerns, clinicians may appraise their effectiveness based on whether they are able to ensure a safe discharge for a patient who is homeless or for whom community resources are unavailable to address their healthcare needs outside of the hospital setting.

Beyond the patient's immediate situation, clinicians may be motivated to address the underlying structural contributors to disparities in access or outcomes of available therapies or healthcare resources. A clinician's sense of doing the right thing may also be challenged, particularly in the face of significant ambiguity and uncertainty. Questions arise: "Am I helping this patient or harming her by the treatments we are providing or not providing? Can I live with the image of myself as a doctor or nurse if I carry out a particular action? Can I live with the choices that I have made on behalf of this patient or family? Can I live with my participation in implementing the choices made by others, be they patients, families, clinicians, or administrators?" Each of these questions reflects a concern about acting in a way that undermines the clinician's sense of personal and professional integrity. When clinicians cannot live up to their personal or professional values by acting in an ethical manner, they can experience moral distress or injury or other consequences in response to their own suffering.

At the core of each concept is the sense of loss—of integrity, self-image, relationships, and hopes for the future—and of grief in the face of loss. For clinicians, this includes threats to their integrity when they cannot resolve fundamental moral or ethical issues. They may feel unable to honor their core commitments to their patients, for example, or incapable of seeing a dignified death as a healing act or in providing care in a fair and equitable manner. The suffering of caregivers can be more personal as they find themselves disconnected from their own needs and desires, from personal or professional relationships, and from the deepest meaning of their lives.

If integrity is the goal, clinicians, and the institutions where they practice, must share a vision of the behaviors and character traits they value. In such an environment, persons of integrity consistently exhibit the virtue of integrity, honoring the integrity of self and others. They understand that integrity encompasses autonomy but is not synonymous with self-determining actions or exerting their will on others. Institutionally, healthcare organizations and leaders will allocate resources and prioritize an ethics infrastructure that enables ethical action, proactively identifies lapses in ethical behavior, and removes impediments to integrity preserving care. This will include new models of care delivery and human resource allocation that enable clinicians to serve in accordance with their values, training, and commitments.

Finding a Path Forward

While it might be attractive to attempt to extinguish all suffering from the work of clinicians, it is unrealistic and, on several levels, undesirable. Contrary to contemporary Western views of suffering as negative and without value, befriending ourselves and our suffering can lead to an awareness that has the potential to transform moral adversity that arises in clinical practice. It takes us back to our roots as healers by embracing deep notions of clinicians—and their patients—as integrated, holistic beings rather than divorced from mind, body, and spirit. Exploring the nature and sources of suffering illuminates how integral it is to clinical practice. Giving language to recognize and respond to it allows opportunities for widespread individual, professional, and systemic interventions. Many clinicians experience a sense of relief when they realize that their suffering is not unique and that they are no longer isolated in their suffering. It is part of a larger dialogue within healthcare to help clinicians to re-connect to the core values and meaning of their work. By recognizing our own suffering, we can begin a process of transforming our practice at the bedside and beyond. Once we recognize our suffering and accept it as our current reality, we can harness internal and external resources to meet it, release it, or possibly transform it. Accepting our suffering does not imply complacency or giving up. It is possible to accept the reality, even if we don't like it, and simultaneously engage in making it better.

How clinicians respond to their own suffering mirrors their responses to the suffering of the patients and families they serve. Ideally, suffering for and with our patients invites compassion and allows us to open our hearts and use our skills for the benefit of those patients and their families. If we can respond to our own suffering with compassion and non-judgment, we will similarly respond to the sufferings of patients and families.[38] Still, clinicians are sorely lacking skills in self-compassion, renewal, and the cultivation of resilience and wellbeing.[40] Attending to these issues is foundational to the creation of a healthy workplace and a robust workforce.[39,40,41,42,43] It is clear that we must understand ethical commitments in a broader context that goes beyond relationships with others to include one's relationship with oneself and the broader moral ecosystem. Simultaneously, individuals must join with leaders, organizations, policymakers, and others to dismantle the systemic impediments to integrity and ethical practice.

Acknowledging the suffering, naming it, giving voice to it, and bearing witness to our suffering are important steps toward creating an environment of integrity. Suffering for and with our patients will always be a dimension of clinical practice. Our challenge is how to care for ourselves so that we can continue to care for others without disproportionately taking on burdens that are not ours to carry. Creating a culture of self-stewardship is another important dimension of addressing caregiver suffering. Without an acute awareness of need for self-compassion,[44] clinicians will struggle to embody a new ethic of self-respect and compassion. No longer is it optional for clinicians to disregard their deepest needs; they must address their own suffering. This professional mandate invites us to consider ways to transform our professional norms to honor values of wholeness, appropriate boundaries, self-respect, and integrity. Clinicians themselves must take the initiative to develop new professional accountabilities and reward them often and visibly.

Clinicians must also partner with the institutions where they practice to create a practice environment that is grounded in integrity. With the shortage of clinicians escalating, institutions must consider the impact of caregiver suffering on the workforce. Denial of its existence and failure to respond to the legitimate suffering of clinicians will further erode the professions. Recent attention is being paid to the issues of clinician burnout that provide a needed platform for system-wide reforms[42,43,44,45,45,46,47] Clinicians must unite to advocate for practice models that celebrate and respect the contributions of clinicians and nurture their physical, emotional, spiritual and moral well-being[38,40,48] These efforts must be coupled with deep and enduring culture change. The responsibility for the magnitude of change that is needed cannot rest on the shoulders of clinicians alone. Expecting clinicians to bear this responsibility is likely to exacerbate the resentment and disengagement that pervade many healthcare organizations and contribute to patterns of mal-alignment of values and oppression that have dominated society and the delivery of health services. It will require individuals who are balanced, clear, and buoyant to engage with leaders who are able to align fundamental values toward meaningful and sustainable solutions. These changes are not easy or quick; the patterns within organizations and professions, society and globally, will need to be systematically dismantled to create the kind of culture that fosters human flourishing by all.

Building this new culture will require new approaches and new strategies for ethical practice. Anchored in integrity, moral resilience holds the power to transform suffering in healthcare alongside systemic reforms. The pages that follow offer a map to the future and detailed descriptions of the concepts, framework, and actions needed as guides on this journey of change and transformation.

References

1. Hauerwas S. Suffering presence: theological reflections on medicine, the mentally handicapped and the church. Notre Dame, IN: University of Notre Dame Press; 1986.
2. Hauwerwas S. Suffering presence. Edinburgh, UK: T & T Clark; 1988.
3. Makowski SK, Epstein RM. Turning toward dissonance: lessons from art, music, and literature. J Pain Symptom Manage. 2012;43:293–298.
4. Peter EH, Macfarlane AV, O'Brien-Pallas LL. Analysis of the moral habitability of the nursing work environment. J Adv Nurs. 2004;47:356–364.
5. Pavlova A, Paine S-J, Sinclair S, O'Callaghan A, Consedine NS. Working in value-discrepant environment inhibits clinicians' ability to provide compassion and reduces well-being: a cross-sectional study. J Intern Med. 2023; 293(6):704–723..
6. Reich WT. Speaking of suffering: a moral account of compassion. Soundings. 1989; 72:83–108.
7. Hanna D. The lived experience of moral distress: nurses who assisted with elective abortions. Res Theory Nurs Pract. 2005;19(1):95–124.
8. Burston AS, Tuckett AG. Moral distress in nursing: contributing factors, outcomes and interventions. Nurs Ethics. 2012;20(3):312–324.
9. Rushton CH, Kaszniak AW, Halifax JS. A framework for understanding moral distress among palliative care clinicians. J Palliat Med. 2013;16(9):1074–1079.
10. American Medical Association. Code of medical ethics. Chicago, IL: AMA; 2017.
11. American Nurses Association. Code of ethics for nurses with interpretive statements. Silver Spring, MD: ANA; 2015.
12. National Association of Social Workers. Code of Ethics of the National Association of Social Workers [Internet]. Washington, DC: NASW; 2017. Available at https://www.socialworkers.org/About/Ethics/Code-of-Ethics/Code-of-Ethics-English.
13. Barnard D. The promise of intimacy and the fear of our own undoing. J Palliat Care. 1995;11:22–26.
14. Kearney M. Mortally wounded. New York: Scribner; 1996.
15. Rushton CH. The baby K case: ethical challenges of preserving professional integrity. Pediatr Nurs. 1995;21:367–372.
16. Rushton CH, Thomas TA, Antonsdottir IM, et al. Moral injury and moral resilience in health care workers during COVID-19 pandemic. J Palliat Med. 2021;25(5):712–719,
17. Spilg E, Rushton C, Phillips J, et al. The new frontline: Exploring the links between moral distress, moral resilience, and mental health in healthcare workers during the COVID-19 pandemic. BMC Psychiatry. 2022;22(19):1–12.
18. Nelson KE, Hanson GC, Boyce D, et al. Organizational impact on health care workers' moral injury during COVID-19: A mixed-methods analysis. J Nurs Adm. 2022;52(1):57–66.

19. de Vries J, Timmins F. Care erosion in hospitals: problems in reflective nursing practice and the role of cognitive dissonance. Nurse Educ Today. 2016;38:5–8.
20. Rushton CH. The baby K case: ethical challenges of preserving professional integrity. Pediatr Nurs. 1995;21:367–372.
21. Potter J, Shields S, Breen R. Palliative sedation, compassionate extubation, and the principle of double effect: an ethical analysis. Am J Hosp Palliat Care. 2021 Dec;38(12):1536–1540.
22. Truog RD, Campbell ML, Curtis JR, Haas CE, Luce, JM, Rubenfeld GD, et al. Recommendations for end-of-life care in the intensive care unit: a consensus statement by the American College of Critical Care Medicine. Crit Care Med. 2008;36:953–963.
23a. Bosslet GT, Pope TM, Rubenfeld G, Lo B, Truog R, Rushton C, Curtis JR, Fords DW, Osborne M, Misak C, Au DH, Azoulay E, Brody B, Fahy B, Hall J, Kesecioglu J, Kon AA, Lindell K., White D. An official ATS/AACN/ACCP/ESICM/SCCM policy statement: Responding to requests for potentially inappropriate treatments in intensive care units. Am J Respir and Critl Care Med. 2015;191(11):1318–1330.
23. Schneiderman LJ, Gilmer T, Teetzel HD, Dugan DO, Blustein J, Cranford R, et al. Effect of ethics consultations on nonbeneficial life-sustaining treatments in the intensive care setting: a randomized controlled trial. J Am Med Assoc. 2003;290:1166–1172.
24. Rushton CH, Thomas TA, Antonsdottir IM, et al. Moral injury and moral resilience in health care workers during COVID-19 pandemic. J Palliat Med. 2021; forthcoming.

Rushton, C. H., Thomas, T., Antonsdottir, I., Nelson, K, Boyce, D., Vioral, A., Swavley, D., Ley, C., Hanson, G. (2021) Moral Injury, Ethical Concerns and Moral Resilience in Health Care Workers during COVID-19 Pandemic, Journal of Palliative Medicine, 25(5), 712-719 https://doi.org/10.1089/jpm.2021.0076
25. Williamson V, Murphy D, Greenberg N. COVID-19 and experiences of moral injury in front-line key workers [Review of COVID-19 and experiences of moral injury in front-line key workers]. Occup Med. 2020;70(5):317–319.
26. Azoulay E, De Waele J, Ferrer R, et al. Symptoms of burnout in intensive care unit specialists facing the COVID-19 outbreak. Ann Intensive Care. 2020;10(1):1–8.
27. Ulrich CM, Rushton CH, Grady C. Nurses confronting the coronavirus: Challenges met and lessons learned to date. Nursing outlook. 2020;68(6): 838–844..
28. Cribb A. Integrity at work: managing routine moral stress in professional roles. Nurs Philos. 2011;12(2):119–127.
29. Pavlova A, Paine S-J, Sinclair S, O'Callaghan A, Consedine NS. Working in value-discrepant environment inhibits clinicians' ability to provide compassion and reduces well-being: a cross-sectional study. J Intern Med. 2023;293(6):704–723,
30. Schlak AE, Rosa WE, Rushton CH, et al. An expanded institutional and national-level blueprint to address nurse burnout and moral suffering. Nurs Manage. 2022;53(1):16–27.

31. Nelson KE, Hanson GC, Boyce D, et al. Organizational impact on health care workers' moral injury during COVID-19: A mixed-methods analysis. *J Nurs Adm*. 2022;52(1):57–66.
32. Swavely D, Weissinger G, Holtz H, Aldi T, Alderfer M, Lynn L, Rushton C. (2022) The impact of traumatic stress, resilience, and threats to core values on nurses during a pandemic. Journal of Nursing Administration. 52(10).
33. Haidt J, Graham J. When morality opposes justice: Conservatives have moral intuitions that liberals may not recognize. Social Justice Res. 2006;20(1):98–116.
34. Singh KD. The grace in dying: how we are transformed spiritually as we die. San Francisco, CA: Harper San Francisco; 2000.
35. Lake ET, Narva AM, Holland S, et al. Hospital nurses' moral distress and mental health during COVID-19. J Adv Nurs. 2021;78(3):799–809.
36. Benishek LE, Kachsalia A, Daugherty Biddison L, Wu AW. Mitigating health-care worker distress from scarce medical resource allocation during a public health crisis. Chest. 2020;158:2285–2287.
37. Garros D. Austin W, Dodek P: How can I survive this? Coping during COVID-19 pandemic. Chest 2021;159: 1484–1492.
38. Rushton CH, Reder E, Hall B, Comello K, Sellers DE, Hutton N. Interdisciplinary interventions to improve pediatric palliative care and reduce health care professional suffering. J Palliat Med. 2006;9:922–933.
40. Wijdenes K L, Badger TA, Sheppard KG. Assessing compassion fatigue risk among nurses in a large urban trauma center. J. Nurs. Administr. 2019;49:19–23.
39. Vollers D, Hill E, Roberts C, Dambaugh L, Brenner ZR. AACN's healthy work environment standards and an empowering nurse advancement system. Crit Care Nurse. 2009;29:20–27.
40. American Association of Critical-Care Nurses. AACN standards for establishing and sustaining healthy work environments. 2nd ed. Aliso Viejo, CA: AACN; 2016.
41. National Academy of Medicine. National plan for health workforce well-being. Washington, DC: National Academies Press; 2022.
42. Office of the Surgeon General. Addressing health worker burnout. The US Surgeon General's Advisory on Building a Thriving Health Workforce. Washington, DC: Office of the Surgeon General; 2022.
43. Office of the Surgeon General. The US Surgeon General's Framework for Workplace Mental Health & Well-Being. Washington, DC: Office of the Surgeon General; 2022.
44. Pavlova A, Paine S-J, Sinclair S, O'Callaghan A, Consedine NS. Working in value-discrepant environment inhibits clinicians' ability to provide compassion and reduces well-being: a cross-sectional study. J Intern Med. 2023;293(6):704–723..
45. The Johnson Foundation. A gold bond to restore joy to nursing: a collaborative exchange of ideas to address burnout [Internet]. Racine, WI: Johnson Foundation; February 2017. Available at http://www.qpatientinsight.com/uploads/2/0/7/1/20710150/nurses_at_wingspread__final.022217.pdf.

46. National Academy of Medicine. Action collaborative on clinician well-being and resilience [Internet]. Washington, DC: NAM; 2017. Available at https://nam.edu/initiatives/clinician-resilience-and-well-being/
47. Perlo J, Balik B, Swensen S, Kabcenell A, Landsman J, Feeley D. Institute for Healthcare Improvement white paper: framework for improving joy in work [Internet]. 2017. Available at http://www.ihi.org/resources/Pages/IHIWhitePapers/Framework-Improving-Joy-in-Work.aspx
48. National Academies of Sciences, Engineering, and Medicine. Supporting the health and professional wellbeing of nurses. In The future of nursing 2020–2030: charting a path to achieve health equity. Washington, DC: National Academies Press; 2021, 301–354.

2

What Is Moral Distress?

UNDERSTANDING CONTEXT, SOURCES, AND CONSEQUENCES

Alisa Carse, Tessy A. Thomas, and Cynda Hylton Rushton

OF THE MANY forms of moral suffering experienced by healthcare professionals (HCPs)—perhaps none has received as much attention as "moral distress." The challenges of moral distress have emerged as a growing concern among HCPs; they have also been the focus of a significant body of research and analysis in clinical bioethics. An alarming number of HCPs report frustration, anguish, and despair in their attempts to provide ethical, patient-centered care in a healthcare system wrought with moral failings*. Finding themselves on the front lines in high-stakes circumstances, often characterized by suffering and uncertainty, many HCPs struggle to sustain integrity and compassion in their work in the face of exhaustion, time pressure, resource constraints, and the profound limitations of their own power to effect needed changes in the systems of healthcare in which they work. The COVID-19 pandemic has both revealed and exacerbated many existing stresses. Under current conditions, too many HCPs are opting to leave their chosen profession in order to preserve their moral integrity and well-being.[1,2,3,4] Although moral dilemmas and other challenges of complex moral decision-making are an inescapable part of healthcare practice, there has been a palpable increase in the frequency

* Portions of this chapter are from: A. Carse and C. H. Rushton (2017). "Harnessing the promise of moral distress," *Journal of Clinical Ethics*, 28, pp. 15–29. Copyright 2017 by the Sage Publishing. Adapted with permission.

Alisa Carse, Tessy A. Thomas, and Cynda Hylton Rushton, *What Is Moral Distress?* In: *Moral Resilience*. Second Edition. Edited by: Cynda Hylton Rushton, Oxford University Press. © Oxford University Press 2024.
DOI: 10.1093/oso/9780197667149.003.0003

and intensity of moral distress, leading many HCPs to experience hopelessness, existential and professional identity crises, and a sense of moral failure. Thus, ongoing exploration and understanding of moral distress and its impact and costs is necessary to guide the development and implementation of strategies to mitigate its lasting consequences.[7]

The Concept of Moral Distress

The term "moral distress" was coined over three decades ago to refer to the anger, frustration, and anxiety of nurses who believed their moral integrity was compromised by constraints and pressures making it difficult or impossible for them to do the right thing.[5,6] Moral distress is now recognized as a growing reality across healthcare disciplines and roles.[7,8,9,10,11,12,13,14] Numerous studies suggest that its effects extend to physicians, pharmacists, respiratory therapists, social workers, psychologists, administrators, chaplains, students, and many other allied health professionals.[7,8,14,15,16,17,18,19,20,21,22,23] It is widely acknowledged that unmitigated moral distress is a key source of escalating rates of professional burnout, turnover, and teamwork erosion, contributing significantly both to a decrease in the quality of patient care and to poor patient outcomes.[24,25,26,27,28,29] As awareness of moral distress has grown, the concept itself has come to have diverse, and sometimes conflicting, meanings.[30,31,32,33,34] Some characterize moral distress as a state of psychological disequilibrium that emerges when one feels unable to act in alignment with one's own considered moral judgments and commitments because of social or institutional pressures or constraints. Others broaden the characterization of moral distress to include a range of psychological impediments to acting with integrity, such as fear, despair, anxiety, and anger, especially when these are themselves responses to morally challenging clinical environments. Concerned that "moral distress" has become an umbrella term for a variety of importantly distinct kinds of moral and psychological stress,[31,32] some have called for a refinement of the term,[33,34,35] others for significantly new conceptualizations,[35,36] and still others for an abandonment of the concept altogether.[31,37]

We believe it is useful to retain the concept of moral distress, in part because concerns organized around the concept have served as a crucial focal point in drawing attention to a troubling epidemic of moral suffering among HCPs. Moreover, naming and identifying moral distress is crucial if we are to constructively address it in better supporting HCPs' moral integrity and resilience. For the purposes of this discussion, we expand upon Jameton's and other scholars' definitions of moral distress. In the healthcare context, moral distress is a phenomenon that occurs when *any* healthcare professional recognizes an ethical problem, feels the responsibility to respond to it, but cannot act or speak up in a way that is consistent with their professional integrity.[5,33,38] We thus understand moral distress as a distinctive kind of moral suffering, one fundamentally tied to a sense of imperiled integrity.[33,39] Paradigmatically, moral distress involves the anguished judgment that one has violated a core value commitment, failed to fulfill a core value commitment, or in some other significant way fallen morally short under conditions of constraint or duress. Moral distress is not, however, always tied directly to an experience of personal or professional moral failure or deficiency. Sometimes it consists in moral uncertainty or anticipatory anxiety in the face of constraints, pressures, or moral concerns that are experienced as challenging or threatening to one's integrity.[33] It can also involve situations in which one is concerned about being complicit in wrongdoing, or uncertain or anxious about contributing to, or supporting, an ethical lapse—perhaps on the part of an organization where one works or with which one is affiliated.[40] As we will explore, moral distress, like other forms of moral suffering, can manifest in a wide array of states, including anguish, anxiety, frustration, anger, guilt, grief, and shame, among others. These states may just be the tip of the iceberg and illuminate the moral-psychological symptoms of having one's deeper core integrity threatened, challenged, or violated. The sources of moral distress can be both social and institutional and, as is increasingly recognized, psychological, including notably the "residue" of insufficiently resolved forms moral distress itself[38,41]—affective states and emotions carried into new situations that can diminish HCPs' moral resilience and responsiveness leading to escalations of distress, now widely known as the "crescendo effect."[38] We will discuss the cumulative nature of moral distress, the role of anticipatory distress, and the crescendo effect in some detail later.

It is important to recognize that HCPs cannot avoid experiences of moral distress entirely given the inherent moral complexities of the healthcare professions.[42] The combination of illness, vulnerability, uncertainty, cultural and social differences and value conflicts, power differentials, resource limitations, and other factors, make some moral distress inevitable. Thus, the objective cannot be to eradicate moral distress; instead, it must be to address and mitigate the modifiable conditions that precipitate moral distress by better supporting HCPs' ability to sustain moral integrity as they navigate moral challenges and pressures on the front lines. Crucially, moral distress emerges in the dynamic relationship between the individual HCPs and the system or organization in which they practice, develop, and learn. Addressing moral distress thus requires attending to a multiplicity of individual, relational, organizational, institutional, and moral-psychological factors as they interact in eroding or supporting HCPs' experiences of effective moral agency and integrity.

While much attention has been given in the literature to the negative impact of moral distress on the psychological well-being of HCPs and the quality of patient care, we want to stress that moral distress is not itself a sign or symptom of individual failure. Most fundamentally, moral distress signals fidelity to, and investment in, moral commitments one believes are threatened or compromised. It is the troubled call of conscience. Heeding this call requires that HCPs be able to sustain connection to their core values and commitments within an organizational culture that provides safety and supports their basic goodness and integrity. We must find better ways of supporting HCPs' moral agency and voice and providing them the opportunity and authority to contribute to needed reform within the teams, organizations, and systems in which they work. The epidemic of moral distress invites us to think more fully about what is entailed in sustaining moral integrity and how HCPs can be better supported and empowered in doing so. If the growing epidemic of moral distress reveals anything, it is that one can do one's best to be true to one's own ethical principles and commitments yet find oneself disempowered and silenced—unable to effectively uphold the moral standards to which one is committed or to give effective voice to moral concern or protest because of external pressures and constraints. Given the high moral stakes of clinical work, and the fundamental expectation that those who do this work will do so with utmost moral integrity and conscientiousness, it is a serious problem that so many HCPs find their own personal and professional integrity challenged by the conditions in which they practice. Too often when this happens, the moral distress experienced is inflected by a sense of personal deficiency and failure, despite the pressures and constraints encountered. It is thus urgent that we more fully understand and address the complex sources and costs of moral distress, especially those contributing to its detrimental persistence and escalation.

The Sources of Moral Distress and Its Impact

The sources of moral distress have been widely studied in nurses and, more recently, physicians, but there is growing research into the moral distress of students, social workers, respiratory therapists, chaplains, pharmacists, and other health professionals.[6,7,8,14,19,20,21,22,23,43,44,45,46,47,48] While moral distress is experienced by a wide variety of HCPs, studies reveal differences across professions, both in the key sources of moral distress and in its frequency and intensity,[44,46] likely a reflection of differences in roles and authority.[49] Nurses in general, for example, report a high frequency and intensity of moral distress in situations in which they are obligated to carry out physicians' orders for tests and treatments they regard as unnecessary[44] or to follow a family's wishes for continued life support when they believed it is not in the best interest of the patient.[8] Nurses in psychiatric and critical care settings report especially acute moral distress around restricting patients' freedom—for example, in participating in the involuntary hospitalization, seclusion, or confinement of patients,[50] or in restraining or coercively medicating patients.[51] Physicians report especially frequent and intense moral distress in witnessing their patients' care suffer because of a lack of provider continuity and, like nurses, in engaging in extensive lifesaving action they believe will only prolong a patient's dying.[44,45] For social workers, a significant source of moral distress is providing less-than-optimal care due to cost reduction pressures from administrators or insurers, or in circumstances of inadequate social support.[7,44] Key sources of moral distress for hospital chaplains are participating in discharging patients they do not believe are ready for discharge, and issues of social justice, such as treating undocumented patients differently than US citizens.[7] In the United Kingdom, pharmacists identify situations in which they are prohibited by law from dispensing controlled drugs that would serve the patient's best interests or cannot provide medications because of shortages.[52] These examples highlight the scope of circumstances that produce moral distress among HCPs.

The intensity of the moral distress reported is often independent of the frequency of the morally distressing situations.[7,53,54,55] Crucially, studies reveal that even when instances of moral distress are infrequent, the intensity of the distress experienced can put HCPs at risk,[8,11,56,57,58] even influencing their decisions about remaining in their role or in their profession.[8,44,59]

Both the frequency and intensity of moral distress vary across practice settings.[54,60] Moral distress is particularly prevalent and intense in high-risk contexts such as critical care,[14,18,49,61,62,63,64,65,66,67,68,69,70] oncology,[71,72,73,74,75,76,77,83] neonatology/pediatrics,[45,57,78,79,80,81,82,83,84] and emergency care.[85,86,87,88] Recent studies of the unprecedented 2019 coronavirus pandemic and the moral distress experiences of HCPs illuminate the commonality of shared lived experiences within healthcare—high patient mortality, patient acuity, and volume; limited resources; personal safety concerns; rapid policy changes; witnessing patients dying alone; generalized uncertainty; imbalance of staffing needs, roles, and responsibilities, a paradigm shift from prioritizing individualized patient care to prioritizing collective needs; the battle of mis-information; and lack of organizational support, among other factors—all of which contribute to increased moral distress, burnout, and HCPs leaving their profession[11,89,90,91,92,93,94] due to constant challenges, threats, and violations of HCPs' integrity. To be clear, the challenges of the 2019 pandemic are not altogether new ones; the pandemic has acutely exacerbated and dramatically exposed chronic challenges HCPs have faced for decades.

The sources of moral distress reflect the inescapable moral complexity of many clinical situations, including the fact that conscientious and thoughtful HCPs, patients, and families can struggle with uncertainty, feel constrained by the pressures and limitations of time and resources, and disagree about ethically appropriate interventions and optimal outcomes. The 2019 pandemic has highlighted these elements. Healthcare professionals often struggle to balance their own moral commitments, the moral obligations of their profession, and the economic and legal priorities of their teams and organizations with their primary obligation to privilege the interest of their patients. Moral distress can thrive in such circumstances, despite one's best efforts.[45,50,53,54,79,80,81,85,95,96,97,98,99,100,101,102,103,104]

Even pre-pandemic, HCPs across disciplines and roles reported chronic concern about the allocation of scarce resources and the impact of constrained resources, including staffing, on their ability to provide safe, quality, and ethically grounded care. As one ICU physician laments, "The patient was expected to die soon, but that didn't happen. Then you have to . . . transfer a patient to the ward, who'll only go there to die. . . . But we do need that bed."[90,105(p7)] The 2019 pandemic significantly exacerbated these concerns.[12,106,107,108] In the current healthcare environment with the ongoing pandemic and multiple-virus threats, staff and resource concerns are likely to continue and to escalate, adding to the urgency and difficulty of designing systems that can support ethical practice.

Moral distress is also frequently rooted in conflicting ethical commitments and value judgments between HCPs; among HCPs, patients, and families; and among HCPs and clinical teams in relation to institutionalized protocols and policies they believe bind them. As a physician in training states: "We spend a lot of time at the end of life in the ICU torturing our patients, and so I can't in good conscience say that our current system really seems to serve the best interests of the patient because we torture them before they die, even though we know that they are going to die."[109(p96)] Conflicts concern many difficult and complex ethical issues, including the appropriate use of technology; allocating scarce resources; overcoming mis-information about preventative care options such as vaccines;[110,111,112] end-of-life care; disparate perspectives on the goals of care; the boundaries of ethical treatment more generally; patient or surrogate decision-making that prolongs death; inadequate informed consent; and management of pain.[6,44,45,46,64,72,79,81,96,113,114,115,116,117,118,119,120,121,122] The 2019 coronavirus pandemic has created new threats to trust, particularly among HCPs, patients and their families, and society more broadly. Some of these threats may have been unavoidable, however: "The preexisting distrust in science was exacerbated by conflicting messages, questionable treatments reported in research publications, concerns about political interference in public health recommendations and decisions regarding the efficacy of therapeutics, and pseudoscience and conspiracy theories."[123] Subsequently, HCPs are experiencing incivility from the very population of patients and families they are trying to advocate and care for; furthering their moral angst and challenging their commitment to their chosen professions.[124,125,126]

In the critical care setting, patients' healthcare issues tend to be extremely complex, requiring ongoing judgments and decision-making around questions that each stakeholder may view differently.[49,60] This can result in ineffective team communication,[6,8,45,120,127,128,129] inconsistent treatment plans, and lack of continuity.[8,44] An emergency department nurse shares the source of her moral distress: "A patient from the nursing home came in not doing well, near that code moment. There was no family. The physician decided not to intervene since there was no family there. He would have done more if family would have been there advocating for the patient."[89(pp237-238)]

Some of the troubling ethical questions that often generate moral distress in the neonatal and pediatric settings include these: "Should the healthcare team follow a family's wish to continue life support, even when it is not in the best interest of the child?" or "Should extensive life-sustaining actions be initiated in order to prolong dying?"[45,72,80,81,115] One nurse describes her experience, saying, "I have seen a 23–24-weeker given full resuscitation and full treatment at parent's insistence when the baby was obviously in very poor condition, and appeared to be suffering greatly, only to die on the ventilator. This situation distressed me greatly."[78(p.738)] Similarly, HCPs are concerned about the ability of stressed and frightened parents to make informed decisions.[77] When innovative treatments result in chronic or critical illness, moral distress is intensified when no one will decide to stop.[81,115] These questions can be difficult to address, given the complexities that surround the communication, decision-making, and management for children with life-threatening or life-limiting illnesses, which can involve complex treatments such as extracorporeal membrane oxygenation and dialysis.[8,57,80,130,131,132,133] Furthermore, moral distress can arise from a gamut of clinical experiences that includes staffing level concerns, incivility and microagressive interactions with patients and their families, increasing mental health crises, and social justice issues plaguing society.[14,68,134,135,136,137,138,139,140]

Moral distress is also shown to stem from the use of advanced technology,[62,141] time constraints when providing care to patients who are rapidly declining,[142,143] highly aggressive care,[79,114,116,144] and concerns that the care being provided is medically ineffective or futile.[7,63,123,145,146] This last concern is a significant factor among ICU nurses, who identify carrying out physicians' orders for futile care as a frequent and intense source of moral distress.[118,124,147,148]

In each of these examples and in many others, HCPs are confronted with situations that challenge, threaten, or violate one or more of their core values.[33,149] When moral distress is not recognized or effectively addressed, there are immediate, and also often more sustained and recalcitrant, moral costs.

The Contours and Costs of Moral Distress

In a collection of personal narratives of moral distress, nurses, physicians, psychologists, and other healthcare professionals share stories of moral pain and anguish.[150,151] The language is striking. Healthcare professionals write of "deep sadness";[152(p211)] "lasting regret";[153(p100)] and "despair."[154(p123)] They report "feeling alternately hypocritical and callous";[155] being "on an emotional rollercoaster";[156(p112)] feeling "an overwhelming sense of dread";[17(p94)]; and "suffering from nightmares, headaches, fear, anxiety, depression, difficulty concentrating, and problems of self-esteem."[156(p113)] Recalling a morally distressing situation, one clinician writes: "Parts of my body felt as though they didn't belong to me, and my words seemed to come out of a mouth that wasn't mine and hang in the air between me and the patient as though spoken by someone else."[157(p116)] Another reflects that "even now, a year later . . . I feel a physical weight on my chest, and sometimes it's hard to breathe."[154(p124)] Many of these narratives bring us into visceral contact with what it is like to feel trapped, constrained, pressured, or disoriented in a situation that acutely challenges one's ability to sustain moral integrity despite one's best efforts.[150] While the specific sources of moral distress vary, there are themes and challenges that are shared. In what follows, we explore a number of themes we believe drive to the heart of the challenges of moral distress: the experiences of moral powerlessness, frustration, and anger; of voicelessness and isolation; and of shame. We also explore common risks of insufficiently addressed moral distress, looking in particular at the perils of diminished moral responsiveness. We highlight the dynamic and cumulative character of moral distress, the way it can itself diminish the capacity of HCPs to respond with composure and clarity to new morally distressing situations, thereby compounding the experience of moral distress, often bringing into the mix experiences of personal moral deficiency, shame, and hopelessness. Making positive and lasting headway in addressing the crisis of moral distress will require finding ways to support HCPs in recognizing and addressing these challenges, among other things, by remediating the complex systemic issues that are so often their cause. Without attention to individual, team, and systemic patterns, sustainable and meaningful change will not be possible.

Powerlessness, Frustration, and Anger

In a narrative exploration of her personal experience with moral distress, Susan McCammon, a surgical oncologist, describes her "helplessness and outrage . . . immense, and frightening in its unfamiliarity," when she learns the institution where she practices has, in the wake of a damaging storm, "terminated" care of its uninsured patients.[152(p109)] She questions this decision, moving up the "increasingly reticent and then elusive" line of authority, only to discover she is powerless to combat it. "While this decision was made by the administration," she writes, "its enactment was delegated to the physicians."[152(p109)] Thus, not only were the physicians not involved in the decision to terminate their patients, but they also shouldered the burden of telling their patients that they would no longer be treated."[152(p109)] Carrying out a decision she deems immoral, McCammon also bears the brunt of her patients' terror, grief, and rage. And she grapples with new questions: Should she shift her care to insured patients, whose cancer she has the resources to treat? Should she become a reformer and fight for changes at the national level to the healthcare system whose moral short fallings she copes with daily? "But I don't do those things," she writes; "I hold hands and weep with patients and go home so very tired. I feel guilty for not taking up arms."[152(p111)]

Like many HCPs, McCammon must navigate a situation she has not herself created, confronting choices that are the consequences of others' decisions and of institutional policies she has no direct authority to change. She is expected to acquiesce to, and even carry out, mandates at odds with her own value commitments—commitments she believes lie at the heart of her profession. Continuing to work within the troubled system is a price she pays, at least initially, to remain connected to her patients.

The experience of powerlessness, of being "caught" and pressured to do what one believes to be wrong, or impeded in meeting moral commitments one takes to be fundamental, is a key theme in narratives of moral distress. Moral frustration and anger are often provoked in situations in which one feels constrained or thwarted, unable to do what one believes to be morally necessary or important.[158] This can engender feelings of helplessness and hopelessness, deflating our confidence and undermining our experience of effective moral agency. When our very integrity is at issue—when we believe we cannot be true to our fundamental value commitments and aspirations, the sense of helplessness and hopelessness can give way to anger, even full-blown moral outrage. Anger and outrage can give rise to the urge to protest, to defend one's authority, expertise, or respect-worthiness. In the absence of constructive avenues of protest, redress, and reform—anger can become a disruptive, even destructive force. Sometimes it is expressed directly in outbursts, contentiousness, or straightforward fighting; sometimes more indirectly in interpersonal slights or conduct that is subtly passive-aggressive. These responses can be directed to the actual sources of one's sense of frustration or imperiled integrity, such as the administration, a supervisor, co-workers, or the patients one cares for; they can also be displaced less discriminately onto others, or become internalized in states of depression, simmering resentment, and despair. An emergency department nurse reflecting on her experience with moral distress laments: "I have probably two emotions: No. 1—anger 'cause I wasn't heard or listened [to]. And No. 2, I'm depressed . . . so you have two polars—I'm very mad, you know, I can't have aggression, but I'm also depressed. To have those two emotions is draining—it's very draining."[88(p43)] Patterns of disrespect and interpersonal conflict may contribute to troubling, disruptive behaviors and bullying.[159,160]

While anger can be a destructive force, it is crucial to recognize that it can also be a morally productive force—a healthy and appropriate response that calls needed attention to moral harms and wrongdoings.[161] Realizing the moral potential of anger can depend on having the skills and tools that enable one to recognize one's anger, to accept it without shame, and to express and direct it constructively; it can also require the existence of a receptive environment, in which one's concerns or protests can be voiced and heard, and thoughtfully taken up and addressed with others.

Voicelessness and Isolation

The experiences of powerlessness, frustration, and anger are often connected to feeling silenced or voiceless, especially when one's moral concerns are devalued or dismissed. McCammon's protests, for example, are met with administrative resistance and evasion. In a different case, a clinician conveys her experience of "isolation" and voicelessness during a troubling incident in her clinical unit: "Athough I was [an] active member of the care team to be involved . . . I was relegated to being a quiet bystander, a technician expected to provide the skills, but not the critical reflection, which I still feel makes us physicians."[162(p114)] Yet another clinician reflects on the "strong wall of silence" he experiences in response to administrative bullying and abuse, of the "fear of retaliation" that "prevents professionals from doing what is right—speaking up."[165(p114,163)] Even when no direct retaliation is feared, institutional hierarchies of power and authority can have a profound impact. A nursing student obeys her teacher's sharp command to remain silent about an act she witnessed: "I finished out my rotation without a peep. But in doing so I feel I betrayed the people in my life who have mental illnesses. I betrayed the belief in human rights, which had led me to healthcare in the first place. And I betrayed the patients who come to that hospital seeking help and compassion and are instead treated like criminals."[160(p100)] A palliative care nurse writes,

"[We're] very frustrated. I think we hurt a lot for the patients. It doesn't matter what we tell most of the physicians, about the pain or suffering . . . about how miserable [patients] are with all the treatments they're getting."[164(p711)] More generally, there is a standing risk that expressions of moral distress will be "silenced" unwittingly, by being construed in a reductive way (both by speakers and hearers) as mere lamentations or personal complaints, expressions of subjective inner states of "distress" (e.g., of frustration, anguish, anger, discomfort) rather than as assertions of moral appraisal, concern, or protest, directed to morally troubling features of the circumstances. This can happen when HCPs attempt to call attention to or protest morally troubling conditions or constraints in their work environment and are told "You are just burned out," or "Buck up!" or "If you can't stand the heat, get out of the kitchen!" The experience of voicelessness—whether resulting from others' disregard, dismissal, or misconstrual, or from one's own fear or diffidence—can be demoralizing. The literature provides evidence that HCPs' demoralization and voicelessness can actually harm, even kill, patients.[165] And if voicelessness persists, it can generate silent suffering that carries a keen sense of moral isolation, estrangement, and alienation.[38,166,167,168] All these factors contribute to a psychological unsafe culture for individuals, teams, and organizations, increasing the dangers to patients.[169,170,171,172]

When moral distress is tied to experiences of disempowerment and voicelessness, HCPs often feel frustrated, angry, helpless, and alone, trapped in situations they are unable to alter or exit without undue moral cost. As we have seen, the contours of such situations are diverse. Sometimes moral distress is the anguished response to direct participation in perceived wrongdoing under duress, sometimes to witnessing wrongdoing that one lacks the power to stop. HCPs may feel their integrity is compromised by resource constraints, by others in authority, by conflicts with patients or colleagues that stymie resolution or progress, or by policies they lack the authority to override. One may not, of course, be as powerless and voiceless as one believes oneself to be.[173] But the experience of moral distress highlights our susceptibility to the power and authority of others, to systems we neither design nor control, and to the way others' treatment and regard can limit what we can effectively do—including the moral concern and protest we can effectively voice.

The experiences of powerlessness, voicelessness, and hopelessness so often at the root of moral distress, make clear that we must, in understanding and addressing moral distress, look beyond the individual who is experiencing moral distress to the broader conditions helping to generate the distress. We must also shift away from the all-too-common negative narrative, in which moral distress is tied to "moral weakness";[39] this narrative reinforces a troubling tendency to regard moral distress as evidence of personal moral deficiency, an inability to withstand the challenges and demands of clinical work.[39] It is crucial to recognize that experiencing moral distress is *not* itself a symptom of moral deficiency or failure; it is a sign that one is attuned to ethical pressures or concerns, "an alarm signal when a conscientious person is required to practice in challenging contexts."[174]

At the same time, it is important to recognize that moral distress can take a moral toll on those who experience it, especially when it is intense or long-lasting. Forms of "self-related distress" can accompany moral distress because of the suffering and exhaustion it induces, motivating self-protective actions that further challenge one's ability to sustain a sense of effective moral agency and integrity.[33] Acute or unresolved moral distress can diminish physical, emotional, and moral resilience, which can, in turn, make it difficult and challenging to sustain robust moral responsiveness. This can lead conscientious HCPs to feel moral frustration and failure, disillusionment, and shame, which can, as we will see, contribute to an escalating spiral of moral distress.

Diminished Moral Responsiveness, Disillusionment, and Shame

The moral demands of clinical work can make the moral toll of moral distress especially poignant and concerning. Patients and their loved ones are often vulnerable, not just to the technical knowledge and skill but also to the expressive quality of care they receive, the sense that their experience of illness is understood and honored, and that those caring for them are respectful, compassionate, attentive, and trustworthy. Empathic understanding and communication can play a critical role in the discernment and responsiveness at the heart of clinical excellence, enabling HCPs and patients to communicate effectively and to build and sustain trusting alliances often essential for effective treatment.[175,176,177,178] More generally, the ability to attune to the emotions and perspectives of those central to and affected by a clinical case—including other colleagues on the treatment team—can be crucial to assessing and responding to ethical challenges and working collaboratively in forging shared resolutions.

The effective navigation of ethically challenging clinical situations requires a constellation of capacities, enabling one to detect and interpret the morally salient dimensions of situations one is in, identify ethically justified responses, even when they entail moral cost or compromise; and execute action in an emotionally balanced, morally grounded, and compassionate manner.[10,179,180] Healthcare professionals in whom these capacities are compromised may overlook morally salient factors and miss occasions for moral action. They may carry unreflective assumptions and projections into new situations, in ways that distort perception and impede their ability to sensitively track the impact of their decisions on patients and others.[181] They may find it difficult to work constructively with conflict or to engage collaboratively in forging shared resolutions to ethical challenges. In the clinical context, empathy and compassion are the countermeasures to potentially serious harms. When they are diminished or absent, there is risk of skewed perception, communication breakdown, and damage to or loss of trust.

Consider the distraught patient responding to a frightening diagnosis with anger and recrimination, directed against his nurses or physicians. Perhaps his anger is the expression of an irascible personality. Or perhaps it is the public face of his shame in being dependent and fragile, a burden to his family.[191] Understanding this patient's state and its determinants can be crucial to gaining his trust, securing the information needed to make an accurate clinical diagnosis, and rallying his participation in the treatment plan. In the context of a team of morally distressed clinicians, such a patient can quickly be labeled "difficult," signaling those caring for him to adopt a defensive stance and igniting their own unacknowledged fears and vulnerabilities. The clinical team may, out of self-protection, engage more "woodenly" with the patient, avoid his room, or attribute negative motives and character traits to him, closing off forms of open and empathic engagement that could help diminish his shame, quell his anger, allay his fear, and begin to build trust.

In clinical environments, the same factors that make moral discernment and responsiveness crucial, can also make them difficult to achieve. Persistent exposure to suffering can lead to empathic over-arousal[182] and secondary trauma, challenging HCPs' ability to regulate their emotions and maintain composure. Time pressures, exhaustion, uncertainty, conflict, and simple distraction can challenge emotional resilience and fortitude. A physician observes: "There [are] 16 patients on your service and a lot of families that want to sit down and hear about what's going on. It's tiring and draining. And then if you get into these battles about end-of-life it gets really exhausting. It does wear me out. I get tired. There are times when I've had enough."[183(p366)]

Healthcare professionals who carry anticipatory and unresolved moral distress into the clinical encounter may find it doubly difficult to achieve the mix of flexibility, openness, emotional equanimity, and stability they need. Negative emotional arousal can become overwhelming and unbearable, leading to a range of behaviors aimed at alleviating one's own distress.[192,184] These include "flight," avoidance and/or abandonment of patients, colleagues, and others; "fight," expressions of anger, contentiousness, cynicism, and other forms of aggression and resistance; and "freeze," emotional disengagement, shutting-down, numbing, and disconnecting, sometimes in ways that produce a "robotic" task-orientation.[10,185,186] One nurse who did not agree with the family's view of the patient's quality of life expresses how she copes: "I basically become indifferent. Close my mouth. Because my opinion in those situations matters but it doesn't. . . . [I]f a family is [steadfast] on an idea it's not my place to change their beliefs. So basically, I just become very objective, [focusing on] numbers, infections, . . . very methodical; I pull my emotional side out of it and I am then just a nurse taking care of a patient and helping the family, but just being the nurse"[183(p362)] Healthcare professionals suffering from persistent moral distress often lament that they have "lost heart," are "simply going through the motions," or just "don't care anymore." All these reactions significantly diminish empathic attunement and compassion, risking conduct that is emotionally remote, even callous. When attunement is diminished and compassion lost, trust more easily erodes, and misunderstandings and conflicts more easily emerge and solidify. This can imperil the alignment of purpose so important to collaboration between patient, family, and clinical team. The persistence of such behaviors also reflects the culture of the teams and organizations where HCPs practice that led to the denial or disregard of their experiences and in some cases normalization of such behaviors as the cost of caring.

Shame

Chronic, unmitigated, or repeated experiences of moral distress often generate an ongoing sense of deficiency—of what Sandra Bartky identifies as a form of shame, "manifest in a pervasive sense of personal inadequacy . . . a species of psychic distress occasioned by a self, or a state of the self-apprehended as inferior, defective, or in some way diminished."[187(p85)] Conscientious HCP may respond with especially acute shame to signs of their own diminished moral responsiveness or moral disengagement, considering these to be moral failings for which they are responsible. Crucially, shame need not entail the belief that one has done something wrong. Too often, HCPs feel shame when they are not able to resolve difficult situations, secure desired outcomes for patients, or prevent others' wrongdoing. While in many instances these factors are beyond their control, shame nevertheless arises. In high-stakes clinical environments, making mistakes of *any* type, including moral ones, can ignite self-criticism; it can also draw critical judgment from others.

Bartky highlights the "profoundly disempowering" drive for "secrecy and concealment" induced by shame, which undercuts the possibility of solidarity with others, even those who may be struggling in similar ways. This can intensify the experience of helplessness, hopelessness, and isolation.[187(p90)] The sense of isolation coupled with feeling voiceless and powerless can compound the despair and hopelessness so often associated with chronic moral distress. Without physically and emotionally safe space to acknowledge individual and collective fears and vulnerabilities, shame can metastasize within individuals, spilling out and infecting teams, organizations and the people they are meant to serve.

Often in the grip of moral distress, especially when it is chronic or sustained, one becomes the victimized person, the "walking wounded," as a sense of moral injury or grievance take over. Experiences of helplessness, hopelessness, and emotional depletion can induce feelings of loss and disillusionment—alienation from aspirations that once informed one's professional identity and grounded engagement in purposeful and trusting collaboration with colleagues. It can be increasingly difficult to sustain confidence, courage, and hope. Clinicians aware of the detrimental moral effects of their own moral distress may experience a compounded sense of deficiency and shame, which in turn may contribute to an escalating dynamic of moral distress and the distinctive patterns of moral suffering it brings.

The Cumulative Dynamic of Moral Distress

There are both short- and long-term consequences of moral distress. Although the evidence is inconclusive regarding the full range of responses characterizing moral distress, the literature suggests that moral distress has significant and often far-reaching impact. Figure 2.1 contains a selected list of moral distress responses.[9,29,36,44,50,62,64,68,69,123,180,188,189,190,191,192,193,194,195]

Repeated instances of unprocessed moral distress can begin to accumulate in our bodies, psyches, and minds.[18] Although the intensity of the distress may dissipate to some degree after an acutely distressing event is over, there is often "moral residue"[38,41]—unresolved moral distress, including feelings of uncertainty, guilt, frustration, and anxiety—that leave HCPs vulnerable to what Epstein and Hamric have called the "crescendo effect," an escalating accumulation of moral distress over time.[38,196] The anticipatory distress and the moral residue that ensues can be rooted in regret or guilt. Sometimes regret and guilt are tied to the recognition that one has

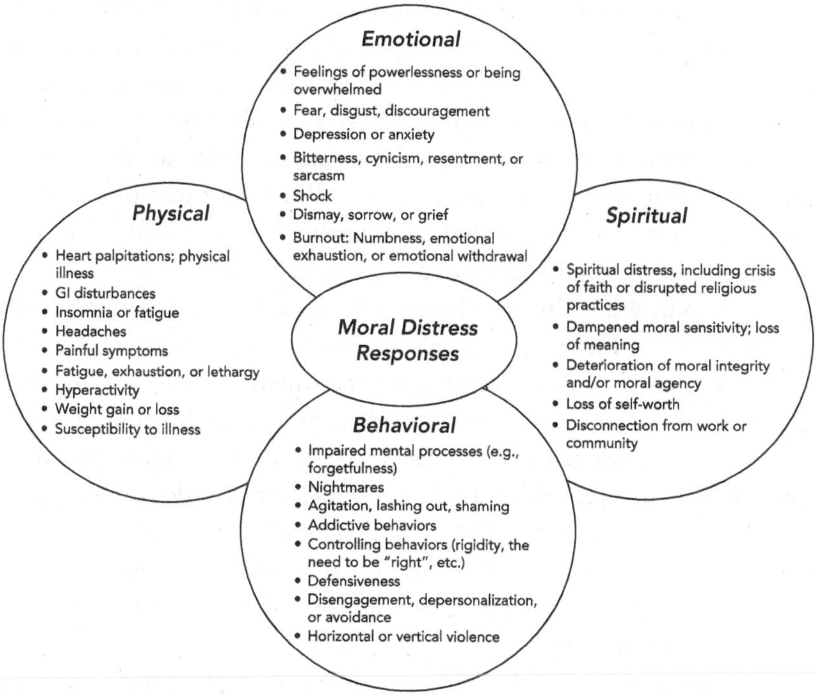

FIGURE 2.1. Moral Distress Responses.

allowed one's integrity to be compromised in response to external pressures; other times they result from doing the best one can in a highly constrained situation, in which any path forward will leave important moral values or commitments unmet.[41] Along with moral residue, there may be physical, emotional, spiritual, and cognitive residue. Physical symptoms accompanying the distress include exhaustion, alterations in weight, appetite, joint and muscle disorders, gastrointestinal symptoms, headaches, or high blood pressure, and these can persist.[88] As one Emergency Department nurse described her response to moral distress, " 'My body's given up on eating, like I long since have not been hungry anymore. Then at the end of the night, when I [urinate], it's orange, and I think, 'Oh my God, my kidneys are going to shut down.' What we're doing to our bodies to take care of other people's bodies and I get upset . . .' "[88(p43)]

Negative emotions and states triggered by moral distress, such anger, fear, frustration, and hopelessness, can have harmful effects, both on the individual experiencing moral distress and on others with whom the individual interacts. Cognitive preoccupation and perseveration can occur as HCPs continue to attempt to reconcile forms of dissonance that accompany the morally distressing event, finding it difficult to release the unresolved or unanswered questions or ruminating about the situation, unable to let go of the negative or difficult aspect of a case. Persisting preoccupation and rumination can lead HCPs to overlook the positive or meaningful aspects of a morally distressing case and thereby further amplify the dissonance and distress experienced. This pattern can hardwire negativity into the nervous system by creating the conditions for negative memory activation when a similar but undifferentiated case arises in the future.[10]

Unresolved moral distress can also provoke denial of the situation or one's role in it. While this may be an effective defense mechanism in the short term, over time it can erode one's engagement, moral responsiveness, and integrity. As one emergency department nurse described, "You just put the blinders on and you pretend . . . pretend that it doesn't bother you."[89 (p238)] Another states: "We just ignore it. I have another patient to care for. And we just move on."[89(p238)] However, the denial eventually catches up. "It starts a negative cycle specifically for the nurse because when you pretend the first time, it makes it easier to pretend the second time. And then it becomes a non-issue and you stop thinking about it and you become numb."[89(p238)]

It is crucial to grasp the cumulative and dynamic nature of moral distress. When compounded by new distressing situations, frustration, anger, anxiety, and shame can simmer and build. Moral distress carries over into new situations through embodied memory, shaping perceptions, appraisals, and responses. Unresolved, it leads to myriad "symptoms";[9,44,197] it can also insidiously begin to "change who you are." When moral distress remains unacknowledged or unaddressed over time, it can begin to erode integrity and character in ways that create dissonance between one's behavior and one's identity as a professional. An Emergency Room nurse reported: "When you are experiencing [moral distress], you don't want to come to work. You try to distance yourself from your patients. You try to be cold and uncaring, but you know you really aren't that way."[89(p238)]

Jameton[198] distinguishes "initial moral distress" from "reactive moral distress," the long-lasting painful emotions, or "moral residue"[41] carried in the aftermath of distressing situations, which, if insufficiently addressed can lead to integrity compromising patterns like the "flight, fight, and freeze" reactions noted earlier. When unresolved or persistent, moral distress can erode resilience, leaving HCPs vulnerable to disruptive and disabling escalations of distress. Empirical evidence reveals that when triggers of distress are repeated, or new morally challenging situations are encountered, the impact is often cumulative, elevating the residual baseline of somatic and emotional dysregulation, producing a "crescendo effect" that increases with intensity as new situations are encountered.[38,215] This is exacerbated when new distressing situations resemble earlier ones, thus activating memory, heightening the sense of frustration and powerlessness, and generating anxiety as one anticipates new distressing situations around the bend. There is also risk that both conflicts generating moral distress and solidarity arising from shared distress can lead to a damaging intensification of negative energy, a litany of reasons to feel hopeless, further entrenching resentment or deflating efforts to seek needed reform.

Unresolved moral distress may enhance susceptibility to burnout, a state of emotional, physical, or mental exhaustion, often characterized by cynicism and doubt, mistrust, and a loss of the experience of shared moral purpose.[199] It can also generate a sense of inefficacy, diminishing one's experience of personal competence and accomplishment.[199,200] Research has confirmed this association.[201,207] Work situations that involve serving others, that are emotionally demanding, and in which one is persistently under pressure from high, and at times, unrealistic expectations, create the conditions for burnout.[13,84,202,203,204,205]

Repeated attempts to give voice to ethical concerns, often reflected in HCPs' laments of "why are we doing this?" and unsuccessful attempts to bring about desired outcomes for patients can lead to a depletion of energy, leaving HCPs feeling drained and exhausted. The exhaustion can prompt efforts to distance oneself. Depleted HCPs often distance themselves by depersonalizing patients, actively ignoring the unique human characteristics of those they serve, labeling them instead as "the CABG in room 27" or referring to them as "frequent flyers" or "drug seekers." Exhaustion and discouragement can also lead to cognitive distancing whereby HCPs can become cynical about or indifferent to the needs of the people they serve. This can manifest in responses such as "this patient is just taking up a ventilator that could be used by someone who we can actually help!" Depersonalizing, cynicism, and other modes of emotional and moral disengagement can converge to erode a HCP's sense of self-efficacy and integrity. As highlighted in the prior sections, an erosion of the sense of effective moral agency can lead to feelings of failure, shame, and hopelessness. In these ways and others, unaddressed moral distress can contribute to escalating rates of burnout, decreased job satisfaction, and even departure from the profession.[200,206]

Mitigating Moral Distress and Fostering Moral Resilience

Crucially, moral distress does not always trace to identifiable crises. Sometimes it emerges more gradually, beginning with vague moral discomfort, or the dawning awareness, for example, that the pressure to cut corners—to discharge patients before they are ready or to perform interventions for which one is insufficiently trained—has become morally intolerable; or an anguished realization that one is becoming impatient, irritated, and cynical, losing the sense of connectedness and generosity once present in one's work. What is then at stake is less a direct violation or betrayal of one's principles or value commitments than a gradual erosion of one's sense of moral integrity and effectiveness. This is important because it can make it more challenging to notice and address moral distress before it escalates in destructive ways.

Whether dramatic or gradual, moral distress itself can further disrupt composure, diminish resilience, and impede effective moral agency. It is an inherently dynamic phenomenon that can spiral in destructive ways.

This is a dynamic we believe is crucial and possible to interrupt. In 2019, the National Academy of Medicine produced a report focusing on system approaches to addressing clinician burnout that included moral distress as a contributing factor to burnout that challenged healthcare, education, and organizational leaders and stakeholders to undertake the empirical work needed to mitigate moral distress and support HCP's moral well-being.[207] The American Nurses Association and the American Journal of Nursing held summits to address moral distress by cultivating moral resilience.[208,209] To tend to these complexities, Communities of Practice were proposed as a foundational process to guide development of interventions.[210] A Community of Practice can be formed by a group of people with a shared passion, common interests or concerns, who have the goal of learning how to do something better or to create change as they interact regularly. Through regular interactions of Communities of Practice, members share knowledge, drive strategy, innovate, and solve problems. More recently, scholars have proposed utilizing Communities of Practice as a critical approach to addressing moral distress in healthcare.[211,212] We support this innovative proposal because we envision how the collective human capital and knowledge gained through connections established within an ethical community of practice can help support, sustain, and bolster its members' integrity and resilience in the face of endemic moral challenges.

Stemming the escalating dynamic of moral distress will require authentic collective engagement with moral distress. It will also, crucially, require recognizing the moral energy and investment revealed by moral distress—the "call of conscience"—so it can be redirected in ways that support HCPs' integrity, bolster their resilience, and fortify and empower their efforts to bring needed reforms to the systems in which they work. It will also require ongoing effort to ameliorate the systemic conditions at the root of so much of the moral distress suffered.

The experience of moral distress provides an important prototype of moral suffering in the clinical context. Examining its impact on HCPs and considering ways to mitigate its detrimental effects and address its deeper sources, both individually and collectively—within teams and organizations—can help create generative and safe spaces in which to explore and address related dimensions of moral suffering. This is crucial if we are to devise strategies that will support all those who work in the complex world of healthcare.

References

1. Abbasi J. Pushed to their limits, 1 in 5 physicians intends to leave practice. JAMA. 2022;327(15):1435–1437.
2. LeClaire M, Poplau S, Linzer M, et al. Compromised integrity, burnout, and intent to leave the job in critical care nurses and physicians. Crit Care Explor. 2022;4(2):e0629.
3. Raso R, Fitzpatrick JJ, Masick K. Nurses' intent to leave their position and the profession during the COVID-19 pandemic. JONA: J Nurs Adm. 2021;51(10):488–494.
4. Falatah R. 2021. The impact of the coronavirus disease (COVID-19) pandemic on nurses' turnover intention: an integrative review. Nursing Reports. 2021;11(4):787–810.
5. Jameton, A. Nursing practice: the ethical issues. Englewood Cliffs, NJ: Prentice-Hall, 1984.
6. Hamric AB, Borchers CT, Epstein EG. Development and testing of an instrument to measure moral distress in healthcare professionals. AJOB Prim Res. 2012;3(2):1–9.
7. Houston S, Casanova MA, Leveille M, et al. The intensity and frequency of moral distress among different healthcare disciplines. J Clin Ethics. 2013;24:98–112.
8. Whitehead PB, Herbertson RK, Hamric AB, et al. Moral distress among healthcare professionals: Report of an institution-wide survey. J Nurs Scholarsh. 2015;47(2):117–125.
9. Oh Y, Gastmans C. Moral distress experienced by nurses: A quantitative literature review. Nurs Ethics. 2015;22:15–31.
10. Rushton CH, Kaszniak AW, Halifax JS. Addressing moral distress: Application of a framework to palliative care practice. J Palliat Med. 2013;16:1080–1088.
11. Riedel PL, Kreh A, Kulcar V, et al. A scoping review of moral stressors, moral distress and moral injury in healthcare workers during COVID-19. Int J Environ Res Public Health. 2022;19(3):1666.
12. Lake ET, Narva AM, Holland S, et al. Hospital nurses' moral distress and mental health during COVID-19. J Adv Nurs. 2022;78(3):799–809.
13. Lamiani G, Borghi L, Argentero P. When healthcare professionals cannot do the right thing: A systematic review of moral distress and its correlates. J Health Psychol. 2017;22(1):51–67.
14. Epstein EG, Whitehead PB, Prompahakul C, et al. Enhancing understanding of moral distress: The measure of moral distress for health care professionals. AJOB Empir Bioeth. 2019;10(2):113–124.
15. Austin WJ, Kagan L, Rankel M, Bergum V. The balancing act: psychiatrists' experience of moral distress. Med Health Care Philos. 2008;11:89–97.
16. Carpenter C. Moral distress in physical therapy practice. Physiother Theory Pract. 2010;26:69–78.

17. One A. What power do I have? A nursing student's concerns lead to a passion for ethics. Narrat Inq Bioeth. 2013;3:93–95.
18. Thomas TA, Mccullough LB. Resuscitations that never end: Originating from unresolved integrity-related moral distress. JAMA Pediatr. 2016;170:521–522.
19. Ong RSR, Wong RSM, Chee RCH, et al. A systematic scoping review moral distress amongst medical students. BMC Med Educ. 2022;22(1):1–21.
20. Foster W, McKellar L, Fleet J, Sweet L. Moral distress in midwifery practice: A concept analysis. Nurs Ethics. 2022;29(2):364–383.
21. Captari LE, Hydinger KR, Sandage SJ, et al. Supporting chaplains on the frontlines of the COVID-19 pandemic: A mixed-method practice-based pilot intervention study. Psychol Serv. 2022;20(1):6–18.
22. Trachtenberg S, Tehan T, Shostak S, et al. Experiences of moral distress in a COVID-19 intensive care unit: A qualitative study of nurses and respiratory therapists in the United States. Nurs Inq. 2023;30(1):e12500.
23. Lynch D, Forde C. "Moral distress" and the beginning practitioner: Preparing social work students for ethical and moral challenges in contemporary contexts. Ethics Soc Welf. 2016;10(2):94–107.
24. Schwenzer KJ, Wang L. Assessing moral distress in respiratory care practitioners. Crit Care Med. 2006;34:2967–2973.
25. Sundin-Huard D, Fahy K. Moral distress, advocacy and burnout: theorizing the relationships. Int J Nurs Pract. 1999;5(1):8–13.
26. Kok N, Van Gurp J, van der Hoeven JG, et al. Complex interplay between moral distress and other risk factors of burnout in ICU professionals: findings from a cross-sectional survey study. BMJ Qual Saf. 2023;32:225–234.
27. Shoorideh FA, Ashktorab T, Yaghmaei F, Alavi Majd H. Relationship between ICU nurses' moral distress with burnout and anticipated turnover. Nurs Ethics. 2022;15(1):64–76.
28. Christodoulou-Fella M, Middleton N, Papathanassoglou ED, Karanikola MN. Exploration of the association between nurses' moral distress and secondary traumatic stress syndrome: Implications for patient safety in mental health services. Biomed Res Int. 2017;1908712.
29. Austin CL, Saylor R, Finley PJ. Moral distress in physicians and nurses: Impact on professional quality of life and turnover. Psychol Trauma. 2017;9(4):399.
30. Hanna DR. Moral distress: The state of the science. Res Theory Nurs Pract. 2004;18(1):73–93.
31. McCarthy J, Deady R. Moral distress reconsidered. Nurs Ethics. 2008;15(2):254–262.
32. Pauly BM, Varcoe C, Storch J. Framing the issues: Moral distress in health care. HEC Forum. 2012;24(1):1–11.
33. Thomas TA, Mccullough LB. A philosophical taxonomy of ethically significant moral distress. J Med Philos. 2015;40(1):102–120.

34. Kolbe L, de Melo-Martin I. Moral distress: What are we measuring? Am J Bioeth. 2023;23(4):46–58.
35. Campbell SM, Ulrich CM, Grady C. A broader understanding of moral distress. Am J Bioeth. 2016;16(2):2–9.
36. Musto LC, Rodney PA, Vanderheide R. Toward interventions to address moral distress: navigating structure and agency. Nurs Ethics. 2015;22(1):91–102.
37. Johnstone M, Hutchinson A. 'Moral distress'—time to abandon a flawed Nursing construct? Nurs Ethics. 2015;22(1):5–14.
38. Epstein EG, Delgado S. Understanding and addressing moral distress. OJIN. 2010;15(3):Manuscript 1.
39. Carse A, Rushton CH. Harnessing the promise of moral distress: A call for reorientation. J Clin Ethics. 2017;28(1):15–29.
40. Morley G. What is "moral distress" in nursing? How can and should we respond to it? J Clin Nurs. 2018;27(19-20):3443.
41. Webster GC, Baylis FE. Moral residue. In SB Rubin, L Zoloth, editors, Margin of error: The ethics of mistakes in the practice of medicine. Hagerstown, MD: University Publishing Group, 2000: 217–230.
42. Pellegrino ED. The metamorphosis of medical ethics: A 30-year retrospective. JAMA. 1993;269(9):1158–1162.
43. Rodney P, Kadychuk S, Liaschenko J, et al. Moral agency: relational connections and support. In JL Storch, P Rodney, R Starzomski, editors, Toward a moral horizon: Nursing ethics for leadership and practice. Toronto, Canada: Pearson, 2013:160–187.
44. Allen R, Judkins-Cohn T, deVelasco R, et al. Moral distress among healthcare professionals at a health system. JONAS Healthc Law Ethics Regul. 2013;15(3):119–120.
45. Trotochaud K, Coleman JR, Krawiecki N, McCracken C. Moral distress in pediatric healthcare providers. J Pediatr Nurs. 2015;30:908–914.
46. Dodek PM, Wong H, Norena M, et al. Moral distress in intensive care unit professionals is associated with profession, age, and years of experience. J Crit Care. 2016;31(1):178–182.
47. Berger JT. 2014. Moral distress in medical education and training. J Gen Intern Med. 2014;29:395–398.
48. Sasso L, Bagnasco A, Bianchi M, et al. Moral distress in undergraduate nursing students: A systematic review. Nurs Ethics. 2016;23(5):523–534.
49. Flannery L, Ramjan LM, Peters K. End-of-life decisions in the intensive care unit (ICU)—Exploring the experiences of ICU nurses and doctors—A critical literature review. Aust Crit Care. 2016;29:97–103.
50. Ohnishi K, Ohgushi Y, Nakano M, et al. Moral distress experienced by psychiatric nurses in Japan. Nurs Ethics. 2010;17:726–740.
51. Deady R, McCarthy J. A study of the situations, features, and coping mechanisms experienced by Irish psychiatric nurses experiencing moral distress. Perspect Psychiatr Care. 2010;46(3):209–220.

52. Astbury JL, Gallagher CT. (2017). Development and validation of a questionnaire to measure moral distress in community pharmacists. Int J Clin Pharm. 2017;39(1):156–164.
53. Pauly B, Varcoe C, Storch J, Newton L. Registered nurses' perceptions of moral distress and ethical climate. Nurs Ethics. 2009;16:561–573.
54. Corley MC, Minick P, Elswick RK, Jacobs M. Nurse moral distress and ethical work environment. Nurs Ethics. 2005;12:381–390.
55. Piers RD, Van den Eynde M, Steeman E, et al. End-of-life care of the geriatric patient and nurses' moral distress. J Am Med Dir Assoc. 2012;13(1):80.e7–.e13.
56. Sporrong SK, Höglund A, Arnetz B. Measuring moral distress in pharmacy and clinical practice. Nurs Ethics. 2006;14:416–427.
57. Prentice T, Janvier A, Gillam L, Davis PG. Moral distress within neonatal and paediatric intensive care units: A systematic review. Arch Dis Child. 2016;101:701–708.
58. Ulrich C, O'Donnell P, Taylor C, et al. Ethical climate, ethics stress, and the job satisfaction of nurses and social workers in the United States. Soc Sci Med. 2007;65:1708–1719.
59. Dyo M, Kalowesb P, Devriesb J. Moral distress and intention to leave: A comparison of adult and paediatric nurses by hospital setting. Intensive Crit Care Nurs. 2016;36:42–48.
60. O'Connell CB. Gender and the experience of moral distress in critical care nurses. Nurs Ethics. 2015;22:32–42.
61. Larson CP, Dryden-Palmer KD, Gibbons C, Parshuram CS. Moral distress in PICU and neonatal ICU practitioners: a cross-sectional evaluation. Pediatr Crit Care Med. 2017;18(8):e318–e326.
62. Thomas TA, Thammasitboon S, Balmer DF, et al. A qualitative study exploring moral distress among pediatric resuscitation team clinicians: challenges to professional integrity. Pediatr Crit Care Med. 2016;17(7):e303–e308.
63. St Ledger U, Begley A, Reid J, et al. Moral distress in end-of-life care in the intensive care unit. J Adv Nurs. 2013;69(8):1869–1880.
64. Gutierrez KM. Critical care nurses' perceptions of and responses to moral distress. Dimens Crit Care Nurs. 2005;24(5):229–241.
65. Özden D, Karagözoğlu Ş, Yıldırım G. Intensive care nurses' perception of futility: Job satisfaction and burnout dimensions. Nurs Ethics. 2013;20:436–447.
66. Elpern EH, Covert B, Kleinpell R. Moral distress of staff nurses in a medical intensive care unit. Am J Crit Care. 2005;14:523–530.
67. Salari N, Shohaimi S, Khaledi-Paveh B, et al. The severity of moral distress in nurses: A systematic review and meta-analysis. Philos Ethics Humanit Med. 2022;17(1):13.
68. Sonis J, Pathman DE, Read S, Gaynes BN. A national study of moral distress among US internal medicine physicians during the COVID-19 pandemic. PLOS One. 2022;17(5):e0268375.

69. McAndrew NS, Leske J, Schroeter K. Moral distress in critical care nursing: The state of the science. Nurs Ethics. 2018;25(5):552–570.
70. Fumis RRL, Junqueira Amarante GA, de Fátima Nascimento A, Vieira Junior JM. Moral distress and its contribution to the development of burnout syndrome among critical care providers. Ann Intensive Care. 2017;7(1):1–8.
71. Pavlish C, Brown-Saltzman K, Jakel P, Fine A. The nature of ethical conflicts and the meaning of moral community in oncology practice. Oncol Nurs Forum. 2014;41(2):130–140.
72. Cohen JS, Erickson JM. Ethical dilemmas and moral distress in oncology nursing practice. Clin J Oncol Nurs. 2006;10:775–783.
73. Lazzarin M, Biondi A, Mauro SD. Moral distress in nurses in oncology and haematology units. Nurs Ethics. 2012;19:183–195.
74. Lievrouw A, Vanheule S, Deveugele M, et al. Coping with moral distress in oncology practice: Nurse and physician strategies. Oncol Nurs Forum. 2016;43:505–512.
75. Hlubocky FJ, Taylor LP, Marron JM, et al. A call to action: Ethics committee roundtable recommendations for addressing burnout and moral distress in oncology. JCO Oncol Pract. 2020;16(4):191–199.
76. Pergert P, Bartholdson C, Blomgren K, Sandeberg M. Moral distress in paediatric oncology: Contributing factors and group differences. Nurs Ethics. 2019;26(7-8):2351–2363.
77. Mehlis K, Bierwirth E, Laryionava K, et al. High prevalence of moral distress reported by oncologists and oncology nurses in end-of-life decision making. Psychooncol. 2018;27(12):2733–2739.
78. Molloy J, Evans M, Coughlin K. Moral distress in the resuscitation of extremely premature infants. Nurs Ethics. 2015;22:52–63.
79. Green J. Living in hope and desperate for a miracle: NICU nurses perceptions of parental anguish. J Relig Health. 2015;54(2):731–744.
80. Cavinder C. The relationship between providing neonatal palliative care and nurses' moral distress: An integrative review. Adv Neonatal Care. 2014;14(5):322–328.
81. Sauerland J, Marotta K, Peinemann MA, et al. Assessing and addressing moral distress and ethical climate part II: Neonatal and pediatric perspectives. Dimens Crit Care Nurs. 2015;34(1):33–46.
82. Cavaliere TA, Daly B, Dowling D, Montgomery K. Moral distress in neonatal intensive care unit RNs. Adv Neonatal Care. 2010;10:145–156.
83. Austin W, Kelecevic J, Goble E, Mekechuk J. An overview of moral distress and the paediatric intensive care team. Nurs Ethics. 2009;16:57–68.
84. Mills M, Cortezzo DE. Moral distress in the neonatal intensive care unit: What is it, why it happens, and how we can address it. Front Pediatr. 2020;8:581.
85. Fernandez-Parsons R, Rodriguez L, Goyal D. Moral distress in emergency nurses. J Emerg Nurse. 2013;39:547–552.

86. Robinson R, Stinson CK. Moral distress: A qualitative study of emergency nurses. Dimens Crit Care Nurs. 2016;35(4):235–240.
87. Zavotsky KE, Chan GK. Exploring the relationship among moral distress, coping, and the practice environment in emergency department nurses. Adv Emerg Nurs J. 2016;38:133–146.
88. Wolf LA, Perhats C, Delao AM, et al. "It's a burden you carry": Describing moral distress in emergency nursing. J Emerg Nurs. 2016;42:37–46.
89. Guttormson JL, Calkins K, McAndrew N, et al. Critical care nurse burnout, moral distress, and mental health during the COVID-19 pandemic: A United States survey. Heart Lung. 2022;55:127–133.
90. Thomas TA, Davis FD, Kumar S, et al. COVID-19 and moral distress: A pediatric critical care survey. Am J Crit Care. 2021;30(6):e80–e98.
91. Rushton CH, Thomas TA, Antonsdottir IM, et al. Moral injury and moral resilience in health care workers during COVID-19 pandemic. J Palliat Med. 2022;25(5):712–719.
92. Kok N, van Gurp J, Teerenstra S, et al. Coronavirus disease 2019 immediately increases burnout symptoms in ICU professionals: a longitudinal cohort study. Critical Care Med. 2021;49(3):419–427.
93. Cacchione PZ. Moral distress in the midst of the COVID-19 pandemic. Clin Nurs Res. 2020;29(4):215–216.
94. Anderson-Shaw LK, Zar FA. COVID-19, moral conflict, distress, and dying alone. J Bioeth Inq. 2020;17(4):777–782.
95. Kleinknecht-Dolf M, Frei IA, Spichiger E, et al. Moral distress in nurses at an acute care hospital in Switzerland: Results of a pilot study. Nurs Ethics. 2015;22:77–90.
96. Rice EM, Rady MY, Hamrick A, et al. Determinants of moral distress in medical and surgical nurses at an adult acute tertiary care hospital. J Nurs Manag. 2008;16:360–373.
97. Silén M, Svantesson M, Kjellström S, et al. Moral distress and ethical climate in a Swedish nursing context: Perceptions and instrument usability. J Clin Nurs. 2011;20:3483–3493.
98. Woods M, Rodgers V, Towers A, Grow SL. Researching moral distress among New Zealand nurses: A national survey. Nurs Ethics. 2015;22:117–130.
99. Zuzelo PR. Exploring the moral distress of registered nurses. NursEthics. 2007;14:344–359.
100. Browning AM. Moral distress and psychological empowerment in critical care nurses caring for adults at the end of life. Am J Crit Care. 2013;22:143–152.
101. Corley MC, Elswick RK, Gorman M, Clor T. Development and evaluation of a moral distress scale. J Adv Nurs. 2001;33:250–256.
102. Ganz FD, Wagner N, Toren O. Nurse middle manager ethical dilemmas and moral distress. Nurs Ethics. 2015;22:43–51.

103. Vaziri MH, Tabatabaei S, Merghati-Khoei E. Moral distress among Iranian nurses. Iran J Psychiatry. 2015;10:32–36.
104. Sommerbakk R, Haugen DF, Tjora A, et al. Barriers to and facilitators for implementing quality improvements in palliative care—Results from a qualitative interview study in Norway. BMC Palliat Care. 2016;15:1–17.
105. Oerlemans AJM, van Sluisveld N, van Leeuwen ESJ, et al. Ethical problems in intensive care unit admission and discharge decisions: A qualitative study among physicians and nurses in the Netherlands. BMC Med Ethics. 2015;16:1–10.
106. Endacott R, Pearce S, Rae P, et al. How COVID-19 has affected staffing models in intensive care: A qualitative study examining alternative staffing models (SEISMIC). J Adv Nurs. 2022;78(4):1075–1088.
107. Morley G, Grady C, McCarthy J, Ulrich CM. Covid-19: ethical challenges for nurses. Hastings Cent Rep. 2020;50(3):35–39.
108. Grimm CA. Hospital experiences responding to the COVID-19 pandemic: results of a national pulse survey March 23–27, 2020. US Department of Health and Human Services, Office of Inspector General. Published 2020. Accessed March 23, 2023. https://oig.hhs.gov/oei/reports/oei-06-20-00300.pdf.
109. Dzeng E, Colaianni A, Roland M, et al. Moral distress amongst American physician trainees regarding futile treatments at the end of life: A qualitative study. J Gen Intern Med. 2015;31:93–99.
110. Loomba S, de Figueiredo A, Piatek SJ, et al. Measuring the impact of COVID-19 vaccine misinformation on vaccination intent in the UK and USA. Nat Hum Behav. 2021;5(3):337–348.
111. Troiano G, Nardi A. Vaccine hesitancy in the era of COVID-19. Public Health. 2021;194:245–251.
112. Gowda C, Dempsey AF. The rise (and fall?) of parental vaccine hesitancy. Hum Vaccin Immunother. 2013;9(8):1755–1762.
113. De Villers MJ, DeVon HA. Moral distress and avoidance behavior in nurses working in critical care and noncritical care units. Nurs Ethics. 2013;20:589–603.
114. Mobley MJ, Rady MY, Verheijde JL, et al. The relationship between moral distress and perception of futile care in the critical care unit. Intensive Crit Care Nurs. 2007;23(5):256–263.
115. Sannino P, Giannì ML, Re LG, Lusignani M. Moral distress in the neonatal intensive care unit: an Italian study. J Perinatol. 2015;35(3):214–217.
116. Hamric AB, Blackhall L. Nurse-physician perspectives on the care of dying patients in intensive care units: Collaboration, moral distress, and ethical climate. Crit Care Med. 2007;35:422–429.

117. Karanikola MNK, Albarran JW, Drigo E, et al. Moral distress, autonomy and nurse-physician collaboration among intensive care unit nurses in Italy. J Nurs Manag. 2014;22:472–484.
118. Papathanassoglou EDE, Karanikola MNK, Kalafati M, et al. Professional autonomy, collaboration with physicians, and moral distress among European intensive care nurses. Am J Crit Care. 2012;21:e41–e52.
119. McClendon H, Buckner EB. Distressing situations in the intensive care unit: A descriptive study of nurses' responses. Dimens Crit Care Nurs. 2007;26:199–206.
120. Henrich NJ, Dodek PM, Alden L, et al. Causes of moral distress in the intensive care unit: A qualitative study. J Crit Care. 2016;35:57–62.
121. Kon AA, Shepard EK, Sederstrom NO, et al. Defining futile and potentially inappropriate interventions: A policy statement from the society of critical care medicine ethics committee. Crit Care Med. 2016;44:1769–1774.
122. Ferrell BR. Understanding the moral distress of nurses witnessing medically futile care. Oncol Nurs Forum. 2006;33:922–930.
123. Baker DW. Trust in health care in the time of COVID-19. JAMA. 2020;324(23):2373–2375.
124. El Ghaziri M, Johnson S, Purpora C, et al. Registered nurses' experiences with incivility during the early phase of COVID-19 pandemic: Results of a multistate survey. Workplace Health Saf. Mar 2022;70(3):148–160.
125. Shoorideh FA, Moosavi S, Balouchi A. Incivility toward nurses: a systematic review and meta-analysis. J Med Ethics Hist Med. 2021;14:15.
126. Ungerleider S, Warren S. Nurses get spit on, kicked, assaulted. Stop hurting us. We are here to help you. USA Today, January 10, 2022. Accessed March 23, 2023. www.usatoday.com/story/opinion/voices/2022/01/10/covid-nurses-assaulted-pandemic/9117731002/?gnt-cfr=1.
127. Abbasi M, Nejadsarvari N, Kiani M, et al. Moral distress in physicians practicing in hospitals affiliated to medical sciences universities. Iran Red Crescent Med J. 2014;16:e18797.
128. Trautmann J, Epstein E, Rovnyak V, Snyder A. Relationships among moral distress, level of practice independence, and intent to leave of nurse practitioners in emergency departments. Adv Emerg Nurs J. 2015;37:134–145.
129. de Boer J, van Rosmalen J, Bakker AB, van Dijk M. Appropriateness of care and moral distress among neonatal intensive care unit staff: Repeated measurements. Nurs Crit Care. 2016;21:e19–e27.
130. Chiswick M. End of life decisions in chronic lung disease. Semin Fetal Neonatal Med. 2009;14:396–400.
131. Shankar V, Costello JP, Peer SM, et al. Ethical dilemma: Offering short-term extracorporeal membrane oxygenation support for terminally ill children who are not candidates for long-term mechanical circulatory support or heart transplantation. World J Pediatr Congenit Heart Surg. 2014;5:311–314.

132. Lantos J, Warady BA. The evolving ethics of infant dialysis. Pediatr Nephrol. 2013;28:1943–1947.
133. Boss RD, Geller G, Donohue PK. Conflicts in learning to care for critically ill newborns: "It makes me question my own morals." J Bioeth Inq. 2015;12:437–448.
134. Fox-Robichaud A, Edmund L, Martin CM. Gender differences in career satisfaction, moral distress, and incivility: a national, cross-sectional survey of Canadian critical care physicians. Can J Anaesth. 2019;66(5):503–511.
135. Blackler L, Scharf AE, Chin M, Voigt LP. Is there a role for ethics in addressing healthcare incivility? Nurs Ethics. 2022;29(6):1466–1475.
136. Paul-Emile K, Smith AK, Lo B, Fernández A. Dealing with racist patients. NEJM. 2016;374:708.
137. Berlinger N, Berlinger A. Culture and moral distress: what's the connection and why does it matter? AMA J Ethics. 2017;19(6):608–616.
138. Hem MH, Gjerberg E, Husum TL, Pedersen R. Ethical challenges when using coercion in mental healthcare: a systematic literature review. Nurs Ethics. 2018;25(1):92–110.
139. Kam S, Kang J. Addressing microaggressions in the health care workplace: Giving trainees a voice. Acad Med. 2022;97(6):772–773.
140. Olcoń K, Gulbas LE. "Their needs are higher than what I can do": Moral distress in providers working with Latino immigrant families. Qual Soc Work. 2021;20(4):967–983.
141. Helft PR, Bledsoe PD, Hancock M, Wocial LD. Facilitated ethics conversations: A novel program for managing moral distress in bedside nursing staff. JONAS Healthc Law Ethics Regul. 2009;11(1):27–33.
142. Kinoshita S. Respecting the wishes of patients in intensive care units. Nurs Ethics. 2007;14:651–664.
143. Atabay G, Çangarli BC, Penbek Ş. Impact of ethical climate on moral distress revisited: Multidimensional view. Nurs Ethics. 2014;22:103–116.
144. O'Neill BJ, Kazer MW. Destination to nowhere: a new look at aggressive treatment for heart failure—a case study. Crit Care Nurse. 2014;34:47–55.
145. Robinson, R. Registered nurses and moral distress. Dimens Crit Care Nurs. 2010;29:197–202.
146. Aghabarary M, Nayeri ND. Nurses' perceptions of futile care: A qualitative study. Holist Nurs Pract. 2016;30:25–32.
147. Kovanci MS, Akyar I. Culturally-sensitive moral distress experiences of intensive care nurses: a scoping review. Nurs Ethics. 2022;29(6):1476–1490.
148. Asayesh H, Mosavi M, Abdi M, et al. The relationship between futile care perception and moral distress among intensive care unit nurses. J Med Ethics Hist Med. 2018;11.
149. American Nurses Association. Code of ethics for nurses with interpretive statements. Silver Spring, MD: ANA, 2015.

150. This section draws from, and develops, material from Carse (2013) and Carse and Rushton (2017). Carse A. Moral distress and moral disempowerment. Narrat Inq Bioeth. 2013;3:147–151. Carse A, Rushton CH. Harnessing the promise of moral distress: A call for reorientation. J Clin Ethics. 2017;28:15–29.
151. Rushton CH, Boss R, One A, et al. The many faces of moral distress among clinicians. Narrat Inq Bioeth. 2013;3:89–93.
152. McCammon S. "Can they do this?": dealing with moral distress after third-party termination of the doctor-patient relationship. Narrat Inq Bioeth. 2013;3109–112.
153. Hensel J. To nurse better. Narrat Inq Bioeth. 2013;3:98–100.
154. Volpe RL. Please help me. Narrat Inq Bioeth. 2013;3:122–124.
155. Hallett K. The sanctity of life—The sanctity of choice. Narrat Inq Bioeth. 2013;3:95–98.
156. Murray JS. Moral distress: the face of workplace bullying. Narrat Inq Bioeth. 2013;3:112–114.
157. Nathanson E. A threat to selfhood: Moral distress and the psychiatric training culture. Narrat Inq Bioeth. 2013;3:115–117.
158. Rushton CH. Principled moral outrage: an antidote to moral distress? AACN Adv Crit Care. 2013; 24:82–89.
159. Nyberg AJ, Moliterno TP, Hale Jr. D, et al. Resource-based perspectives on unit-level human capital: a review and integration. J Manag. 2012;40(1):316–346.
160. Lachman VD. Ethical issues in the disruptive behaviors of incivility, bullying, and horizontal/lateral violence. Medsurg Nurs. 2014;23(1):56–58, 60.
161. Cherry M. The case for rage. New York: Oxford University Press, 2021
162. Mack C. When moral uncertainty becomes moral distress. Narrat Inq Bioeth. 2013;3:106–109.
163. Spenceley S, Witcher CSG, Hagen B, et al. Hall, B., Sources of moral distress for nursing staff providing care to residents with dementia. Dementia. 2015;0:1–20.
164. Oberle K, Hughes D. Doctors' and nurses' perceptions of ethical problems in end-of-life decisions. J Adv Nurs. 2001;33:707–715.
165. Maxfield D, Grenny J, McMillan R, et al. Silence kills. The seven crucial conversations for healthcare. Aliso Viejo, CA: American Association of Critical Care Nurses, 2005: 4–9.
166. Austin W, Rankel M, Kagan L, et al. To stay or to go, to speak or stay silent, to act or not to act: Moral distress as experienced by psychologists. Ethics Behav. 2005;15:197–212.
167. McCarthy J, Gastmans C. Moral distress: A review of the argument-based nursing ethics literature. Nurs Ethics. 2015;22:131–152.
168. Reich WT. Speaking of suffering: A moral account of compassion. Soundings. 1989;72:83–108.

169. Edmondson A. Psychological safety and learning behavior in work teams. Adm Sci Q. 1999;44(2):350–383.
170. DeKeyser GF, Berkovitz K. Surgical nurses' perceptions of ethical dilemmas, moral distress and quality of care. J Adv Nurs. 2012;68:1516–1525.
171. Quillivan RR, Burlison JD, Browne EK, et al. Patient safety culture and the second victim phenomenon: connecting culture to staff distress in nurses. Jt Comm J Qual Patient Saf. 2016;42(8):377–386.
172. Sherf EN, Parke MR, Isaakyan S. Distinguishing voice and silence at work: Unique relationships with perceived impact, psychological safety, and burnout. Acad Manag J. 2021;64(1):114–148.
173. Berger JT, Hamric AB, Epstein E. Self-inflicted moral distress: opportunity for a fuller exercise of professionalism. J Clin Ethics. 2019;30(4):314–317.
174. Garros D, Austin W, Carnevale FA. Moral distress in pediatric intensive care. JAMA Pediatr. 2015;169:885–886.
175. Halpern J. From idealized clinical empathy to empathic communication in medical care. Med Health Care Philos. 2014;17:301–311.
176. Halpern J. What is clinical empathy? J Gen Intern Med. 2003;18:670–674.
177. Halpern JH. Concern to empathy: humanizing medical practice. Oxford: Oxford University Press, 2001.
178. Carse A. The moral contours of empathy. Ethical Theory Moral Pract. 2005;8:169–195.
179. Carse A. Impartial principles and moral context: Securing a place for the particular in ethical theory. J Med Philos. 1998;23:1–17.
180. Rushton CH, Kaszniak AW, Halifax JS. A framework for understanding moral distress among palliative care clinicians. J Palliat Med. 2013;16:1074–1079.
181. Lützén K, Blom T, Ewalds-Kvist B, Winch S. Moral stress, moral climate, and moral sensitivity among psychiatric professionals. Nurs Ethics. 2010;17:213–224.
182. Eisenberg N. Empathy-related emotional responses, altruism, and their socialization. In RJ Davidson, A Harrington, editors, Visions of compassion. Oxford: Oxford University Press, 2002: 131–164.
183. McAndrew NS, Leske JS. A balancing act: experiences of nurses and physicians when making end-of-life decisions in intensive care units. Clin Nurs Res. 2015;24:357–374.
184. Batson CD, Early S, Salvarani G. Perspective taking: imagining how another feels versus imagining how you would feel. Pers Soc Psychol Bull. 1997;23:751–758.
185. O'Rourke ME. Choose wisely: Therapeutic decisions and quality of life in patients with prostate cancer. Clin J Oncol Nurs. 2007;11:401–408.
186. Catlin A, Volat D, Hadley MA, et al. Conscientious objection: a potential neonatal nursing response to care orders that cause suffering at the end of life? study of a concept. Neonatal Netw. 2008;27:101–108.

187. Bartky SL. Femininity and domination: studies in the phenomenology of oppression: thinking gender. New York: Routledge, 1990.
188. Corley MC. Nurse moral distress: A proposed theory and research agenda. Nurs Ethics. 2002;9:636–650.
189. Wilkinson JM. Moral distress in nursing practice: Experience and effect. Nurs Forum. 1987;23:16–29.
190. LaSala, C. A. (2009). Moral accountability and integrity in nursing practice. Nurs Clin North Am. 2009;44:423–434.
191. Hardingham LB. Integrity and moral residue: Nurses as participants in a moral community. Nurs Philos. 2004;5:127–134.
192. Rushton CH. Caregiver suffering in palliative care for infants, children & adolescents: a practical handbook. Baltimore, MD: Johns Hopkins University Press, 2004.
193. Burston AS, Tuckett AG. Moral distress in nursing: Contributing factors, outcomes and interventions. Nurs Ethics. 2012;20:312–324.
194. American Association of Critical Care Nurses (AACN) from AACN Ethics Work Group. The 4 A's to rise above moral distress. Aliso Viejo, CA: AACN, 2004.
195. Hyatt J. 2017. Recognizing moral disengagement and its impact on patient safety. J Nurs Reg. 2017;7(4):15–21.
196. Epstein EG, Hamric AB. Moral distress, moral residue, and the crescendo effect. J Clin Ethics. 2009;20:330–342.
197. Rushton CH, Caldwell M, Kurtz M. Moral distress: A catalyst in building moral resilience. Am J Nurs. 2016;116:40–49.
198. Jameton A. Dilemmas of moral distress: Moral responsibility and nursing practice. AWHONNS Clin Issues Perinat Womens Health Nurs. 1993;4:542–551.
199. Maslach C, Schaufeli WB, Leiter MP. Job burnout. Ann Review Psychol. 2001;52:397–422.
200. Moss M, Good VS, Kleinpell R, Sessler CN. An official critical care societies collaborative statement: burnout syndrome in critical care healthcare professionals: a call for action. Crit Care Med. 2016;44:1414–1421.
201. Antonsdottir, I., Rushton, C. H., Nelson, K. E., Heinze, K. E., Swoboda, S. M., Hanson, G. C. Burnout and moral resilience in interdisciplinary healthcare professionals. Journal of Clinical Nursing.2021, 00, 1–13.
202. Corley MC. 1995. Moral distress of critical care nurses. Am J Crit Care. 1995;4(4):280–285.
203. Giannetta N, Sergi R, Villa G, et al. Levels of moral distress among health care professionals working in hospital and community settings: a cross sectional study. In Healthcare (Vol. 9, No. 12, p. 1673). MDPI, 2021.
204. Emple A, Fonseca L, Nakagawa S, et al. Moral distress in clinicians caring for critically ill patients who require mechanical circulatory support. Am J Crit Care. 2021;30(5):356–362.

205. Maffoni M, Argentero P, Giorgi I, et al. Healthcare professionals' moral distress in adult palliative care: a systematic review. BMJ Support Palliat Care. 2019;9(3):245–254.
206. Varcoe C, Pauly B, Webster G, Storch J. Moral distress: tensions as springboards for action. HEC Forum. 2012;24:51–62.
207. National Academies of Sciences, Engineering, and Medicine; National Academy of Medicine; Committee on Systems Approaches to Improve Patient Care by Supporting Clinician Well-Being. Taking action against clinician burnout: a systems approach to professional well-being. Washington, DC: National Academies Press; 2019.
208. Rushton CH, Schoonover-Shoffner K, Kennedy MS. A collaborative state of the science initiative: transforming moral distress into moral resilience in nursing. Am J Nurs. 2017;117(S2): S2–S6.
209. American Nurses Association (ANA) Professional Issues Panel on Moral Resilience. Exploring moral resilience toward a culture of ethical practice: a call to action report. American Nurses Association. Published 2017. Accessed February 21, 2023. https://www.nursingworld.org/~4907b6/globalassets/docs/ana/ana-call-to-action--exploring-moral-resilience-final.pdf.
210. Cruess RL, Cruess SR, Steinert Y. Medicine as a community of practice: implications for medical education. Acad Med. 2018;93(2):185–191.
211. Delgado J, Siow S, de Groot J, et al. Towards collective moral resilience: the potential of communities of practice during the COVID-19 pandemic and beyond. J Med Ethics. 2021;47(6):374–382.
212. Epstein EG, Haizlip J, Liaschenko J, et al. Moral distress, mattering, and secondary traumatic stress in provider burnout: a call for moral community. AACN Adv Crit Care. 2020;31(2):146–157.

3

Mapping the Path of Moral Adversity

Cynda Hylton Rushton

OVER THE PAST three decades, our orientation to the moral suffering experienced by clinicians working in stressful healthcare environments has been framed primarily in terms of the concept Jameton termed "moral distress."[1,2,3,4,5] Reviewed at length in Chapter 2, studies conducted within this conceptual framework, have added immeasurably to our understanding of moral suffering and what must be done to address the adverse effects of moral distress on clinician well-being, retention, and recruitment, and the quality of patient care. In the current epidemic of moral distress,[6] clinicians struggle to practice in ways aligned with their personal and professional values and commitments.

An Alternative Orientation

Clearly, we need to explore approaches that empower and support clinicians in sustaining their moral integrity under conditions of constraint and duress and take principled action to redress the systemic factors that regularly and persistently undermine individual clinicians' integrity. While it is true that in some circumstances clinicians may be overwhelmed and dispirited by various types of moral adversity, it is also true that such adversity offers the possibility for constructive and beneficial results. As the Buddhist monk and Zen master Thich Nhat Hanh observes, "If we can recognize suffering, and if we can embrace it and look deeply into its

Cynda Hylton Rushton, *Mapping the Path of Moral Adversity* In: *Moral Resilience*. Second Edition.
Edited by: Cynda Hylton Rushton, Oxford University Press. © Oxford University Press 2024.
DOI: 10.1093/oso/9780197667149.003.0004

roots, then we'll be able to let go of the habits that feed it and, at the same time, find a way to happiness."[7(p15)]

Clinicians do not have a uniform experience of moral adversity. As studies measuring moral distress using multi-dimensional scoring suggest,[5,8,9,10] not everyone experiences the same intensity of negative consequences. We believe that it is possible for clinicians to navigate morally distressing situations in ways that lessen their suffering and produce integrity-preserving results. We hold that, in the wake of moral suffering, clinicians can find meaning, re-affirm their original commitments and values, and release the residual effects of frustration, anger, despair, and shame.[6,11] Embracing such an orientation requires recognizing the moral energy revealed by moral adversity and directing that energy in ways that empower clinicians and foster their personal and professional integrity and resilience, they need to navigate and address complexities of clinical care.[6] While clinicians have individual responsibility for their choices, decisions, and actions, this alternative approach in no way suggests that they are blameworthy for the pervasive and significant contributions of the environments where they practice that may undermine their individual efforts of moral conscientiousness and integrity. Clinicians will be able to fully practice with integrity only if organizations join with them to co-create conditions that allow them to be morally resilient and to deliberately develop systems and processes that enable ethical practice. Figure 3.1 reflects a conceptual typology of moral resilience and ethical practice that illustrates the central role of integrity and the synergistic relationship among the elements of moral resilience and a culture of ethical practice.

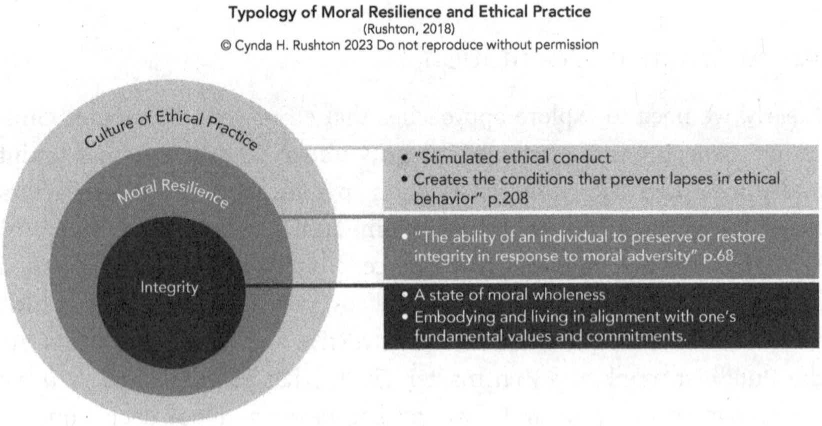

FIGURE 3.1. A typology of moral resilience and ethical practice.

A Conceptual Map of Responses to Moral Adversity

Synthesizing selected moral concepts explored in conceptual and empirical scholarship illustrates core elements that offer promise in refining our understanding of moral adversity and moral resilience as a means for shifting how we experience it. As shown in Figure 3.2, these concepts can be viewed as focal points in a cycle of imperiled integrity in response to moral harms, wrongs, failures, or other forms of moral adversity that initially create moral stress, a neutral state of readiness to respond that will eventually involve an appraisal as positive or negative. Depending on this appraisal and individual capabilities, we postulate that moral stress may be re-balanced, released, or resolved, engaging our moral resilience to respond to moral adversity proactively or prospectively. Alternatively, when the moral stress of imperiled integrity exceeds the individual's capacities and becomes unmanageable or overwhelming, it can instigate a pathway leading to moral suffering.

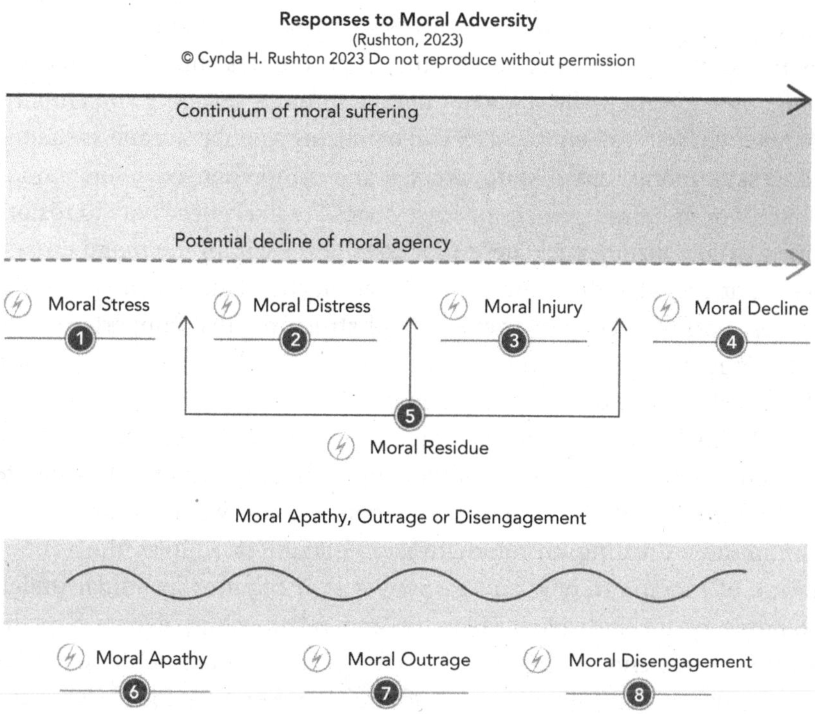

FIGURE 3.2. Responses to moral adversity.

As Figure 3.2 illustrates, there is a continuum of responses to moral adversity. Moral suffering, including moral distress and moral outrage (and potentially other responses), can be experienced as threats of varying degrees of intensity to integrity or well-being, or as an opportunity for learning and transformation. If the moral suffering, such as unrelieved moral distress, is appraised as imperiling integrity and is not sufficiently redressed, its more severe forms can lead to temporary or sustained moral injury, potentially leading to diminished moral agency, moral impairment, or decline.

Alternatively, if the stress or suffering is appraised as moral opportunity and is sufficiently resourced, moral resilience—a process aimed at restoring, preserving, or deepening moral integrity and ultimately cultivating the sustained capacity for principled moral action—may be engaged (Figure 3.3). Embedded in moral resilience is the capacity to engage in a process of moral repair. This capacity will engage interconnected, synergistic skills that have the potential to contribute to processes of preserving, restoring, or deepening moral integrity. If moral suffering occurs, restoring integrity involving moral repair and moral resilience can be instigated or can lead to recalcitrant or persistent forms of moral impairment and decline. When more corrosive forms of moral suffering such as moral injury lead to moral decline, opportunities still exist to recover one's moral agency, efficacy, and integrity through engaging and amplifying one's moral resilient capacity and practicing a deliberate and sustained process of moral repair. More targeted and comprehensive interventions to address the consequences of these states are likely necessary to restore integrity and well-being. These processes occur within the moral ecosystem that includes the culture of ethical practice that encompasses the values, norms, processes, systems, and structures that support an individual's moral agency, dignity, integrity, and moral resilience. These are described in more detail in Chapters 10 and 11.

Admittedly, the process illustrated in Figure 3.2 is not linear and the concepts identified are likely overlapping without bright lines to separate them from one another. The labels help us to locate where we are on this continuum. Creating an alternative orientation to address the various forms of moral adversity and responses to it requires an initial understanding of the individual elements and relationships depicted in the figure. To this end, we describe key elements and examine the interplay among them, starting with moral adversity and ending, ideally, with the restoration of integrity. We offer this map as a catalyst for further refinement and dialogue. Further theoretical and empirical work is needed to

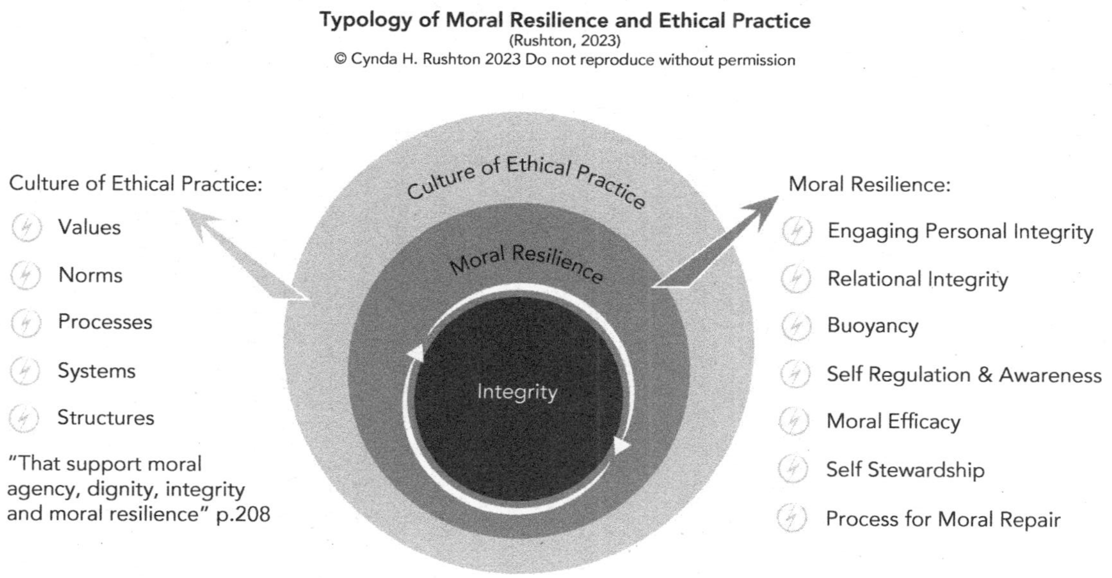

FIGURE 3.3. Elements of moral resilience and ethical practice.

fully define these interconnections and boundaries. An understanding of the moral ecosystem including the organizational context for these individual elements is essential to efforts to design systems that support individuals in addressing the moral adversity embedded in healthcare in integrity-preserving ways.

Moral Adversity

Moral adversity occurs when internal or external circumstances or actions produce morally objectionable, troublesome, or unfortunate circumstances or results that can imperil integrity and well-being, either individually or collectively.[12] There are some forms of moral adversity that accompany particular roles, such as those of clinicians, which we are unable to avoid and are required to face. A spectrum of adversity, ranging from mild to severe, produces consequences that include various forms of moral stress and suffering. Moral adversity takes many forms: the stress manifest in somatic twinges of anxiety related to a moral conflict that we begin to forecast before it occurs; the distress we experience when we are unable to act in accordance with our moral compass; or the despair that accompanies moral injury arising from our participation in moral wrongdoing. It can also manifest as persistent or repeated experiences of diminished or thwarted moral effectiveness—a sustained experience of being unable, under given circumstances, to effectively act in alignment with one's core values and commitments; it can lead to acute moral despair and the correlative experience of being unable to sustain robust moral integrity in a positive sense.[6] It can also manifest in response to moral harms, wrongs, or failures that may or may not be of our own making. The sources of moral adversity also include problematic expectations, working conditions that are inhospitable to ethical practice, internal and external policies that undermine core value commitments, fracture relationships, or create systemic inequities, among others. Often there is a dynamic interplay among these instigators of moral adversity that require targeted inquiry, discernment, and action.

Being afflicted by an instance that challenges, threatens, or compromises our moral core reveals the contours and limitations of our moral capacities and resilience. Sometimes we can proactively detect these situations or prospectively leverage our internal and external resources and address them without undue stress or distress. Other instances render us impotent to change the underlying source of our adversity and lead to varying degrees of impairment, despair, or overwhelming emotions. While stress and distress may cause myriad burdens, they also provide us with the opportunity to enhance our moral capacities, to remain true to our values and commitments in response to situations that challenge or threaten them, to deepen our character, and to strengthen our resolve to live in concert with what matters most. Although we, as individual clinicians, cannot negate the endemic systemic problems that precipitate or intensify moral adversity, moral adversity can create the conditions that allow us to access or cultivate our innate resilient potential, fortify our capacities for resilience, and foster reintegration, understanding, or growth.[13] Given that as humans we tend to orient toward the negative aspects of our experience, overcoming the hardship, loss, and despair we experience will require a substantial shift in our mindsets, responses, and actions if we are to embrace the possibility of a growth-producing alternative. With this foundation we are better able to discern an integrity-preserving pathway to engage in systemic reforms within our sphere of influence and capability and to leverage our collective efforts to dismantle the contributors to degraded integrity.

Imperiled Integrity

As discussed in Chapter 4, integrity is the anchor for moral resilience. It encompasses personal, professional, and relational aspects of integrity. As clinicians, we find ourselves in a range of situations that imperil our integrity in minor and/or profound ways, especially if we experience serious moral harms, wrongs, or failures, associated with varying degrees and forms of moral adversity. The experience of imperiled integrity may manifest itself as anxiety about our ability to sustain compassion during a harried workday, as worry about being unable to avoid a foreseeable moral harm, or as fear associated with the perceived ramifications of taking an ethical stand within a toxic work environment. It may involve the inability to withstand moral harms or threats to integrity reflecting a level of complicity and the inability to trust ourselves to resist doing what is unjustified, thus harming not only the individual but also the broader community. Likewise, our integrity can be imperiled when we abandon our own moral agency in favor of political correctness, abandon our core moral commitments in deference to authority or organizational or regulatory requirements, or (perhaps more insidiously and corrosively) associate with persons who model or sanction behaviors contrary to personal or professional norms. When our integrity is compromised or diminished, we are more susceptible to corruption by others and more vulnerable to lapses in what we believe to be morally or ethically correct attitudes or actions.

Integrity can also be imperiled in response to a moral crisis where a clinician is faced with inconsistency in the unjust application of ethical principles or values in caring for a particular patient or, over time, caring for patients with similar clinical profiles, or when systemic inequities limit access to clinically indicated treatments or resources. Depending on the attending physician in charge of the case, for example, there may be widely divergent treatment plans for similar patients—aggressive treatment for some and early recommendations to withdraw life-sustaining treatments for others. These differences in approach can also be evident over time for a single patient with the weekly change of attending physicians and the plan of care. As one ICU nurse reflected, "You've got one doctor that's obviously positive about the patient and then, the next day, another doctor that's negative about that patient. And that's hard because it's almost like that person's life is hovering between which doctor is going to be on duty."[14(p28)] These discrepant approaches can create initial moral stress but can also accumulate and intensify, resulting in various forms of moral suffering.

A hallmark of integrity is a commitment to uphold core ethical values, principles, and commitments (all things considered) and to speak up about violations of these values and principles; this may involve executing unpopular decisions and, when appropriate, conscientiously objecting to ethically compromising situations despite resistance in a fair, respectful, and modulated manner. It does not imply apathy, disregard, or indifference to everyday ethical challenges or troublesome or egregious situations. On the contrary, clinicians must take steps to determine personal and collective thresholds of accommodation in situations of moral adversity and define norms governing when action is permissible or justified. This requires the environment in which we act and speak to be supportive of and receptive to our efforts. When relational circumstances erect powerful deterrents to speaking about and acting on one's conscientious moral judgments, both individual and collective integrity are undermined. Both forms of integrity are described in more detail in Chapter 4.

When integrity is imperiled in some way in response to moral adversity, the path forward may be punctuated by a variety of responses affecting body, mind, and spirit. We postulate that several processes may be activated along a spectrum. Prominent among these is generalized moral stress that may lead to moral residue that can contribute to moral suffering, including moral distress or injury that in turn can lead to more permanent states such as moral impairment or decline. Other prominent responses to moral adversity include moral apathy, outrage, or disengagement.

Moral Stress

Clinicians are exposed to myriad stressors every day. The stressors associated with the managerial aspects of clinical work, the physical labor of caregiving, competing demands for time and expertise, or the emotional toll of confronting suffering are commonplace. Cribb describes these as expected, especially within stressed systems, but not necessarily crisis points.[15] Stress is inevitable and normal for all humans. Although widely considered detrimental to human well-being, stress can have both positive and negative consequences depending on a variety of genetic, biologic, emotional, and cognitive factors including one's appraisal of the stressor as a threat or an opportunity. Although the narrative surrounding stress typically tends to isolate the negative aspects rather than engage the potential for positive enrichment, stress, as Hans Selye suggests, is not always negative.[16] It can be beneficial stress. or *eustress,* a state of positive orientation toward a stressor that fuels self-efficacy and motivation for action. In the short term, it can heighten awareness; prepare the body, mind, and emotions for responsiveness; and instigate connection and relationship. Moreover, eustress is associated with hope, meaning, engagement, and a positive correlation with life satisfaction and well-being.[17] Moral "eustress" is defined as "a sense of well-being, which in turn, enhances the individual's moral potential."[18(p45)] When we are in a state of moral balance, it is possible to accurately perceive the moral/ethical contours of the situation, effectively exercise moral agency, discern integrity-preserving actions, and have the energy to enact decisions that reflect character, values, and commitments.

In this context, moral stress is defined as a state of arousal in response to real or potential threats or challenges to one's integrity arising from moral adversity. The moral alarm system can manifest as a quivering of awareness in the body of potential threats to important values or commitments and help focus attention on the features of the situation that are most salient. Leveraging the potential for eustress, we can fine-tune the definition of moral stress to signify a situation that taxes but does not deplete one's resources and leaves one's moral agency and integrity intact, albeit bruised. Moral stress may be activated in response to moral uncertainty, where one is unsure which path is morally obligatory or desirable or which moral concerns or principles ought to be prioritized[19] or when conscience is activated.[20] It may occur in a variety of circumstances: when there is dissonance between moral values or commitments within a process of understanding or discerning the moral contours of the situation; when there is anticipatory anxiety about how one might navigate a complex ethical concern or deal with the collateral consequences of the decisions of others; or when there are moral disagreements about which values or principles apply or the morally justified course to take but does not include moral culpability. Moral stress may also be manifest as the strain experienced in response to a perceived conflict between personal moral values and professional requirements.[21] In such instances, expectations or requirements to act in a particular way are prescribed, but the ethical justification for doing so may be unclear or contested. Other authors have narrowed the focus exclusively on the systemic contributors to moral stress.[22] In each of these examples, the moral stress does not necessarily create a crisis point because the consequences are anticipated or proportionate to the potential harm or wrong, but the person is nonetheless burdened by them.[15]

While moral stress may have negative consequences, viewing it as a state of receptivity, curiosity, balanced awareness, and non-judgment that initiates moral attunement, inquiry and action offers a more neutral starting point. It serves to alert us to vulnerabilities in upholding our moral obligations[23] and is associated with a more positive mindset and enhanced ability to detect our own "moral blindness."[24] When moral stressors are appraised as a constructive challenge and an opportunity for learning and growth, and clinicians perceive themselves as having the requisite capacities included in moral resilience to modulate the effects of the stress, detrimental consequences can be modulated or potentially eliminated.

Consider the oncology fellow caring for an elderly man with metastatic cancer, declining functional status, and quality of life who persistently rejects suggestions to shift the focus of his care toward palliation. After talking with the patient, the oncology fellow notices feeling unsettled as he orders another round of chemotherapy. He finds himself wondering if the patient truly understands the extent of his disease and his prognosis. Could a lack of understanding be compromising the patient's autonomy to make informed decisions about his treatment? The fellow shares his concern with the patient's nurse, who suggests the patient may need more time to accept his prognosis and reports he has confided that he is worried about what will happen to his wife if "things don't go well." The fellow acknowledges his uncertainty and unrest about doing the right thing for the patient; writes an order for the palliative care social worker to see the patient to clarify his understanding and assess his preferences for continued interventions; and asks the chaplain to visit with the patient to determine if there are unmet spiritual needs.

In this case, the goal is to find and maintain an optimum balance of moral stress (eustress) by recognizing the presence of a moral challenge, discerning, and mobilizing action despite uncertainty, anxiety, or unrest. The presence of a stress response does not imply that the fellow is violating an ethical standard or commitment. It could alert him of a potential or impending moral compromise and lead to further inquiry, discernment, or engagement of others to address the concern before such a violation occurs. At this juncture, there is an opportunity to shift the appraisal of the event that is perceived as imperiling integrity to one of possibility, not threat, and to recognize the signals of stressed capacities in responding to it. Viewing oneself as capable of responding to and being effective in one's professional role, despite the stress, can enable clearer discernment, engage self-stewardship practices, release energy, and motivate action. Doing so engages our capacities of moral resilience. Conceptualizing the process of imperiled integrity in this way creates an avenue for prevention, heightened awareness, and proactive principled action. If the source of the moral stress is identified, it may be possible to reduce or re-balance the moral stress by utilizing internal or external resources such as pausing to re-focus attention, taking care of basic needs (eating, sleeping, exercising, socializing), or other practices to reduce the impact of the situation and to motivate action aimed at addressing and potentially remediating the source of the stress.[20] It may also involve engaging a vital element of moral resilience: re-appraisal of one's assumptions or understandings of the boundaries of one's moral responsibility or moral agency in the situation or examining one's responses to the situation if their intensity exceeds what is warranted.

Proactive engagement of additional resources to assist in addressing the source of the moral stress or relieving it can be enhanced by engaging in constructive dialogue with colleagues, participating in forums to explore ethical tensions, or seeking consultation with others. As Lützén and Kvist[23] posit, moral stress is not only an individual process; it also becomes an interpersonal process when a group of clinicians share and respond to a common experience and perceive the source of their stress in a similar manner. Leveraging the individual and collective experience of the situation creates an opportunity for learning and growth and offers a way to demonstrate one's integrity in relationship to others. Others have argued that moral eustress enables the "alignment among the stated and unstated organizational values and practices, and the interactive capacity of the individual and the organization to assess, interact, and resolve progressively more complex organizational issues."[17(p45)] Mobilizing moral stress to identify the systemic sources of moral adversity offers a means for creating new patterns that decrease the likelihood of recurrence and to engage leaders and others in designing solutions. It must be acknowledged that there are some moral stressors created by systemic policies, structures, and decisions that are not easily amenable to intervention, such as structural injustices, patterns of disempowerment, economic drivers, budgetary constraints, and so on. These stressors, while predictable and often recalcitrant, can also accumulate and intensify.

When the capacity to modulate the moral stressor, through adaptation and coping, is exceeded, or when the physical, emotional, or cognitive systems are overwhelmed and disabled, negative consequences ensue.[25,26,27] When the moral stress of imperiled integrity exceeds the individual's capacity for balance and inquiry and becomes unmanageable or overwhelming, it can potentially lead to moral suffering, including moral distress or injury and other consequences. At such a juncture, the limits of one's moral capacities may also be temporarily or permanently stretched, overwhelmed, or disabled.

Moral Suffering, Moral Distress, and Moral injury

Moral Suffering

As discussed in Chapter 1, moral suffering is the anguish experienced in response to moral adversity, harms, wrongs, or failures, or unrelieved moral stress. As an embodied state, it is activated when we witness, participate in, or directly precipitate situations that produce a wide range of negative moral outcomes. It can also arise when we fail to uphold important moral values or in some other way fall short from a moral point of view; in these situations, the response commonly includes the activation of conscience signifying a threat to one's integrity. Somatic signals often arise before cognitive awareness of their source. Clinicians who work in situations where there are pressures for efficiency, throughput, or inadequate staffing may acutely or chronically experience moral suffering in response to the dissonance between their professional values and their organizational mandates or inconsistencies in behaviors, thoughts, and action related to how dying people are treated.[28,29,30,31,32,33] They may also experience it in response to threats by superiors when moral concerns are expressed or obstacles are erected that create compromises to professional norms.[21,34] Most fundamentally at stake are one's moral values and commitments that can be ignored, challenged, or violated, leading to a loss of self-esteem, self-confidence, or moral wholeness. It can also be precipitated in response to moral betrayal and unresolved moral dissonance that can lead to various forms of moral alienation, fatigue, or indifference or in extreme situations "soul pain."[35]

While we acknowledge moral adversity as a reality in clinical practice, we hold that the moral suffering it produces has the potential for cultivating greater insight, strengthening character, and fostering moral perseverance and growth. We agree that, as Dorothy Soelle suggests, "suffering is a form of change that a person experiences; it is a mode of becoming."[36(p98)] This life-affirming view of moral suffering offers us the means for letting go of what has bound us in the past and embracing a new reality or shifting our perspective in ways that releases the anguish surrounding our experience while allowing us to remain steadfastly and responsibly engaged in illuminating and responding to threats and violations of essential moral and ethical values. Embracing this possibility does not imply complacency or denial of the systemic contributions to moral adversity or moral suffering. Restoring wholeness and moral agency gives clinicians the ability to choose their responses and determine integrity-preserving actions to address systemic adversities rather than be rendered powerless. With renewed or restored integrity, they are better able to determine the boundaries of personal or professional authority and responsibility, appraise their level of engagement and organizational investment, make non-reactive decisions, and discern when they have exerted sufficient effort to fulfill their ethical values and commitments.

Moral Distress

As documented at length in Chapter 2, one prominent type of moral suffering is moral distress, broadly understood as the anguish felt in response to a situation in which one has "violated a core value commitment, failed to fulfill a fundamental moral obligation, or in some other significant way fallen morally short under conditions of constraint or duress."[6] Moral distress can also arise more insidiously as persistent anxiety, uncertainty, or anticipatory concern, tied to a sense of imperiled integrity under conditions of constraint or duress.[37,38] The impact of external factors, namely, social and institutional impediments, is commonly acknowledged in the moral distress literature; internal factors are increasingly recognized as significant, especially the "residue" of insufficiently resolved distress carried into new situations.[39] Unrelieved moral stress can lead to moral distress, negatively affecting a person's whole being—physically, psychologically, behaviorally, spiritually, and morally. The intensity and persistence of the distress often reveal the tenuousness and strain of one's capacities to maintain integrity and wholeness. A particular of set of moral consequences can spill over into other areas of one's life and create impediments to principled action and well-being leading to states such as burnout.[40], Post Traumatic Stress Disorder (PTSD), and degraded mental health.[41,42,43] The challenges of sustaining integrity under conditions of constraint and uncertainty readily engage notions of moral agency. Sometimes the moral tension resides in doing what is best for the clinician versus what will serve the patient. How does an exhausted clinician reason about the moral trade-offs between getting rest and nourishment so that they can return the next day refreshed and competent with routinely extending their clinic hours to accommodate the organization's productivity benchmarks? Clinicians must wrestle with how to compromise, speak out, refuse, or exit under conditions of constraint that arise from unequal authority, organizational structures, and societal mandates. Clinicians are moral agents in an imperfect, complex system, where they practice in a moral ecosystem with very real constraints and pressures that can lead to self-betrayal or incentives that propel them to abandon important values or commitments.[6] Often these circumstances are not of their making but nonetheless acutely and chronically erode their integrity, well-being, and work engagement.

Clinicians of integrity do not escape moral distress or moral suffering; they engage with it. They recognize the ethical conflicts and dilemmas in difficult situations and strive to bring their values and commitments to bear on the moral issues they face without unrealistic expectations of themselves or taking on more responsibility for the outcome than is within their control or authority. They understand that fulfilling their societally constructed and sanctioned authority and professional ethical values is dependent upon a societal and organizational investment in an infrastructure that enables, rather than constrains, their professionalism, integrity, and well-being. Committed to their professional role, they accept the experience of moral distress as a testament to their moral conscientiousness rather than evidence of their moral failing.[6] While it is true that situations of moral adversity can lead clinicians to be overwhelmed with the depleting and disempowering nature of their experiences, the shift from seeing oneself as a victim of the situation to a fully engaged moral agent requires the cultivation of both individual strategies as well as system reforms designed to support individual and collective integrity, as discussed in detail in later chapters.

Moral Injury

If the moral suffering in the form of persistent moral distress is not stabilized or relieved, moral injury can ensue. There is no unified definition of moral injury despite efforts to achieve consensus on the concept.[44] Nancy Sherman defines moral injury as the "experiences of serious inner conflict arising from what one takes to be grievous moral transgressions that can overwhelm one's sense of goodness and humanity."[45(p8)] She continues to explain that "the assertion of moral injury presumes a state of moral wholeness that can be compromised by injury or pathology. In some cases, the moral injury has less to do with specific (real or apparent) transgressive acts than with a generalized sense of falling short of moral and normative standards befitting 'good persons.'"[45(p8)] Like other forms of moral suffering, moral injury incites conscience and impairs moral capability. In contrast to episodes of moral distress and moral outrage, the threat to integrity becomes an actual violation that erodes our moral core and can lead to loss of identity and self-worth, and result in self-destructive habits or choices.[46] We tend to recognize moral injury after it has occurred, when we realize that our individual threshold of conscience violation has been breached; our physical, emotional, and cognitive well-being has been depleted; or our usual protective mechanisms have been overwhelmed or disabled.

In the military context, moral injury results from real or apparent transgressive acts of commission or omission that led to serious inner conflict because the experience is at odds with one's moral compass and conscience. More specifically, moral injury has been defined as "perpetrating, failing to prevent, bearing witness to, or learning about acts that transgress deeply held moral beliefs and expectations."[46(p700)] They can occur in response to severe personal, collective, organizational, or leadership transgressions or betrayals. Others have suggested that moral injury may also encompass situations that "shatter fundamental moral assumptions" and create a profound disorientation, erosion of moral identity, and meaning.[47(p1022)] As with other states of moral suffering, these dimensions may be intertwined with moral distress, moral outrage, or other response to moral adversity. Betrayal-based definitions are reflected in scales used to measure moral injury.[48]

In the clinical setting, various acts of commission or omission set the stage for the development of moral injury. Consider a hypothetical example: a resident physician voices his distress about continuing to resuscitate a patient with multi-system organ failure 300 days post-transplant because of concerns about regulatory sanctions for the transplant program. His comments are disregarded and dismissed, and the resident is obligated to engage in resuscitation efforts that result in broken ribs, anoxia, and further diminished quality of life in favor of "survival" statistics. Following the incident, daily rounds are an ongoing reminder of his role in what he perceives to be a charade to "get the numbers" required by regulatory agencies. Months later the resident finds himself confronted with a similar situation and either "goes through the motions" without moral engagement or erupts with an outburst that results in a referral for "anger management" by his supervisor. As he becomes aware of his scars from the experience, he notices his reliance on sleeping medications at night and stimulants during the day along with a pattern of drinking multiple cocktails each night, often alone in his apartment. The moral injury in this case involves not simply a perpetrator and a victim but also a shared moral code that maintains social order by enforcing certain behavioral norms.[49] The resident physician operates within a culture where expressions of distress or doubt are poorly tolerated or shamed, and protests or resistance to established norms carry a high price for career advancement. Betrayal at both the personal and organizational levels act as a precipitant of his moral injury.

The degree of moral injury "manifests in a constellation of moral states ranging from mildly asymptomatic (moodiness, impatience, lack of empathy) to negative emotions (fear, anger, resentment), and emotional disorders such as depression or numbness to actual emotional trauma. It can also manifest in subclinical states (sleep disturbance, tantrums, bullying, binge eating/drinking), physical symptoms (headaches, hypertension, asthma) to severe, incapacitating physical and emotional dysfunction such as self-harm or substance use disorders."[50(p2344)] It can also cause an "existential disorientation" that breeds guilt and shame." It can lead to erosion of one's moral identity and ignite feelings of unworthiness.[51,52] It is associated with post-traumatic stress disorder (PTSD), depression, anxiety, substance use, suicidality, burnout, and turnover intent.[46,53,54,55,56,57] Moral injury symptoms are commonly assessed in empirical studies.[51] Symptoms and injury can be reversible (often with targeted intervention) or persistent, lasting a lifetime.

Prior to the COVID-19 pandemic it was assumed that most experiences of moral distress in clinical settings did not reach the level of moral injury associated with the trauma of war or other atrocities. Recent data suggest that clinicians experienced significant symptoms of moral injury.[56,57,58,59] Significant moral injury scores have been reported in four in ten nurses.[60,61] Consistent with the military experience, if moral injury is not healed, it can lead to chronic patterns of anger and unregulated moral outrage that result in harm to self or others, directly or indirectly.[46] It can also intensify vulnerability to ongoing moral stressors or situations that imperil integrity and further accumulation of moral residue and suffering.

The concept of moral injury has developed as a means of recognizing, managing, and learning from moral harms, wrongs, or failures or other forms of moral adversity in situations of moral dissonance and unrelenting moral distress. It has been framed as a deeply personal breech of sacred relationships.[62] Increasingly, moral injury is being framed as an organizational failure and as distinct from burnout.[63] Whether these distinctions are valid remain to be empirically investigated. Regardless, moral injury begins as a personal experience in response to intense and corrosive forms of moral adversity and impacts everyone within that ecosystem. Moral injury need not be a permanent state. Through a process of moral repair and other targeted interventions to address underlying conditions, recovery, healing, and restoration to health are also possible. Depending upon the severity of the symptoms, moral injury treatment may require engagement with mental health or other specially trained practitioners to heal the injury. When these occur in tandem with comprehensive systemic reforms to dismantle the conditions and behaviors that produce it, sustainable change is possible. The kinds of sweeping reforms of the healthcare system that are needed will likely take time to accomplish. In the meantime, we can begin to heal the wounds of the people within the system to restore their integrity and well-being.

Moral Residue

Throughout the continuum of responses to moral adversity, as described in chapter 2, unprocessed moral suffering can accumulate in our bodies, hearts, and minds as moral residue. As illustrated in Figure 3.2, it can follow a morally stressful situation or the experience of moral distress or moral injury and may contribute to moral apathy, outrage, or disengagement. When moral distress leads to compromised integrity, Webster and Baylis[64] refer to this as moral residue. They assert, "The experience of compromised integrity that involves the setting aside or violation of deeply held (and publicly professed) beliefs, values, and principles can sear the heart."[63(p223)] It can provoke feelings of uncertainty, guilt, regret, frustration, shame, and anxiety. The intensity and consequences of moral residue vary depending on the circumstances, individual capacities, and systemic structures and support. See Chapter 2 for more details.

Unresolved moral/ethical challenges or decisions contribute to the accumulation of moral residue. Ethical challenges typically involve trade-offs in the balance of benefits and burdens or outcomes; some are avoidable, others are inevitable. These situations occur acutely or chronically when choices among competing values, obligations, or commitments produce residual consequences and unmet obligations despite discernment that result in advancing the "least worst" outcome rather than the most beneficial. There is a difference between having to make hard choices between equally important ethical values and principles, and making choices that violate them in ways that imperil one's integrity. Clinicians can do the right thing, all things considered, and not achieve their desired outcome yet hold themselves responsible for these incommensurable trade-offs. Whether their sense of accountability is accurately attributed does not erase the residue that persists. The residual from these situations can contribute to a growing sense of ineffectiveness, self-recrimination, guilt, shame, and grief.[65]

Moral Decline

If extreme forms of unrelieved moral distress or moral injury are not addressed and sufficiently rehabilitated, the result may be temporary or persistent moral impairment reflected by declines in moral perception, discernment, and action reflective of diminished moral competence, character, or function.[49] It can become a state of "habituated, maladaptive moral impairment" individually or collectively.[49(p2344)] In such a state, the ability to recognize or address ethical conflicts and behave within a range of moral norms declines and may cause individuals to exhibit behaviors or attitudes such as callousness, disregard, apathy, or decreased empathy. It can also result in detrimental patterns of normalizing deviations in moral norms, disabling the call of conscience and one's ability to recognize moral failures or to feel guilt or remorse for decisions, actions, or consequences. In extreme instances, it can even lead to taking pride in misdeeds. As is true in most processes, however, the state of moral decline can hold steady, accelerate, or recede. When moral decline becomes recalcitrant to individual or collective efforts to restore character or moral norms or implement sanctions to address deviations in judgment or behavior, it can become an insidious, metastatic force that infects not only the individual but everyone in his relational field. While this state represents diminished moral capacity, it does not negate the possibility that, under the right circumstances, people can at any time choose to engage in activities aimed at rehabilitating or healing the sources of moral adversity or suffering. We postulate that such efforts are enhanced by work environments that are intentionally designed to foster integrity-preserving actions by clinicians and create safety and trustworthiness through policies, decisions, and behaviors.

Moral suffering can also be manifested in other states such as moral apathy, outrage, or disengagement that can be indicators of moral decline (see Figure 3.2). These responses may be episodic or sustained with varying degrees of intensity and impact. Locating oneself within this typology offers clinicians a space to consider their unique profile of responses, gain insights into their sources, and restore their ability to choose how they express their moral suffering and the potential to invest in strategies to restore their moral perception, engagement, and action. There may be areas of overlap or synergy among these concepts. Each shines a slightly different light on the potential responses to moral adversity and the pathways to address them.

Moral Apathy

Moral apathy refers to degeneration in one's moral sensitivity to recognize and respond to ethical conflicts or dilemmas that results in indifference, denial, or numbness. It pertains to a state of disinterest or lack of concern for one's own or others' moral values or principles. Moral apathy can manifest in a disposition devoid of moral motivation to act or behave in a way that is congruent with personal, professional, or broader societal values.

Moral apathy can be an insidious process, where evidence of disengagement or numbness becomes more prominent over time. Signals of moral apathy are evident in intentionally or unintentionally overlooking morally salient features of clinical work such as the inequities associated with poverty, homelessness, or substance use or in turning away from situations that provoke feelings of futility or ineffectiveness. When these signals become habitual, other responses such as moral disengagement can take hold. Moral apathy can be acute involving a clinical situation that exceeds one's capacities to respond in an integrity-preserving manner or chronic in response to accumulated moral suffering or exhaustion. Clinicians may lament that they are "going through the motions" of their work without perceiving the inherent ethical tensions or conflicts embedded in it. These themes were prominent during the COVID-19 pandemic when clinicians were confronted with an onslaught of patients needing treatment and the reality of insufficient human and material resources such as masks or other equipment. For some it was a response to moral adversity that was associated with their survival.[66] It may be difficult to differentiate moral apathy from an attitude of resignation and numbness as a means of responding to overwhelming conditions, or whether a lack of concern or engagement reflects a conscious choice.

Moral apathy can be intertwined with one's appraisal of the boundaries of one's moral agency to impact the situation that under other circumstances would engage participation rather than disengagement. A common theme in clinician narratives reflects this sentiment in their statements of "there's nothing I can do so as a result I will do nothing or not engage." Feeling shut down or numb or being unable to access emotional energy or empathic concern in response to situations where ethical concerns are present may alert clinicians to the presence of moral apathy or invite exploration of other related states such as burnout or depression. Noticing the intensity and impact of these responses can illuminate opportunities to engage in understanding their source and implement strategies to restore moral agency, moral sensitivity, and moral engagement.

Moral Outrage

The anger* that arises when clinicians perceive that fairness, respect, or other ethical standards have been violated is known as "moral

* The "Moral Outrage" section is from "Principled Moral Outrage: An Antidote to Moral Distress?," by C. H. Rushton, 2013, *AACN Advanced Critical Care, 24*, p. 82– 89. Copyright 2013 by AACN. Adapted with permission.

outrage."[67,68,69] According to Pike, it is "characterized by energy-draining frustration, anger, disgust, and a sense of powerlessness."[70(p351)] The intensity of moral outrage clinicians experience is most likely attributable to their perception of threats; their beliefs, customs, and values; their personal or professional role and identity, self-worth, or integrity.[71] Moral distress or injury does not invariably lead to moral outrage, but outrage may be the outcome when individuals respond to threats with such high intensity that they are bereft of the positive energy needed to resolve their distress. In some instances, they may vent the anger and disgust that fuel their moral outrage at other individuals or groups; and powerful negative emotions may even lead them to the moral condemnation of others.[72] It should be noted that such intense emotions may manifest themselves in a somatic, embodied state, for example, activating the gastroenteric nervous system to produce physical symptoms such as nausea.[73] Recognizing the sources of and responses to moral outrage is key to distinguishing it from other strong emotional responses that may involve projection, rationalization, displacement, or reaction formation.[70]

Consider a critical care clinician working in a unit where decision-making for surgical patients is shared between the critical care team and the surgical team, who struggle with the daily advancement of aggressive therapies to treat a patient in multi-system organ failure without acknowledging the high likelihood of ongoing suffering and death. She may feel frustrated at not being able to achieve the desired outcome for a patient and blame other clinicians or specialists for their inability to achieve their goals. She may direct her anger or outrage toward the administration of the institution, the government, or the policymaker who create external barriers to what clinicians perceive as quality patient care. These sources of strong reactions need to be differentiated to determine whether moral outrage is, in fact, the source of the response.

Characteristically moral outrage arises from our conscience, character, and core moral commitments.[74] It is a justified response to morally transgressive decisions or acts and is appropriate in situations that compromise a clinician's important ethical values, standards, or commitments. Emotional responses to egregious situations can fuel the insights one needs to discern the moral contours of a situation, to evaluate the ethically permissible or ethically required actions to address the concern, and to motivate and sustain the courage to persevere in the face of resistance.

The expression of moral outrage is not without risk. It requires rigorous inquiry and exacting self-regulation on the part of the clinician who speaks out to avoid or reduce detrimental consequences.[75] For the clinician and all the parties involved, the strong drive to protect deeply held values may propel them toward "absolutism, either/or thinking, power struggles, and blaming or disconnection."[73(p83)] In some situations, the clinician may express an excessive or disproportionate level of outrage or, in others, err in identifying what exactly caused it. Conflicts are inevitable in the practice environment, and interdisciplinary team members may disagree with one another or find themselves at odds with patients or their families or their leaders. Some will justify their anger toward an individual or group by giving it moral sanction and adopting an arrogant or self-righteous stance or by morally disengaging. A clinician's expressions of moral outrage may be met by anger on the part of another clinician or group, or by silence or by moral indifference or unconcern. The fallout in either case is that, in future instances, clinicians may fail to speak out about moral issues or may choose to overlook issues raised by others.[73]

When moral outrage remains unexpressed, unregulated, unheard, and unresolved, it can do potentially irreparable damage across the clinical environment. Despite the risk of detrimental consequences, we stand to gain from the regulated expression of moral outrage. When mindful and conscientious, it can fuel insights and actions that benefit not only ourselves but also other clinicians, patients, and their families, the organization where we practice, and greater society.[75]

Moral Disengagement

Throughout the continuum of moral stress and moral suffering, moral disengagement may be another response to moral adversity. Moral disengagement is a process whereby individuals or groups disengage from their moral standards to justify their engagement in actions that are contrary to them without shame, remorse, or self-censure. Moral disengagement occurs by recasting the immoral conduct as morally justified, diffusing responsibility, or blaming the victim of the harmful act by dehumanizing or distorting the harmful consequences of behaviors, or actions on them.[76,77]

Consider neonatologist Paulina Wexton who has practiced more than twenty years in a variety of clinical settings.[78] During this time, she has regularly confronted tragic and ethically challenging situations. Dr. Wexton was drawn to the field of neonatology after being troubled by high infant mortality rates in her rural hometown. She defied the odds and was the first woman in her county to go to medical school. Early on in her career,

Dr. Wexton was adamant about doing all she could to give every baby in her care the best chance for a good life and dedicated herself to finding ways to improve mother-infant bonding. But now, after ten years working in a busy, resource-strapped neonatal unit, Dr. Wexton is often frustrated and exhausted. She is especially distressed about the growing number of infants in her unit born to substance abusing mothers (ISAM). Her focus and priorities have shifted, and she finds herself drawn to administrative roles in which she doesn't, as she puts it, "have to deal with the dysfunctional families and dwindling funding." She has come to dread the weeks when she must be "on service," working directly with patients. Her hospital is in another reorganization with looming budget cuts to support services in her department. Given recent cuts in Medicaid funding in her state, the resources that are available to support substance use disorder recovery, especially for pregnant mothers, is becoming more limited. While the example of Dr. Wexton is theoretical, it is based on actual clinical encounters. On the one hand, Dr. Wexton may be described as "burned out," but upon a closer look, she also evinces what might be called "moral disengagement."

Bandura[76,79] describes moral disengagement as a coping strategy, a way to avoid self-condemnation and a sense of failure one might otherwise experience when one has acted in ways that violate or fall short of one's own moral standards. Within clinical practice, moral disengagement can emerge as a gradual process in which both self-awareness and self-sanctioning that would normally accompany compromises of integrity or violations of ethical standards are slowly eroded. A drift in one's own moral conduct may go unnoticed, becoming accepted and normalized, diminishing the distress it would otherwise provoke. Physicians like Dr. Wexton, for example, might at the beginning of their careers be deeply distressed by institutional and governmental pressures to discharge infants of substance abusing mothers (ISAM) and troubled by concerns about the infants' safety. They may start out energetically attempting to voice these concerns in advocating for their patients through local channels or national organizations. Persistent pressure and disappointment may, however, over time, leave them feeling powerless and despairing. And they may then come slowly to rationalize their own participation in the troubled system by adopting a "disengaged" mindset, claiming, for example, that "if it weren't for the unbridled substance use in our city that no one is addressing, these babies wouldn't be at risk; these ISAM mothers are hopeless 'druggies' who will never get help." They may, that is, come to see the mothers as "the problem," thereby deflecting attention from limitations of their own involvement in the situation impacting the mother and baby. Or they may think it is up to the Department of Children and Family Services to figure out a home environment that is safe for a baby, minimizing their own accountability because, in the end, "it's a legal issue, and something I can't control." These statements may be factually true and partially explain the reality, but they overlook the deeper moral concerns that are at play. While there are other explanations for such shifts in orientation, moral disengagement can be a way to assuage one's distress and self-condemnation, especially under conditions of exhaustion, frustration, and despair. Dr. Wexton's response may not qualify as an unethical response to a complex problem; it can signify the ethical drift that occurs as the process begins to normalize behaviors that would otherwise be regarded as morally suspect or unjustified. Although moral disengagement begins as a personal experience, it is deeply intertwined with systemic patterns that contribute to the complexity and potential for unmet expectations, obstructions to progress, and betrayal. When individual moral disengagement spreads to an entire team or organization, new norms of behavior become part of the fabric of the organization; they become solidified without ongoing reflection or challenge.

Bandura's conception of moral disengagement[77,80] is used to illustrate a potential fallout of moral suffering. Bandura's analysis illuminates some common psychological processes that clinicians in situations like Dr. Wexton's employ when repeatedly confronted with morally distressing or injurious situations they feel powerless to change. Our analysis is not designed to harshly judge Dr. Wexton's behavior or character but to illustrate the myriad ways that moral disengagement can manifest in clinicians, leaders, and others engaged in healthcare or society. A similar process may unfold when the focus of one's moral suffering is on leaders or organizations rather than a patient or population. One facet of moral disengagement involves re-defining those elements of one's conduct that threaten one's moral core, even assigning them positive value as a way of rendering them more acceptable. Given Dr. Wexton's initial interest in mother/infant bonding, for example, she is likely aware that pregnancy may offer a period of great potential for a mother to engage in treatment for her substance use disorder, especially if she is approached with empathy and respect. It is likely that early in her career this is what motivated her focus and how she approached her patients. Over time, dismissive language such as "these ISAM mothers are just hopeless druggies" can camouflage and distort the moral implications of behaviors that dehumanize the mother. Labeling a mother in this way suggests that she is undeserving of respect and support because of her substance use disorder, and the harm it does her baby is her own doing, something for which she is principally responsible. Repeating these phrases and associated narratives not only impacts Dr. Wexton's care, but it also spreads to other members of the team and eventually to the patient. These factors can be magnified when coupled with unrecognized or unacknowledged gender, race, or other biases that reflect patterns of inequality, disrespect, and injustice. The response to circumstances that erode the moral core of our work can begin as normalized labeling of patients in this way as part of our handoffs or charting and can become internalized, un-reflected beliefs. Dr. Wexton may attempt to rationalize her growing disinclination to attempt to understand the mothers' circumstances and health conditions, explore their efforts to address their substance use problem, or take seriously their constraints in securing a stable home situation for their infants. She may come to justify her withdrawal from or indifference toward substance using mothers and their babies by framing the mothers as morally deficient in their inability to fulfill their responsibilities to their infants and seeing the moral failure as theirs, a failure for which they are alone blameworthy and responsible. This in turn may enable her to justify her own conduct, to see it, not as abandonment, but as a refusal to participate in enabling drug abusing mothers to sustain their addiction.

Another dimension of moral disengagement involves relinquishing responsibility for, or in some way minimizing or disregarding, one's own role in bringing about detrimental consequences. If, for example, Dr. Wexton claims that she "doesn't have anything to do with discharge decisions of the Department of Children and Family Services; they are out of [her] control" she may be employing a strategy that relieves her of the burden of the decision about a safe discharge by placing the sole responsibility on the governmental agency. While it is true that the department does have final decision-making authority, the clinicians involved in the baby's care have moral authority and responsibility to contribute their assessment fairly and steadfastly and to make recommendations based on their knowledge of the facts of the case. Whether the department acts on their recommendations is separate from the exercise of moral agency to bring the issues to the attention of those with the authority to address them. Doing so does not diminish the responsibility of the governmental agency to fulfill its mandate or to advocate for sufficient resources to do so.

Similarly, minimizing or disregarding detrimental consequences of one's actions can be a way to compartmentalize and avoid the pain of acknowledging one's role in a troubling process. In cases like Dr. Wexton's, it can minimize distress to focus on the immediate task of discharging an infant without considering the longer-term consequences of the unstable situation into which the infant is discharged. In reality, there are many reasons that neonatologists and other neonatal clinicians may be unaware of the ultimate outcomes of their efforts for the babies and families they care for. Harmful consequences are easier to disregard, however, when clinicians neither know about nor witness the long-term impact of their decisions. Moral disengagement as a strategy of self-protection can motivate incuriosity about, and disconnection from, the consequences of one's actions within contexts in which one feels overwhelmed, frustrated, and hopeless in bringing about optimal or even morally decent outcomes.

Moral disengagement in various forms can be witnessed in clinicians in many specialties and healthcare settings. These situations are not created by clinicians nor do clinicians have the sole responsibility to address them. Many clinicians have exhausted themselves attempting to make ineffective and harmful systems work. As outlined in the case, there are complex healthcare organization, government, and societal factors at play that are beyond the scope of authority or influence of clinicians, like Dr. Wexton, that erode their integrity and moral agency. Within this ecosystem there are myriad interconnected policies and structures that have direct bearing on the way clinical care is delivered that require accountability by healthcare leadership, policymakers, insurers, educators, and others. We have used Dr. Wexton's case to illustrate a hypothetical situation in which mechanisms of moral disengagement can lead to a gradual erosion of moral standards over time, especially in well-meaning but exhausted or frustrated clinicians who have come to feel powerless in a system that continually "demands" moral compromises of them. Crucially, moral disengagement is one way clinicians cope with the difficult and painful forms of moral suffering—in effect, by dissipating the affective distress through gradual divestment of moral awareness and concern, served by rationalization, deflection, and displacement of moral responsibility and blame. Gradually divesting moral concern and involvement as one disengages, and becoming increasingly distant and dissociated from the actual moral implications of what one is doing, are ways of dealing with moral suffering. Dealing with moral suffering in this way, however, often comes at a steep price to clinicians themselves. When clinicians become aware that they've slipped into a pattern of disengagement, this itself can compound their moral suffering; it can also contribute to troubling forms of shame, guilt, and unworthiness.

Moral apathy, outrage, and disengagement are common responses to moral adversity, especially when it results in moral suffering. These illustrations are not indictments of clinicians' responses but rather a possible explanatory frame to assist clinicians to locate themselves within the context of their experiences and to invite self-honest and compassionate discernment to understand the contours of their responses and potential pathways to reclaim or fortify their moral agency and integrity. Doing so does not diminish the importance of large-scale systemic changes needed to reduce the incidence and impact of healthcare system and societal patterns that produced the conditions for moral adversity to thrive.

Moral Resilience

Defined as "the capacity of an individual to sustain or restore his or her integrity in response to moral adversity,"[81(p112)] moral resilience includes regaining moral stability and balance in the wake of the experience of imperiled integrity. Moral resilience is posited as a necessary ingredient in responding to moral stress and a vital countermeasure to the despair provoked in response to moral suffering instigated by moral conflicts, dilemmas, or internal or external constraints. It leverages our biological, psychological, and social ecological resources to regain balance and harness the necessary resources to respond to moral adversity in integrity preserving and wholesome ways. In the face of negative arousal, morally resilient clinicians are those who, in the face of the negative arousal and heightened moral sensitivity associated with moral adversity, can shift their appraisal from viewing their response as evidence of moral insufficiency to viewing that response as a signal of moral conscientiousness. This shift acknowledges that the individual is aware of the tension, disagreement, or conflict between various courses of action, notices it, and is propelled into a process of inquiry to understand the nuances, context, boundaries of ethical permissibility, personal and professional responsibility, and consequences of possible courses of action on self and others. Aware individuals possess the moral competence to discern what is at stake, the justification for various moral trade-offs, and the degree of alignment with their personal and professional values and commitments. They acknowledge their own limitations as well as the interpersonal and institutional pressures and constraints inherent in clinical practice, thereby leveraging their inherent resources and energy toward constructive solutions. Being morally resilient does not imply complacency or diminishment of the moral stakes and consequences or one's responsibility to take action to address violations of moral principles or norms. On the contrary, moral resilience provides the foundation for wise, principled action that does not rely exclusively on the authority of others to preserve or restore integrity. It requires exercising the full range of moral options including those that challenge the status quo, illuminate lapses in ethical norms and behavior, and leverage principled moral outrage. Moral resilience is also reflected as conscientious inaction or choosing to bear witness to the situation rather than engaging in more aggressive measures.

We posit that morally resilient clinicians are better able to navigate the inevitable moral stress and ethical conflicts they confront without detrimental or lingering moral residue; in some instances they can grow despite their moral suffering. This does not imply that morally resilient clinicians engage in morally complex situations or confront moral adversity and remain unscathed by the experience. On the contrary, many will experience a spectrum of mild to severe consequences and yet are able to integrate their experiences into their lives and work with restored or deepened integrity while learning to constructively address moral disagreement or conflict and system reforms. Our research has demonstrated a pattern of responses to moral adversity that suggest moral resilience is a protective resource to mitigate the harmful consequences of moral suffering.[82]

Moral resilience is fundamentally oriented toward personal, professional, and relational integrity and offers clinicians an important anchor when they must make ethical choices that require trade-offs that will necessarily cause harm or suffering to specific people or groups of people they are serving. Congruent with our understanding of integrity as including relational integrity, moral resilience is cultivated both intra-personally and interpersonally, ideally within a culture that supports ethical practice. Moral resilience is comprehensively explored in Chapter 6 (see Figure 3.3).

Moral Repair

One of the crucial elements of moral resilience is the capacity for moral repair, both individually and collectively. "Moral repair is a process of moving from the situation of loss and damage to a situation where some degree of stability in moral relations is restored." [47(p6)] As a process, it involves devising and using methods for moral repair that are focused on stabilizing or restoring moral agency, physiology, and "moral relationships by restoring or creating trust and hope in a shared sense of values and responsibility."[47(p27)] Congruent with notions of relational integrity, a clinician of integrity is committed to ongoing exploration and engagement in a variety of strategies aimed at moral repair as a dimension of moral resilience. However, it is critical to acknowledge that despite one's intentions and efforts toward moral repair, the process of restoration or re-creation is not always possible, especially in cases where serious harm and wrongs have occurred that are resistant to interventions to heal them, or one continues to practice in an environment that is adversarial or unsupportive.

There is a series of entry points into the process of moral repair in response to moral adversity and the resultant moral suffering including moral distress or injury. A fundamental component of moral repair is discerning the level of repair that is needed. Depending on the locus of the threat or violation of integrity, moral repair can be internal, interpersonal, or directed at systemic reforms. Individually focused interventions are aimed at restoring integrity, moral agency, and well-being, while interventions involving interpersonal moral repair focus on relationships with others including inter-professional colleagues, supervisors, leaders and potentially the people we serve. Moral repair may be needed at a broader level of organizational and systemic intervention when the root cause of imperiled integrity is linked to systemic norms, policies, culture, or external constraints. Typically, both levels are necessary and desirable.

Moral repair can also involve personal reconciliation in the face of interpersonal or systemic pressures and constraints that cannot otherwise be productively addressed. In such cases, moral repair may be more fundamentally first-personal and individual involving, for example, acknowledging and accepting one's limited authority and moral agency with compassion and honesty, minimizing personal harms, expanding one's capacity to distinguish the contours of personal and professional responsibility, examining one's own behavior and decision-making and reconnecting to one's fundamental nature. Individual factors may intensify the experience of moral suffering, such as one's capacity to trust oneself and others.[83] Previous experiences may limit one's vision of possible responses in the current situation or diminish self-esteem and moral confidence. Unprocessed moral suffering may accumulate and intensify and sustain the response to moral adversity. Contextual features such as culture, previous trauma, religion, and gender must be considered in designing individual methods of moral repair. The process of moral repair is supported by the cultivation of the components of moral resilience and facilitated by a means for addressing the moral threats to integrity and transgressions that one participates in or witnesses. Clinicians will likely need help in discerning the best way to respond to the range of situations of compromised integrity including actual participation in moral wrongdoing. A range of strategies for moral repair is described at length in Chapter 8, including such innovations as the use of narratives to cognitively re-frame ethically painful experiences and participation in programs developed to foster resilience.[84] The power of these individual strategies stands to increase exponentially within a collective culture designed to support ethical practice, described in Chapters 10 and 11.

Processes aimed at moral repair do not necessarily erase the suffering, isolation, and anguish experienced by the individual or group.[47] There may be some violations of integrity that cannot be undone or rehabilitated despite intentional care, skill, and responsibility. Rather, such processes are an invitation to the affected individuals to acknowledge their experience, give voice to it, and have it validated by others. Since our moral agency is developed through socialization, many people rely on moral bonds and solidarity with others (family, friends, and colleagues) to develop and clarify their notions of moral integrity. When clinicians experience feelings of moral culpability or moral suffering, their need for connections with those in their social network intensify as they attempt to reconnect their personal values with shared social and professional values. Facilitated sessions to debrief ethically complex and challenging situations in a psychologically safe environment can build solidarity and relational integrity among team members.[85]

Clinicians may need support to grieve the violation of an essential value, to reconcile the dissonance created in their views of themselves, and to find some level of vindication, such as an apology, reparation, or a personal acknowledgment of effective moral agency.[86] Access to chaplains or mental health professionals with expertise in processing grief offer clinicians additional resources. If they are experiencing personal moral culpability, social rituals may be necessary to acknowledge the deviant behavior or action and define the consequences or restitution that is necessary to restore the person's place within the social order.[47] For clinicians, this might include mechanisms such as mortality and morbidity review, after action reviews, or formal apologies that are aimed at locating the locus of responsibility and/or culpability. Without mechanisms for people to make restitution for actions they perceive to be morally culpable, they can carry an unrelenting and often overwhelming burden that undermines their ability to function as a whole and responsible moral agent. A parallel can be drawn from the arena of patient safety and the importance of having a process for errors to be acknowledged and to provide support to the second victims of such errors[87] and to offer apologies when errors have been made.[88]

For some clinicians, evidence of change in policies, practices, or relationships is part of the healing process; for others, healing comes with restored integrity, personal growth, and strengthened moral resilience. A potential outgrowth of moral repair can be the cultivation of greater empathy and compassion, together with enhanced moral attunement and discernment. Collectively, the process of moral repair can illuminate suppressed assumptions, fuel moral progress, promote healing, and contribute to systemic reforms that address the root causes of moral distress, outrage, or injury. It can also illuminate the patterns within teams, organizations, and the broader society that solidify individual patterns of choices, behaviors, and actions that either enable or disable individual and collective integrity. Moral repair is a necessary component of an ethical practice environment. It must include both individual and systemic resources and shared accountability to create integrity preserving environment for delivering healthcare for everyone.

Restored Integrity

Constructing a conceptual framework to address moral adversity and suffering and support moral resilience requires attention to the elements and processes identified in Figures 3.1–3.3. The human reality of suffering renders moral adversity an intrinsic part of the clinical environment and, as such, can imperil clinician integrity. In a workplace beset by multiple constraints and constant pressures, moral stress is inevitable. It can be the prelude to moral suffering, distress, outrage, injury, and decline. These painful and debilitating phenomena affect far too many clinicians; they deplete our professional ranks, ultimately depriving patients, and society, of the safe, quality care they deserve.[89]

This need not be so. There is an alternative approach, described in the chapters that follow. Acknowledging the current reality, Chapter 4 describes integrity as the anchor for moral resilience; and the chapters that follow offer strategies and structures that promote moral repair and foster moral resilience. This alternative approach sets forth the ways clinicians and healthcare organizations can come together to align—and thereby strengthen—individual and collective efforts to design and create a culture of ethical practice.

Acknowledgement

Dr. Alisa Carse contributed to the conceptualization of many of the concepts included in chapter. Her conceptualization and analysis of moral disengagement is greatly appreciated.

References

1. Houston S, Casanova MA, Leveille M, Schmidt KL, Barnes SA, Trungale KR, et al. The intensity and frequency of moral distress among different healthcare disciplines. J Clin Ethics, 2013;24:98–112.
2. Jameton A. Nursing practice: the ethical issues. Englewood Cliffs, NJ: Prentice-Hall; 1984.
3. Oh Y, Gastmans C. Moral distress experienced by nurses: a quantitative literature review. Nurs Ethics. 2015;22:15–31.
4. Rushton CH, Kaszniak AW, Halifax JS. A framework for understanding moral distress among palliative care clinicians. J Palliat Med. 2013;16:1074–1079.
5. Whitehead PB, Herbertson RK, Hamric AB, Epstein EG, Fisher JM. Moral distress among healthcare professionals: report of an institution-wide survey. J Nurs Scholar. 2015;47:117–25.
6. Carse A, Rushton CH. Harnessing the promise of moral distress: a call for re-orientation. J Clin Ethics. 2017;28:15–29
7. Hanh, TN. No mud, no lotus: the art of transforming suffering. Berkeley, CA: Parallax Press, 2014.
8. Allen R, Judkins-Cohn T, deVelasco R, Forges E, Lee R, Clark L, Procunier M. Moral distress among healthcare professionals at a health system. JONAS Healthc Law Ethics Regul. 2013;15:111–118.
9. Hamric AB, Borchers CT, Epstein EG. Development and testing of an instrument to measure moral distress in healthcare professionals. AJOB Prim Res. 2012;3:1–9.
10. Epstein EG, Whitehead PB, Prompahakul C, Thacker LR, Hamric AB. Enhancing understanding of moral distress: the measure of moral distress for health care professionals. AJOB Empir Bioethics. 2019;10(2):113–124.
11. Musto LC, Rodney PA, Vanderheide R. Toward interventions to address moral distress: navigating structure and agency. Nurs Ethics. 2015;22:91–102.

12. Halfon MS. Integrity: a philosophical inquiry. Philadelphia, PA: Temple University Press; 1989.
13. Young PD, Rushton CH. A concept analysis of moral resilience. Nurs Outlook. 2017; 65:579–587.
14. Heland M. Fruitful or futile: intensive care nurses' experiences and perceptions of medical futility. Aust Crit Care. 2006;19:25–31.
15. Cribb, Alan. Integrity at work: managing routine moral stress in professional roles. Nurs Phil. 2011; 12(2):119–127.
16. Selye H. Confusion and controversy in the stress field. J Human Stress. 1975;1:37–44.
17. O'Sullivan G. The relationship between hope, eustress, self-efficacy, and life satisfaction among undergraduates. Soc Indic Res. 2011;101:155–172.
18. Rambur B, Vallett C, Cohen JA, Tarule J. The moral cascade: distress, eustress and the virtuous organization. J Organizational Moral Psychol. 2010;1:1–14.
19. DeTienne KB, Agle BR, Phillips JC, Ingerson MC. The impact of moral stress compared to other stressors on employee fatigue, job satisfaction, and turnover: an empirical investigation. J Bus Ethics. 2012;110(3):377–391.
20. Glasberg A-L, Eriksson S, Dahlqvist V, Lindahl E, Strandberg G, Söderberg A, et al. Development and initial validation of the stress of conscience questionnaire. Nurs Ethics. 2006;13:633–648.
21. Cronqvist A, Lützén K, Nyström M. Nurses' lived experiences of moral stress support in the intensive care context. J Nurs Manage. 2006;14:405–413.
22. Owens J, Singh G, Cribb A. Austerity and professionalism: being a good healthcare professional in bad conditions. Health care analysis: HCA: J Health Phil, and Policy. 2019;27(3):157–170.
23. Lützén K, Kvist BE. Moral distress: a comparative analysis of theoretical understandings and inter-related concepts. HEC Forum. 2012;24:13–25.
24. Johnstone M. Bioethics: a nursing perspective. 3rd ed. Sydney, Australia: Harcourt Australia; 1999.
25. Crum AJ, Salovey P, Achor S. Rethinking stress: the role of mindsets in determining the stress response. J Pers Soc Psychol. 2013;104:716–33.
26. Fevre ML, Kolt GS, Matheny J. Eustress, distress and their interpretation in primary and secondary occupational stress management interventions: which way first? J Managerial Psychol. 2006;21:547–565.
27. Gibbons C, Dempster M, Moutray M. Stress and eustress in nursing students. J Adv Nurs. 2008;61:282–290.
28. de Vries J, Timmins F. Care erosion in hospitals: problems in reflective nursing practice and the role of cognitive dissonance. Nurse Educ Today. 2016;38:5–8.
29. Truog RD, Campbell ML, Curtis JR, Haas CE, Luce JM, Rubenfeld GD, et al. Recommendations for end-of-life care in the intensive care unit: a consensus statement by the American College of Critical Care Medicine. Crit Care Med. 2008;36:953–963.

30. Schneiderman LJ, Gilmer T, Teetzel HD, Dugan DO, Blustein J, Cranford R, et al. Effect of ethics consultations on nonbeneficial life-sustaining treatments in the intensive care setting: a randomized controlled trial. JAMA. 2003;290:1166–1172.
31. Garros D, Austin W, Dodek P. How can I survive this? Coping during COVID-19 pandemic. Chest. 2021;159:1484–1492.
32. Ulrich C, Rushton C, Grady C. Nurses confronting the coronavirus: challenges met and lessons learned to date. Nursing Outlook. 2020;68:838–844.
33. Mantri S, Song YK, Lawson JM, et al. Moral injury and burnout in health care professionals during the COVID-19 pandemic. J Nerv Mental Dis. 20211;209:720–726.
34. Haidt J, Graham J. When morality opposes justice: conservatives have moral intuitions that liberals may not recognize. Soc Justice Res. 2006;20(1):98–116.
35. Kearney M. Mortally wounded: stories of soul pain, death and healing. New York: Touchstone; 1996
36. Soelle D. Suffering. Philadelphia, PA: Fortress Press; 1975.
37. McCarthy J, Deady R. Moral distress reconsidered. Nurs Ethics. 2008;15:254–262.
38. Morley G, Bradbury-Jones C, Ives J. What is 'moral distress' in nursing? a feminist empirical bioethics study. Nursing ethics. 2020;27(5):1297–1314
39. Epstein E, Delgado S. Understanding and addressing moral distress. Online J Issues Nurs [Internet]. 2010;15(1). Available at http://dx.doi.org/10.3912/OJIN.Vol15No03Man01.
40. Moss M, Good VS, Gozal D, Kleinpell R, Sessler CN. An official critical care societies collaborative statement: burnout syndrome in critical care healthcare professionals: a call for action. Crit Care Med. 2016;44:1414–1421.
41. Powell CAJ, Butler JP. (2022). The role of moral distress on physician burnout during COVID-19. International journal of environmental research and public health. 2022;19(10):6066.
42. Norman SB, Feingold JH, Kaye-Kauderer H, Kaplan CA, Hurtado A, Kachadourian L, Feder A, Murrough JW, Charney D, Southwick SM, Ripp J, Peccoralo L, Pietrzak RH. Moral distress in frontline healthcare workers in the initial epicenter of the COVID-19 pandemic in the United States: relationship to PTSD symptoms, burnout, and psychosocial functioning. Depression and anxiety. 2021;38(10):1007–1017.
43. Spilg E, Rushton C, Phillips J, Kendzerska T, Saad M, Gifford W, Gautam M, Bhatla R, Edwards J, Quilty L, Leveille C, Robillard R. The new frontline: exploring the links between moral distress, moral resilience, and mental health in healthcare workers during the COVID-19 pandemic. BMC Psychiatry. 2022;22(19):1–12.
44. Griffin BJ, Purcell N, Burkman K, Litz BT, Bryan CJ, Schmitz M, Villierme C, Walsh J, Maguen S. Moral injury: an integrative review. Journal of traumatic stress. 2019;32(3):350–362.

45. Sherman N. Afterwar: healing the moral wounds of our soldiers. Oxford: Oxford University Press; 2015.
46. Litz BT, Stein N, Delaney E, Lebowitz L, Nash WP, Silva C, Maguen S. Moral injury and moral repair in war veterans: a preliminary model and intervention strategy. Clinical psychology review. 2009;29(8):695–706.
47. Fleming WH. Complex moral injury: shattered moral assumptions. Journal of religion and health. 2022;61(2):1022–1050.
48. Nash WC, Marino Carper TL, Mills MA, Au T, Goldsmith A, Litz BT. Psychometric evaluation of the Moral Injury Events Scale. Military Medicine. 2013;178(6):646–652.
49. Walker MU. Moral repair: reconstructing moral relations after wrongdoing. Cambridge: Cambridge University Press; 2006.
50. Thompson LJ. Moral injury. In Encyclopedia of business ethics and society (Vol. 10, pp. 2340–2343). Thousand Oaks, CA: Sage; 2018.
51. Mantri S, Lawson JM, Wang Z, Koenig HG. Identifying moral injury in health-care professionals: the Moral Injury Symptom Scale-HP. J Relig Health. 2020 Oct;59(5):2323–2340.
52. Rushton C, Turner K, Brock R, Braxton J. The invisible moral wounds of the pandemic: are we experiencing moral injury? AACN Adv Critical Care. 2021;35(1): 119–125.
53. Antonsdottir I, Rushton C, Nelson K, Heinze KE, Swoboda SM, Hanson GC. Burnout and moral resilience in interdisciplinary healthcare professionals. Journal of Clinical Nursing. 2022;31(1–2):196–208. https://doi.org/10.1111/jocn.15896.
54. Hall NA, Everson AT, Billingsley MR, Miller MB. Moral injury, mental health and behavioural health outcomes: a systematic review of the literature. Clinical Psychology & Psychotherapy. 2022;29(1): 92–110.
55. Lesley M. Psychoanalytic perspectives on moral injury in nurses on the front-lines of the COVID-19 pandemic. Journal of the American Psychiatric Nurses Association. 2021;27(1):72–76.
56. Mantri S, Lawson JM, Wang Z, Koenig HG. Prevalence and predictors of moral injury symptoms in health care professionals. Journal of Nervous & Mental Disease. 2021a;209(3):174–180.
57. Mantri S, Song YK, Lawson JM, Berger EJ, Koenig HG. Moral injury and burn-out in health care professionals during the COVID-19 pandemic. Journal of Nervous & Mental Disease. 2021b;209(10):720–726.
58. Rushton CH, Thomas T, Antonsdottir I, Nelson K, Boyce D, Vioral A, Swavley D, Ley C, Hanson G. Moral injury, ethical concerns and moral resilience in health care workers during COVID-19 pandemic. Journal of Palliative Medicine. 2021;25(5):712–719
59. Ritchie K, D'Alessandro-Lowe AM, Brown A, Millman H, Pichtikova M, Xue Y, Altman M, et al. The hidden crisis: understanding potentially morally

injurious events experienced by healthcare providers during COVID-19 in Canada. International Journal of Environmental Research. 2023.

60. Rushton C, Nelson K, Antonsdottir I, Hanson G, Boyce D. Perceived organizational effectiveness, moral injury, and moral resilience among nurses during the COVID-19 pandemic: Secondary analysis. Nursing Management, 2022;53(7):12–22.
61. Fitzpatrick JJ, Pignatiello G, Kim M Jun, J, O'Mathúna DP, Duah HO, Taibl J, Tucker S. Moral injury, nurse well-being, and resilience among nurses practicing during the COVID-19 pandemic. JONA: Journal of Nursing Administration, 2022;52(7/8): 392–398.
62. DeMarco M. Moral injury and the agony and power of love. Psychology Today. September 22, 2022. https://www.psychologytoday.com/us/blog/soul-console/202209/moral-injury-and-the-agony-and-power-of-love.
63. Dean W, Talbot S, Dean A. Reframing clinician distress: moral injury not burnout. Fed Pract. 2019;36:400–402.
64. Webster GC, Baylis F. Moral residue. In Rubin SB, Zoloth L, editors, Margin of error: the ethics of mistakes in the practice of medicine. Hagerstown, MD: University Publishing Group; 2000.
65. Hardingham LB. Integrity and moral residue: nurses as participants in a moral community. Nurs Phi: Internat J Healthcare Profes. 2004;5(2):127–134.
66. Ulrich C, Rushton C, Grady C. Nurses confronting the coronavirus: challenges met and lessons learned to date. Nursing Outlook. 2020..
67. The "Moral Outrage" section is from "Principled Moral Outrage: An Antidote to Moral Distress?" by C. H. Rushton, 2013, AACN Advanced Critical Care, 24, pp. 82–89. Copyright 2013 by AACN. Adapted with permission.
68. Wilkinson JM. Moral distress in nursing practice: experience and effect. Nurs Forum. 1987;23:16–29.
69. Batson CD, Kennedy CL, Nord L, Stocksy EL, Fleming DA, Marzette CM, et al. Anger at unfairness: is it moral outrage? Eur J Soc Psychol. 2007;37:1272–1285.
70. Pike AW. Moral outrage and moral discourse in nurse-physician collaboration. J Prof Nurs. 1991;7:351–362.
71. Goodenough WH. Moral outrage: territoriality in human guise. Zygon. 1997;32:5–27.
72. Rozin P, Lowery L, Imada S, Haidt J. The CAD triad hypothesis: a mapping between three moral emotions (contempt, anger, disgust) and three moral codes (community, autonomy, divinity). J Pers Soc Psychol. 1999;74:574–586.
73. Schnall S, Haidt J, Clore GL, Jordan AH. Disgust as embodied moral judgment. Pers Soc Psychol Bull. 2008;34:1096–1099.
74. Rushton CH. Principled moral outrage: an antidote to moral distress? AACN Adv Crit Care. 2013;24:82–89.
75. Rushton C, Thompson L. Moral outrage: promise or peril. Nursing Outlook. 2020; 68(5):536–538.

76. Bandura, A. (2011). Moral disengagement. In The encyclopedia of peace psychology, D.J. Christie, ed.
77. Bandura, A. Moral disengagement: how people do harm and live with themselves. New York: Worth; 2016.
78. An unpublished version of this scenario and analysis by Alisa Carse PhD. was adapted for inclusion in this chapter.
79. Bandura A. Selective moral disengagement in the exercise of moral agency. Journal of Moral Education. 2002;31:101–119.
80. Rodney P, Kadychuk S, Liaschenko J, Brown H, Musto L, Snyder N. Moral agency: relational connections and support. In JL Storch, P Rodney, R Starzomski, editors, Toward a moral horizon: nursing ethics for leadership and practice (160–187). Toronto, Canada: Pearson; 2013..
81. Rushton CH. Moral resilience: a capacity for navigating moral distress in critical care. AACN Adv Crit Care. 2016;27:111–119.
82. Rushton CH. Transforming moral suffering by cultivating moral resilience and ethical practice. Amer Jour Crit Care. 2023;32(4):238–248.
83. Reina ML, Reina DS, Rushton CH. Trust: the foundation for team collaboration and healthy work environments. AACN Adv Crit Care. 2007;18:103–108.
84. Nelson HL. Damaged identities: moral repair. Ithaca, NY: Cornell University Press; 2001.
85. Morley G, Horsburgh CC. Reflective debriefs as a response to moral distress: two case study examples. HEC Forum. 2023;35(1):1–20.
86. Lazare A, Levy RS. Apologizing for humiliations in medical practice. Chest. 2011;139(4):746–751..
87. Seys D, Scott S, Wu A, Van Gerven E, Vleugels A, Euwema M, et al. Supporting involved health care professionals (second victims) following an adverse health event: a literature review. Int J Nurs Stud. 2013;50(2):678–687.
88. Lazare A. Apology in medical practice: an emerging clinical skill. JAMA. 2006;296(11):1401–1404.
89. Fry-Bowers E, Rushton C. Reimagining nursing's social contract with the public. American Nurse Journal. 2023.

4

Integrity

THE ANCHOR FOR MORAL RESILIENCE

Cynda Hylton Rushton

CLINICIANS ARE REGULARLY called to act in accordance with their personal and professional moral compasses—and to do so with integrity. Such occasions go largely unnoticed because they occur in the everyday moments of clinical care; they are not confined to dramatic, high-profile situations punctuated by moral distress and despair.* Yet most clinicians experience a sense of inner harmony when they see that the action aligned with their essential values and commitments and that they have "done their best" in bringing about a beneficial outcome despite resistance or adversity. Such is the case of the nurse who, despite competing obligations to others in his care, intentionally reallocates his time, attention, and expertise to listen to a frightened patient struggling to decide about a risky treatment. Or of the physician who is steadfast in her pursuit of solutions to a complex diagnosis by being willing to question the received view of her colleagues and leveraging new evidence to reveal a new possibility. Clinicians in various roles also seize opportunities to change practice patterns or policies that disproportionately disadvantage groups of patients or create unequitable barriers to access treatment or resources. For clinicians, these everyday choices reflect an orientation toward making intentions, commitments, moral values, and actions congruent and thereby mitigating the energy

* Portions of this chapter are excerpted or adapted from a previous article with permission: Holtz H, Heinze K, Rushton C. Inter-professionals' definitions of moral resilience. J Clin Nurs. August 3, 2017; (1–7).

Cynda Hylton Rushton, *Integrity* In: *Moral Resilience.* Second Edition. Edited by: Cynda Hylton Rushton,
Oxford University Press. © Oxford University Press 2024. DOI: 10.1093/oso/9780197667149.003.0005

drain that accompanies dissonance, compromise of moral values, negative moral emotions, and self-betrayal. They also highlight an inherent moral tension between advancing one's professional interests and those of others including the organization where one practices.

While individuals are accountable for their own moral choices, leaders and organizations must also be accountable for creating the conditions for integrity to flourish and ethical practice to be enabled.[1] It is a misunderstanding to conclude that individual efforts to preserve or restore clinician integrity diminish the corollary responsibility of healthcare organizations to uphold their moral obligations to create systems that restore integrity when it is compromised and to support ethical practice.[2] Strategies for both sectors are described at length in Chapters 10 and 11.

Personal and Professional Integrity

Integrity, or "moral wholeness," is foundational to ethically grounded clinical care. Viewed as a state of balance, harmony, or solidarity, or being undiminished, integrity is a necessary element of human flourishing. Personal and professional integrity are interconnected, and the boundaries between them are nuanced. We must know ourselves intimately—who we *really* are, including our intentions, essential purpose, and commitments as well as our biases, histories, wounds, and less evolved aspects. We must heed "the silent call to our potentiality for being ourselves."[3(p329)] and embody the essential values that drive our choices and actions. Accepting responsibility for being in alignment with our moral compass and the consequences of our action or inaction is inextricably linked to a robust notion of integrity that is manifest in freedom within rightful boundaries.

Living in alignment with one's fundamental values and setting a level below which one will not stoop reflects honesty, sincerity, and integration of moral character and conscience.[4] Acting with integrity is closely tied to protecting the essence of one's values and purpose against forces that may corrupt or degrade them. Integrity arises when intentions, words, thoughts, and actions align and there is fidelity in adherence to ethical commitments, norms, and conscience.[5] When integrity is present, fear can be neutralized and the conditions for compassionate action more fully cultivated. Acting with integrity cultivates self-respect, inner balance, and ease; under conditions of adversity, it may require principled action despite personal consequences and distress to uphold fundamental values, commitments, or responsibilities.

Clinicians of integrity are committed to *being* moral, steadfastly upholding their fundamental moral beliefs and values, discerning the moral features of a particular situation with emotional balance and insight, analyzing various moral points of view, and bringing about the best course of action based upon what they discern to be consonant with those values, commitments, and responsibilities, all things considered, and to the best of their ability. They are aware of the deeper moral values that drive their behavior and choices and are not oblivious to the moral components embedded in everyday practice. At the same time, they are intimately aware of their own personal biases, assumptions, and vulnerabilities. Personal integrity is woven into and depends on how one chooses to pursue one's life and work; it is inextricably tied to one's character, understood as the manifestation of dispositions, habits, and patterns of being, responding, and acting. Virtues such as honesty, fidelity, compassion, trustworthiness, courage, and temperance are strengthened by integrity. Halifax[6] asserts that a person of integrity must also embody gratitude, a stance that reflects open-heartedness, generosity, and humility.

The experience of living with integrity is marked by wholeness, transparency, and stability. Feelings, thoughts, and sensations are vividly present, but one is not limited or driven by them. Integrity manifests as a steady flow of actions that are in alignment with the truth of who one is and what one stands for in life. As a result, one feels balanced, open, and clear, independent yet intimately connected to others and to one's circumstances. It is a state of constant unfolding with the ebb and flow of life's challenges and rewards.

Integrity is not a static state but rather an ongoing process of reflection, refinement, and discernment in response to situations that call our integrity to task. Sustaining integrity is a matter of being true, as best one can, to one's moral principles, ideals, and commitments within the moral complexity and diversity of the clinical world. This can be a daunting challenge. Table 4.1 includes statements that assist in determining areas where integrity is robust and points to areas for strengthening. Admittedly, there are disagreements, differences of moral perspective, and even significant conflicts within moral communities regarding the moral terrain. Nonetheless, commitments to compassion, justice, and respect for the inherent dignity of persons are fundamental values within clinical practice, even though there may be diverse and even conflicting

Table 4.1. Integrity Begins with "I" © C. Rushton

- I know what I stand for.
- I walk the talk—I live my values in each moment.
- I am open and listen wholeheartedly.
- I ask the hard questions.
- I embrace difficult, or potentially unknowable, questions.
- I listen to the call of conscience.
- I know and honor my limits with compassion
- I am courageous in response to moral adversity.
- I inquire and am curious to discover what will serve.
- I speak out for what I stand for.
- I act even when doing so is difficult or consequences unpleasant.
- I am responsible and accountable.

interpretations of how best to honor these commitments. These values are reflected in the Code of Ethics for the American Nurses Association[7] and the American Medical Association[8] and are foundational to notions of relational integrity. Personal and professional integrity are inextricably intertwined. The dimensions illustrated through personal integrity also apply in our professional roles, although conflicts between them can arise that must be reconciled.

If identity and self-concept depend upon the approval or endorsement of views or actions by others, if there is a fear of being judged harshly or alienated from the broader community, acts of integrity may require courage along with internal and external resources to stay true to ourselves when various forms of moral adversity arise. Integrity sometimes requires us to stand alone in the midst of our moral communities to remain true to who we essentially are. At other times, we must stand in solidarity with others in our collective knowing of what we believe to be true. In both instances we are responsible for how we manifest our values and commitments and the skills we employ to do so.

Sustaining integrity does not signify a rigid, dogmatic, or unreflective pursuit of specific ideals, principles, or courses of action.[5] Rather, it requires an ongoing intention and commitment to discover the truth—or falsity—of one's point of view or beliefs.[5] It means exploring relevant evidence to find reasons for and against possible paths of behavior or action, including those that conflict with one's point of view or reveal areas of self-doubt, self-deception, or self-betrayal.[5] Clinicians of integrity may shift their points of view or recalibrate their understandings of the implications of certain fundamental values based on further discernment, experience, or insight. Some may not fully appreciate the depth of their value commitments or steadfast adherence to ethical norms until they are threatened, challenged, or compromised. Clinicians of integrity strive to be conceptually clear, consistent in their analysis, and aware of competing moral claims; they carefully weigh moral considerations against each other.[5] They act upon what they discern to be true to their moral values and commitments and bear the consequences of their convictions even if doing so is inconvenient, unpleasant, or personally costly.[9,10] They have a faith in their values and capacities that enables them to confront personal risks or make sacrifices.[10] Importantly, they are also cognizant that their appraisal of others' integrity is subject to a host of value judgments, subjective understandings, or projections that may lead them to conclude that others who hold different views, within certain boundaries, are wrong and what they, the clinicians, believe is right. While there are egregious examples of fundamental value claims that violate widely accepted norms and values, clinicians of integrity strive to understand points of view that diverge from their own.[10] The pursuit of understanding does not imply endorsement but rather an expression of respect for all persons.

Integrity is not merely doing what is morally or ethically justified but doing so with the properly nuanced knowledge, intention, and attitude. Skillfully enacting one's values and commitments requires ongoing discernment, practice, and opportunities for course corrections along the way. Integrity is not only a moral ideal—it requires commitment and discipline to live the values and principles one espouses rather than to merely profess them. This is closely linked to the notion of moral agency as embodied and visible in choice, action, and character.[11]

Moral Agency

Broadly construed, the concept of moral agency includes considerations of the congruence (or lack thereof) among one's intentions, character, choices, behaviors, and actions as well as one's responsibility for them. It presumes a level of awareness of one's values and conscientiousness that includes the intention to do what is morally justified, and the motivation to do so based on one's values, commitments, and discernment of what is ethically justified. This requires one to "cultivate an honest consciousness; to control tendencies toward unfair partiality; to develop an internally consistent and uncorrupted set of beliefs; to nurture dimensions of the self that fit together and are fitting for a particular time, place and profession; and to manifest a wholeness and solidarity of self that signifies individuality."[12(p1)] These must be coupled with clear boundaries of responsibility that acknowledge one's authority, role, power, and capacities to bring about results or consequences while also defining the appropriate level of effort to achieve the best outcome—again, all things considered. Importantly, the locus of personal integrity is internal; it is not primarily defined by the behaviors or decisions of others. When we define our integrity externally, we risk abandoning our own moral agency, authority, and power to choose for ourselves.[12] Tensions in our professional roles may be exacerbated when the practice ecosystem animates systemic inequities and power imbalances.

Moral agency encompasses more than cognitive judgment. It requires a well-honed conscience; moral sensitivity, perception, and imagination; self-regulatory capacities; ongoing reflection to evaluate one's intentions, motivations, and actions; the ability to devise reasonable solutions to internal conflicts; and steadfast commitment to responsibly enact considered decisions. Moral agency includes both affective (emotional attunement) and cognitive (perspective-taking) empathy that is vital in discerning the moral beliefs of others, perceiving another's distress or suffering, and defining the boundaries of ethically permissible or justified action. The expression or exercise of our personal integrity may be constrained by the professional obligations and commitments defined in our Codes of Ethics and norms of professionalism.[7,8,13]

Clinicians appraise what is morally justified based on values, principles, beliefs, ideals, character, and conscience. This appraisal includes a robust understanding of the contours and nuances required by our professions. Integrity does not imply moral perfection or perfect alignment with principles but rather excellence in fulfilling one's moral commitments, purpose, and professional role, while embracing one's vulnerabilities, limitations, and quest for improvement. Integrity requires ongoing appraisal and course corrections as situations unfold, forgiving one's mistakes and failures while committing to learn from them and adjusting one's responses accordingly.

Sustaining integrity requires inquiry and discernment to determine what is consonant with one's personal and professional moral values, commitments, and responsibilities and what one is fundamentally able to live with, even if it requires action that may compromise other important values or threaten harmony. Integrity requires giving moral concerns priority over non-moral or pragmatic concerns and taking seriously the possibility that exceptions are sometimes justifiable because of overriding moral considerations. In clinical practice this may unfold as a decision to exert pressure on behalf of a patient to align the patient's preferences with treatment decisions despite resistance by other clinicians or organizational policies. In one study, nurses reported that integrity was preserved by ongoing balancing of values and commitments, relationships, and related factors in response to their patients' vulnerability that sometimes led to moral and non-moral compromises.[14]

Integrity also means that clinicians consistently uphold their commitments even in the face of moral adversity and do not abandon them for arbitrary, inconsistent, or unjustified reasons.[5] Consistency does not, however, suggest rigidity; morally justified compromises or concessions are considered under conditions of constraint. Integrity does not imply that one will consistently be successful in bringing about the outcomes that one strives to achieve. Indeed, it is possible to have integrity in one's decision-making and action and still not achieve the intended outcome. For example, a nurse who exerts consistent and deliberate efforts to stop an ethically questionable practice involving resident physicians practicing intubation on newly dead patients without family consent may not be able to stop the practice in the short term[15,16] but will be viewed by some as having integrity because she aligns her actions with her ethical values.[15] In the end, she must discern the alignment with her values and commitments, what she is able to live with and what allows her to "sleep at night."

Threats to Integrity

Humans are continually subject to lapses of integrity. Despite our best efforts, we are all vulnerable under certain circumstances. Myriad conditions arise that may contribute to our acting in ways that are contrary to our moral commitments and moral core. Among these are stress that exceeds our capacity for balance and adaptation, and fear that arises from morally uncertain and challenging clinical situations. Fear is also bred when the culture of practice permits abusive interpersonal behaviors and power relationships or fails to offer mechanisms that reconcile diverse opinions, standards, norms, or policies. Being aware of the circumstances and vulnerabilities that create the conditions for lapses of integrity is vital in taking steps to regain moral wholeness.

When our integrity is imperiled, we may fall prey to abandoning our own personal and professional judgment in favor of another's. Such instances can be exacerbated when there are perceived power imbalances, external public opinion, or pressure, regulatory or legal interpretations, or physical, emotional, or mental exhaustion.[1] Consider, for example, the physician in training who requests clarification of resuscitation status for a patient with multi-system organ failure from her attending physician because of concerns that the harms of instituting resuscitation outweigh the potential benefits to the patient. When confronted by the attending physician's public disregard of her concern, she adopts a stance of apathetic agreement to avoid further humiliation, backlash, or threats to future career advancement. Such moral compromises may be made to pursue, consciously or unconsciously, gain, status, reward, or approval, or to avoid penalties or undesirable consequences; or they are simply less morally demanding.

In these instances, the call of conscience may be particularly vulnerable to being ignored or overridden. The more authoritative or coercive the external demand, the more intensely integrity is threatened.[1] Clinicians may find themselves in situations where they succumb to being cajoled, bullied, embarrassed, or implicitly or explicitly coerced or manipulated to abandon their moral commitments, conscience, or character.

Increasingly, unresolved moral distress is leading clinicians to leave their positions or abandon their professions, in part because of imperiled integrity.[17,18,19,20,21] For clinicians, such decisions come with a heavy personal price. We surmise that few clinicians abandon their profession without serious deliberation, regret, or sense of loss. Some conclude that they were not able to withstand or effectively cope with the ethical conflicts of their role and the cumulative physical, emotional, and spiritual toll. For others it represents their acceptance of the recalcitrant systemic problems that routinely imperil their integrity and have not changed despite their concerted efforts. Frequently such decisions are a last-ditch effort to preserve their own well-being and restore their personal integrity. When a fully trained professional leaves a position within a team, the institution and the profession lose an important and scarce resource that is increasingly difficult to replace.[22,23,24,25,26] Clinicians who decide not to leave still have to bear the inner conflict and dissonance between their values and actions, and some will have to confront value conflicts between their personal and professional commitments. Over time, muting of conscience and unresolved moral distress can ultimately have profound personal and interpersonal consequences[27] (see Chapter 3)

Patterns in which multiple clinicians leave a position or institution may signal toxic or untenable conditions in the practice environment that systematically undermine individual and collective integrity. Such patterns may begin to tarnish the reputation of the profession and the institution where clinicians are exiting. These breaches of organizational commitment must simultaneously be addressed alongside individual efforts to remain whole amid complex and ethically challenging circumstances that impact not only clinicians but also the people they serve.[28]

Integrity can also be undermined when the boundaries of individual or professional moral authority are exceeded, imperiling the integrity of others. For example, the physician who makes a decision that the entire team must implement assumes responsibility for the decision on their behalf and may believe that he has relieved the team members of moral responsibility and questions of conscience. While such a stance could be viewed as beneficent to the other members of the team, it can inadvertently silence the views of others, undermine individual moral agency, erode the integrity of the moral community, and fuel conflict that simmers underneath the surface. Understanding and considering the implications of witnessing or carrying out the decisions of others can illuminate the moral stakes and shared responsibility of not only the physician but the other members of the team.

When faced with morally ambiguous situations where they perceive that moral trade-offs may result in harm, clinicians may try to extinguish uncertainty surrounding treatments or decisions. When interventions do not yield the desired outcomes, they may question whether they "did everything" to help the patient or missed diagnostic or therapeutic options. They may compartmentalize the patient's care into organ systems and scour observations for evidence of progress; they may consider innovative interventions and approaches that have unforeseen consequences and lack formal evaluation.[29,30] If, for example, if clinicians view death as a failure, then doing everything to forestall that outcome, defined by criteria of clinical competence as a threat to their integrity, becomes the modus operandi. In such instances, efforts to avoid "failure" may contribute to clinical practices that result in premature declarations of futility, or, to mitigate the anxiety surrounding the ineffectiveness of their efforts, may result in burdensome over-treatment. To add to the complexity, clinicians may also experience lapses of their integrity when they are responding to patient or family pressure to do something they fundamentally believe is not indicated, will produce more harm than good, or will lead to departures from usual practice patterns.[31] The inability to set limits and boundaries with clarity and compassion can lead to contortions in clinical care that can produce untoward consequences for both clinicians and those they serve.[32]

Unrealistic expectations of ourselves or others can also imperil our integrity as clinicians. When we cannot acknowledge and honor the limits of our knowledge, capacities, or energy, they can lapse into decisions or behaviors that compromise our integrity. Pushing beyond our limits or denying the gaps in our understanding or knowledge creates an impetus to rationalize lapses in conscientiousness or behavior or to become numb, apathetic, or morally disengaged. Similarly, unrealistic expectations of us by patients, families, or others can propel us into situations where we intentionally or unintentionally abandon our essential values to avoid the distress of disappointing others or acknowledging the limits of our knowledge or expertise.

Our integrity is challenged when we witness or confront the many forms of adversity or suffering in clinical practice. There may be myriad factors that threaten our integrity. Table 4.2 summarizes some of the internal and external factors that may undermine integrity. Awareness of these areas of vulnerability offers useful ways to anticipate or proactively address these and other factors.

Conscience

Conscience is "a fundamental moral commitment on the part of a moral agent to moral integrity" and involves our personal "inner" sense of moral standards that help us gauge how our intentions, character, or behaviors align with our moral values and commitments.[33(p144)] It also serves as "a mode of consciousness and thought about one's own acts and their value or disvalue" in situations that may tempt the clinician to deviate from established moral values, commitments, or standards.[34(p137)] Not a static state, conscience reflects an evolving experience of moral reflection and action in navigating situations that engage our moral core.[35] The strength of one's attunement to the boundaries of conscience informs how one modulates, monitors, appraises, and carries out action or deliberative inaction. Activation of conscience often leads to feelings of guilt, remorse, or self-reproach when one has acted contrary to one's moral values or has done an actual moral wrong. These stand in contrast to feelings of internal

Table 4.2. Summary: Selected Factors That May Undermine Integrity

Internal	External
• Inattention to personal needs • Powerlessness • Competing obligations • Value conflicts • Inability to articulate the ethical problem or source of moral suffering • Conscience violations • Lack of knowledge or skill • Lack of competence or confidence • Lack of awareness or self-regulation • Misplaced guilt, blame, shame • Low tolerance for uncertainty or ambiguity	• Institutional policies, priorities, values • Lack of administrative support • Inter- and intra-professional conflicts • Interpersonal disrespect or peer pressure • Unclear responsibility or authority • Professional or organizational culture • Disintegrated models of care delivery • System design or pressures • Legal, regulatory, or financial constraints or incentives

stability, resoluteness, or confidence when one acts in alignment with one's moral values or commitments. It is postulated that the greater the depth of conscience and subsequent alignment with intentions, character, and action, the less stress we experience.[35] The gap between our values and commitments and our actions can instigate a cascade of physiologic, emotional, and cognitive responses that alert us to this gap.

Conscience may be activated when we detect threats to our integrity or struggle to align facts, values, and commitments with the circumstances we find ourselves in or the actions that we choose to take or not take. It can remain active as the discernment process unfolds and the uncertainty, confusion, or dissonance is addressed, is resolved, or persists. Ideally, when one can discover the path of integrity, even if the consequences of doing so are personally or professionally difficult, a sense of ease or harmony will begin to emerge. There may, however, be feelings of regret in the inevitable situations where one acts with utmost integrity to bring about the best outcome but through no fault of one's own does not succeed. In such situations guilt and remorse may be misplaced, causing unnecessary moral suffering, as opposed to situations where one has intentionally or consciously acted contrary to one's conscience.

Conscience is part of an internal radar system that detects prospective or retrospective alignment or malalignment of one's intentions, values, character, and actions. It is the watchdog of one's integrity and honesty and the quality of one's actions. However, conscience can be modulated and influenced by human instincts for survival. When fear or threat arises, conscience can go "offline" and become muted, leading to more primitive behaviors with diminished conscious control. Similarly, dysregulated emotions can overwhelm cognitive processes such as reasoning, causing a clinician to take actions that violate a fundamental moral value, commitment, or responsibility. Reasoning can become faulty when the mind seeks to rationalize behaviors that are contrary to what conscientious judgment would prescribe.[33]

For example, a young oncologist implementing a new clinical research protocol may gloss over the risks of the treatment to increase his enrollment numbers and thereby violate the ethical standard of informed consent. He may reason that the patient or his surrogate is not educated enough to understand the complexities of the protocol and that, in the end, the patient will likely benefit. As a young physician, he may have a target to meet to keep the protocol viable and his funding secure; it is vital to his professional advancement, which in the end will benefit many more patients with cancer. While such concerns are valid and supported by various ethical arguments, how one engages conscience in making explicit the moral trade-offs and reasons for them is a necessary element of integrity-preserving action.

Conscience is relational and socially mediated. While our internal conflicts are vital in determining integrity-preserving decisions, we are also relationally attuned to the appraisal others have of our actions or inactions. There are times when on balance, the appraisal by others of our actions as morally praiseworthy or deficient carries significant weight in how we determine our responses. This can have both beneficial and harmful results. In some instances, the external pressure can be the tipping point that propels us toward action that preserves integrity; in others, external appraisal can lead us to abandon what matters most and allow us to compromise values, commitments, and responsibilities that are foundational to our integrity. The task is to accurately and diligently investigate the implications of adhering to either type of pressure to determine the path that preserves integrity to the greatest extent.

Conscience involves not only with what we do directly but also with what we observe others do—and our struggles with whether we should intervene, and discerning the vehicle of our response. The nursing student whose indoctrination has been that respect is a core value of his profession struggles with the dissonance in these norms because of what he witnesses daily during his clinical rotation. He notices that many of the nurses on the medical unit refer to certain patients as "frequent flyers" or "drug seekers" while routinely discounting their concerns or punctuating their handoff report with thinly veiled racist innuendoes. When he brings up his concern, the response is, "That's just the way it is; don't take it so seriously!" While the student may not engage in the activity himself and may intentionally attempt to reconcile the disrespect by his own actions, his conscience is likely activated in response to the violation of a central norm of the profession and basic human civility.

In clinically difficult cases, we must grapple with appraising and discerning the boundaries of our participation in moral compromises or wrongdoing using conscience as a guide in socially mediated circumstances. For example, Sandy, an experienced neuro-critical care nurse who has cared for many trauma patients with severe head injuries, finds her integrity imperiled as she strives to safeguard the rights of her patient and relieve his suffering in ways that are consistent with his preferences and her professional values. If she protests the decision-making, she may put at risk her relational integrity, cooperation, and relationships with other disciplines as well as team unity and harmony, intensifying her distress. Moreover, she may place herself at risk of organizational pressures focused on patient throughput, budget concerns, and staffing issues that create an additional realm of complexity.

The "Call of Conscience"

The call of conscience can be activated by both one's own choices and the actions or inactions of others. Commonly, it is activated when there is a perceived threat or violation of integrity in response to situations that provoke temptation to deviate from established moral values, commitments, or standards.[34] We can be jolted out of alignment with our integrity by a challenging situation where we must choose among competing interests or values or an interaction with a person that provokes disgust, disregard, or another strong reaction. Or our alignment can become slowly eroded by repeatedly ignoring our sense of truth or by ongoing situational conflicts that prevent our moral code from being honored. The stirring of conscience can also arise as we contemplate the various courses of action in response to a moral or ethical conundrum that renders certain values moot and others prioritized, thereby creating a conflict of conscience.[34]

No matter how we lose connection with our integrity, our nervous system responds with warning signals alerting us to the misalignment.

Conscience engages physical, emotional, mental, and spiritual processes that are activated and reactivated as one detects potential threats or challenges to one's moral core and integrity. Its role is to recognize the gap between one's fundamental moral commitments and what one contemplates doing or what one has chosen to do.[33] When our integrity is threatened, each of us responds with a unique and recognizable pattern—a distinctive moral fingerprint. Mindful awareness and self-attunement can alert us when we are stepping into the uncomfortable stream of thought and action that threatens our morals and troubles our conscience.[36] For some, it may be a flash of heat rising into the chest and head; for others, it takes a variety of forms—irregular and shallow breathing, tightening in the gut or chest, a rapid heartbeat, dry mouth, queasiness, fatigue, or agitation. Concurrently or quite separately, individuals may become easily agitated, angered, saddened, or anxious, or vacillate between emotions without anything that warrants the intensity of emotion, or be susceptible to rapid shifts in emotion. Individuals may also have cognitive signals of unrest, becoming either easily distractible or scattered, or stuck and rigid with a particular point of view. In some cases, they may find their questions and thought patterns proliferate, reflecting dissonance, conflict, or confusion. These cues can instigate discernment, insight, and mindful action or produce moral stress or moral suffering.[37] If the cues that arise from activation of conscience are not heeded, the warning signals can become dulled. They are ever present, but if they are overridden repeatedly, they may become "normalized" or no longer discernible. Chapters 7 and 8 detail the capabilities and strategies that protect our moral integrity and foster our moral resilience.

While conscience is a powerful signal of moral attention, it is not an infallible moral guide. Clinicians of integrity inquire into the truth or falsity of their cognitive moral claims, examine their moral convictions, and pause to investigate the meaning and significance of the call of their conscience. Conscience can be fallible if it relies on incorrect information, dysregulated emotions, projections, or rationalizations, or if it is overwhelmed by external influence. Pangs of conscience may cause people to mistakenly identify the source of the discomfort or to misinterpret its meaning. In some cases, one's conscience is activated because it detects an inconsistent or irrational point of view rather than realizing that one is about to violate an important moral standard. At times, it may reflect a moral certitude that exceeds the facts or available justification.[37] Conscience alone ought not be the final arbiter of moral/ethical discernment and action; it must be constructively and mindfully engaged to discover the path of wisdom and integrity.[37]

Relational Integrity

Personal and professional integrity requires a robust notion of effective moral agency that is embodied—made real by one's actions—and "acknowledges the relational nature and the "embeddedness" of individuals in culture and social practices."[38(p4)] Traditionally tied to autonomy as self-determination and moral authority, moral agency is now being redefined with insights from feminist ethical theory that recognizes its inherently relational, contextual, and interconnected nature. Rodney et al. propose that "moral agency includes rational and self-expressive choice, embodiment, identity, social and historical influences, and autonomous action within wider social structures."[11(p163)] Such an orientation focuses attention on the interrelationship and reciprocity between cultural schema and structures and individual agency.

Being a clinician with moral integrity is not an insular, internal matter, but a mode of *being* ethical that characterizes one's relationships with others. We are not separate from context, relationships, or intersubjectivity within the moral ecosystem. Hence, individual integrity is intertwined with the integrity of that one serve and those one collaborates with to provide care and services as well as the social and organizational context where one practices. It is sustaining *relational integrity* or wholeness that enables a clinician to best preserve personal and professional integrity while being interdependently connected with others whose integrity is also at stake.[39] Clinicians of integrity must consider what they owe each other in the context of healthcare relationships and what commitments and expectations they are willing to enact and hold ourselves and each other accountable for.

As a developmental process, the cultivation of personal integrity is a precondition for relational integrity; one must be able to discern the contours of personal integrity before being able to skillfully engage with the integrity of others. Moral agency in this context is understood as striving for a stance of equanimity—being able to remain true to one's own moral commitments while creating a space of understanding and respect for positions and points of view that are contrary to one's own in service of the integrity of the community one is part of. The ability to do so requires the personal integrity that comes from intimate self-knowledge of "what it means to honor one's own beliefs, without "being self-indulgent or self-centered."[38,(p4)] It requires a clear conception of the ethical contours of professional responsibility as outlined in professional Codes of Ethics, is reflected in openness and flexibility in response to others' values and beliefs while maintaining personal wholeness."[38(p4)] This level of understanding allows clinicians to preserve their personal integrity "while being interdependently connected with others whose integrity is also at stake."[38 (p4)] Professional ethical norms are predicated on the ability to "distinguish one's own views, values, and commitments from those of others."[38(p4)] For the clinician, this means "being true to one's own moral compass while establishing effective engagement and boundaries in relationships and decisions."[38(p4)] Decisions in healthcare settings often involve making challenging determinations that include other people's diverse and at times conflicting opinions, beliefs, and values. The ability to "be flexible, open, and accepting of differences" is paramount.[38(p4.)] One healthcare provider described the authentic evaluation of another as "being able to see, feel and listen to as many different viewpoints as possible without your own agenda clouding the picture."[38(p4)] Being inclusive of other people's views, social context, and interests is a core feature of professionalism and respect for all persons.[39] As clinicians, there are times when our personal values must be temporarily set aside or tempered when our professional responsibilities take precedence. As described earlier, these accommodations may create a troubled conscience or moral suffering.

Clinical practice is fundamentally relational work: its very nature engages vulnerabilities and interdependency that are shared by all human beings.[40] Even though an individual clinician is not dependent on her patient in the way the patient is dependent on her, her clinical engagement takes her directly into engaging with forms of dependency and vulnerability that she shares with her patient and all other human beings.[41] Shared interdependence takes various forms when extended to the integrity of an entire healthcare team. Power and authority imbalances, hierarchical systems, and constraints imposed on clinician choices create distinctive vulnerabilities and dependencies on other members of the team and the organization itself.[41] Personal and relational integrity coexist in a dynamic flow of permeability between them. Sometimes we need to discern the appropriate level of engagement, prioritize independent and interdependent values and commitments, and determine the contours of skillful action.

To be clinicians of integrity we must be engaged with our own vulnerabilities and those of others in such a way that we can discern the boundaries of our experience and obligations flexibly and with enough permeability to authentically appreciate and value the experiences and perspectives of others.[41] Creating harmony among the integral parts of the whole—whether intra-personally or interpersonally among clinicians, patients, families, clinical teams, programs, or services within an institution or health system—contributes to the unity of the whole.[12]

Characteristically, professional integrity in clinical practice is tied to professional moral/ethical norms, obligations, responsibilities, and commitments. As disciplines, nursing and medicine have distinct moral/ethical contours, yet their foundational commitments focus on their covenant with society to serve those who need their services with respect, compassion, and fairness.[41] Our responsibilities are socially construed and bind us to certain commitments that accompany our roles, conduct, and choices within a moral ecosystem. We are called to prioritize the interests of those we serve while tempering our own self-interest and collaboratively leveraging our unique contributions toward our shared goal.[7,41,42] Relational integrity depends upon solidarity of purpose and the presence and contribution of the elements needed for wholeness and functioning of the clinical team, unit, or system. When a team is divided, lacks solidarity, or is weakened by cowardice or ineffective leadership, it can disable the whole enterprise.[12] This requires astute awareness of how our decisions affect others and the interconnection of our individual and collective integrity.

Interprofessional clinicians participate in a shared moral endeavor that includes a basic moral vision of clinical caretaking reflected in professional codes of ethics or the vows they take as they fulfill the requirements for their professional roles, the Nightingale Pledge[41] or Hippocratic Oath.[43] These publicly stated and formal sets of values or rules form the basis for professional codes of ethics. Table 4.3 outlines the core tenets of the Codes of Ethics for Medicine and Nursing. Other disciplines have similar provisions. Our clinical roles demand that we work in service of certain moral commitments such as compassion, justice, and respect for the inherent dignity of all persons. Clinical practice is thus distinctive moral work. It strives, among other things, to realize "goods" or "ends" that can only be

Table 4.3. Basis of ANA and AMA Codes of Ethics

Provision	American Nurses Association Code of Ethics for Nurses	American Medical Association Principles of Medical Ethics
I	"The nurse practices with compassion and respect for the inherent dignity, worth, and unique attributes of every person."	"A physician shall be dedicated to providing competent medical care, with compassion and respect for human dignity and rights."
II	"The nurse's primary commitment is to the patient, whether an individual, family, group, community, or population."	"A physician shall uphold the standards of professionalism, be honest in all professional interactions, and strive to report physicians deficient in character or competence, or engaging in fraud or deception, to appropriate entities."
III	"The nurse promotes, advocates for, and protects the rights, health, and safety of the patient."	"A physician shall respect the law and also recognize a responsibility to seek changes in those requirements which are contrary to the best interests of the patient."
IV	"The nurse has authority, accountability, and responsibility for nursing practice; makes decisions; and takes action consistent with the obligation to provide optimal patient care."	"A physician shall respect the rights of patients, colleagues, and other health professionals, and shall safeguard patient confidences and privacy within the constraints of the law."
V	"The nurse owes the same duties to self as to others, including the responsibility to promote health and safety, preserve wholeness of character and integrity, maintain competence, and continue personal and professional growth."	"A physician shall continue to study, apply, and advance scientific knowledge, maintain a commitment to medical education, make relevant information available to patients, colleagues, and the public, obtain consultation, and use the talents of other health professionals as indicated."

(continued)

Table 4.3. Continued

Provision	American Nurses Association Code of Ethics for Nurses	American Medical Association Principles of Medical Ethics
VI	"The nurse, through individual and collective effort, establishes, maintains, and improves the ethical environment of the work setting and conditions of employment that are conducive to safe, quality health care."	"A physician shall, in the provision of appropriate patient care, except in emergencies, be free to choose whom to serve, with whom to associate, and the environment in which to provide medical care."
VII	"The nurse, in all roles and settings, advances the profession through research and scholarly inquiry, professional standards development, and the generation of both nursing and health policy."	"A physician shall recognize a responsibility to participate in activities contributing to the improvement of the community and the betterment of public health."
VIII	"The nurse collaborates with other health professionals and the public to protect human rights, promote health diplomacy, and reduce health disparities."	"A physician shall, while caring for a patient, regard responsibility to the patient as paramount."
IX	"The profession of nursing, collectively through its professional organizations, must articulate nursing values, maintain the integrity of the profession, and integrate principles of social justice into nursing and health policy."	"A physician shall support access to medical care for all people."

Sources: American Nurses Association. Code of ethics for nurses with interpretive statements. Silver Spring, MD: ANA; 2015.

American Medical Association. Code of medical ethics. Chicago, IL: AMA.

described in moral terms—trust, hope, dignity, healing, compassion—in a context in which universal human vulnerabilities are central.[41] The excellent clinician is by definition a clinician of integrity—one who is committed to moral values tied to fundamental universal human vulnerabilities and who upholds the moral commitments of his or her profession and character.[41]

Sustaining personal and relational integrity requires many distinct "excellences" or virtues that are tied to honoring the moral commitments outlined in professional codes of ethics, not just in theory but also in daily, moment-to-moment clinical practice.[41] This means that clinicians of integrity are committed to an ongoing process of living their values rather than merely professing them. Being committed to compassion, for example, is not just a matter of being personally disposed to be compassionate. It is also a matter of having the courage to speak up about instances of cruelty or indifference that one sees as failures of compassion, to take risks to restore the conditions for compassion to thrive, or to act in a way that inspires others to strengthen their compassion.[41] It may also entail having the resilience to engage in integrity-preserving acts aimed at restoring one's own well-being in the service of compassion.[41] If, for example, a clinician is so exhausted and stressed that she is no longer able to be compassionate in her clinical work, being committed to compassion will require her to do something to revitalize her capacity for compassion.[41] This may take a whole realm of virtues—self-honesty, a willingness and ability to make hard decisions, and discipline to stay the course despite adversity or resistance—to be able to manifest alignment with one's moral ideals, values, and commitments within the reality of one's clinical world.[41] Being compassionate, rather than talking about compassion, requires sustained investment in learning and consistently practicing the skills necessary for compassion to arise in oneself and others.[44] Practices such as the G.R.A.C.E. process support clinicians to enact compassion in their professional roles.[45]

When we act with relational integrity, we create possibility and space for people to connect to and leverage their deepest intentions, commitments, and wisdom. This also means that commitments to moral values such as compassion, justice, and respect for others are not only individual, personal values but also inform group process, clinical practice, and organizational culture and policy. Alignment in this way is needed to support and encourage clinicians to meet their individual and shared moral commitments.

Relational integrity leverages our intimate knowing of ourselves within a relational context where no one is left out and everyone is included that enlarges the sphere of awareness and inclusion. We must sustain integrity not only as individual clinicians but also in relationships to others, including collaborative enterprises among diverse people with diverse perspectives that may disagree, create moral conflicts, and pose limitations of authority tied to roles. This interrelationship is particularly vital when considering the situations that clinicians find themselves in when they must navigate and balance competing obligations to their patients and their surrogates, the institutions where they practice, and the broader society. Healthcare institutions often have complex ethical norms with a diverse and often conflicting array of values, commitments, and principles that are interpreted based on one's position, identity, and responsibility.[1] Clinicians and leaders of healthcare organizations are regularly faced with making conflicting or incommensurate trade-offs; how they resolve them may lead to actions that are congruent with their values or the source of dissonance and distress.

Beyond the walls of healthcare organizations, there are complex social, political, economic, racial, and cultural forces that impact the personal, professional, and relational integrity of clinicians and those they serve. When there is alignment in values, behaviors, policies, and practices the integrity of everyone thrives. Yet the economic drivers of healthcare, focused on efficiency, disproportionate profits, and unbridled capitalism, have created patterns of greed, waste, and perverse incentives that undermine clinician values and the delivery of healthcare.[46] Clinicians see the impact of these themes on patient engagement and outcomes. They witness the impact on patients, who, waiting too long for treatment, limit its effectiveness or reduce the likelihood of benefit. They hear the lament of patients who make financial trade-offs between buying essential medications and putting food on the table for their families. The disparities in access and inequitable distribution of benefits and harms are everyday ethical realities that erode clinicians' ability to provide care and treatment that align with their core professional values. These types of moral adversity are intensified as clinicians attempt to uphold organizational mandates for high patient volume and rapid throughput to meet financial benchmarks, in systems that lack the human, material, or community resources to deliver safe, quality care without overburdening the workforce.

A foundation of clinical practice is the social contract or covenant that outlines clinicians' obligations and commitments to the welfare of society, which encompasses requisite boundaries and accountabilities.[47] Our professional ethics are implemented through socially defined, sanctioned roles and authority. These responsibilities cannot be realized without corollary commitments from, and accountabilities assumed by the people being served, the healthcare organization's culture, and society at large.[45] Inevitably, broader social conditions and expectations enable or hinder clinicians' ability to practice in alignment with their professional and ethical mandates.[48]. These social conditions include reciprocal and respectful relationships with the public. The contours of the social covenant have been evolving. Escalating racial and political division and social unrest brought into focus how the social fabric that surrounds the delivery of healthcare have frayed.[46] Racial, political, and social polarization came into stark display during the COVID-19 pandemic. Our society's fragmentation was evident in conflicts over policies and approaches to limit the spread of disease (i.e., mask mandates, school closures, visitor limitations in healthcare settings, etc.) and attempts to decrease morbidity and mortality (e.g., vaccine mandates, distribution of promising treatments, etc.).[45,46] Polarization emerged in a context of law enforcement and community violence, disparities in access to treatment, and the disproportionate number of deaths among people systemically disadvantaged. Because of competing forces, the social contract or covenant between clinicians and society was overtly and covertly eroded,[45,46] Violence against point-of-care clinicians, especially nurses, became a lightning rod that focused attention on the degradation of basic norms of respectful engagement between clinicians and the people they serve.[49,50] Initially heralded as heroes, clinicians became the target of political rhetoric and disinformation that questioned their fundamental commitment to patients and to their professional identities and purpose. Over time their dedication to patients no longer provided sufficient motivation to continue in their roles in the face of growing shortages of personnel and materials, escalating moral suffering, exhaustion, and work overload. The confluence of these destructive and disorienting forces has challenged our basic notions of professionalism, the meaning of ethical practice in healthcare, and the reciprocal responsibility of society to support healthcare, while honoring the humanity of everyone. These complex and often conflicting elements of the moral ecosystem impact the relational integrity of everyone within it. The interplay of these dynamics is further explored in the following sections and in chapters 10 and 11.

Relational Integrity in Clinical Practice

Consider a clinician who is faced with insufficient family and community resources to ensure a safe discharge for a homeless child needing a complicated medication regimen to treat a recurrent infection, and who must also adhere to the legal and regulatory criteria for discharge when hospital beds are scarce. The clinician's conscience may be ignited in response to her intention to bring about the best outcome for the child, and she may be tempted to cut corners in the clinical protocol to avoid administrative sanctions. The social and economic factors that surround the provision of healthcare are inextricably intertwined, and the clinician has little authority to alter them, despite concerted efforts to bring the issues to the attention of leaders within the organization and beyond. Her own moral agency is called into question as she tries to create congruence between her professional code of ethics and her personal values and actions within the context of institutional policies and resource constraints. In this difficult case, she must dynamically engage the circumstances—the relationships and the organizations—in which she works to define the boundaries of her integrity and to act, as best she can, in alignment with them. Other cases demand that we, as clinicians, endeavor to do the same while acknowledging that there will be situations where the moral/ethical dissonance is unresolvable, the moral residue persistent, and options for integrity preserving action limited. Contextualizing our moral and ethical commitments in this way is consistent with a social ecological view of resilience. Shifts in one aspect of the ecosystem will have an impact on other aspects, and this invites us to consider the interconnectedness of individual and relational integrity.

Without cultivating relational integrity, a singular, self-centered focus can overwhelm, discount, or disable the integrity of others. Arrogance, closed-mindedness, defensiveness, and unyielding resistance to alternative views or criticism suggest an unwillingness or inability to recognize the consequences of adherence to one's single-minded judgment on oneself and others.[1] For example, a liver transplant surgeon expands access to high-risk transplant candidates and commits the entire clinical team to implementing a highly regulated treatment plan focused on one-year survival to ensure the program's viability. Advocating enhanced access and improved quality of life is a laudable moral stance, but it carries with it potential threats to the integrity of others, particularly those who must implement the plan initiated by an individual or dedicated team. This reality carries with it a responsibility to engage in a discernment process so that the moral trade-offs and compromises are explicit and transparent rather than discounted or ignored. Those in authority may believe that their moral point of view takes priority over that of others or represents the views of the entire team. Such a stance may be justified by the belief that the surgeon has ultimate responsibility and accountability for the patient's care. However, it overlooks the moral agency and shared responsibility of the other clinicians involved in the patient's care and usurps their moral authority to speak for themselves, whether they support or oppose the surgeon's point of view.

The Interface Between Personal and Relational Integrity

A more dynamic, relational view of integrity concerns the individual ability to stand for, speak to, and flexibly find meaningful ways of being true to one's own moral compass and the call of conscience while simultaneously honoring and engaging the values, points of view, and integrity of others. This is an inherently social phenomenon: it requires attending to interpersonal dynamics, patterns of empowerment, activation of conscience, and individual and collective voices within institutions. As clinicians of integrity, we must each possess interpersonal capacities and qualities that engage empathy and perspective-taking; we must have the ability to distinguish our own interests, emotions, and motivations from those of others, and to authentically value and respect the humanness of others.[51] Integrity demands that we stand behind our convictions and conscience in the midst of conflict and chaos without crushing or discounting different or contrary points of view. This includes ongoing attempts for mutual understanding as part of a moral community committed to a shared moral vision. In like manner, we must take seriously the objections or doubts of others regarding the merit of our discernment or moral choices and the twinges of our conscience.[1] We must also exercise due process and care when our colleagues question claims of integrity and values[1] or voice dissent from the point of view of others.

Sustaining integrity requires balance and integrity-preserving compromise to find solutions that serve the interests of ourselves and others. Clinicians of integrity can engage in a conscious and principled discernment process to weigh the trade-offs of various options and to mindfully consider the boundaries of their moral agency within their professional role. As a result, acting with integrity does not guarantee achieving what one may regard as the *preferred* outcome. For clinicians, this translates into recognizing the ethical mandates of the professions, the implications of conscience, and the power imbalances that are inherent in the patient–clinician relationship and their dual obligations to patients and the organizations where they practice.[14] At times, integrity goes beyond acting for the sake of duty or the apparent "rightness" of an action when doing so is contradictory to our emotional inclinations, intentions, conscience, or cognitive appraisal.[1]

Clinicians are regularly faced with situations where they must make these distinctions. Consider the night nurse who is completing her third twelve-hour shift and has been caring for an adolescent following a serious car accident that left him paralyzed from the waist down. A former basketball player, he will never walk again. As she is preparing to leave, he summons her to inspect one of his wounds. She knows that the next nurse can easily respond and that her hospital has mandated no overtime, requiring that she punch the time clock within a window of time after her shift ends. Something propels her into the room where she finds the young man holding a picture of his team at his last basketball tournament. When she asks about his concern about his wound, tears begin to stream down his cheeks. He says, "My life is over. I'll never play again." Confronted with a moment of opportunity to connect with her patient's suffering or to obey institutional rules, she must weigh the trade-offs of each to determine which risks she will be able to live with—the gift of being of service in that moment or the consequences of reprimand by her organization for not following protocol.

Organizational integrity requires the solidarity and interconnectedness of individuals within healthcare institutions, the alignment and coherence of organizational policies and decision-making with their professed values, and respect for individual and professional moral commitments. Similar to individual integrity, the integrity of a hospital or healthcare system may be judged by whether it "represents itself truthfully, treats its own and others fairly, is uncorrupted and acts consistently, exhibits a fittingness among the component parts, and expresses a wholeness wherein all essential elements contribute to the whole system."[12,165–166] Without alignment with organizational integrity, individuals within these systems face significant obstacles and risk undermining their own integrity to adhere to organizational mandates and norms. As illustrated above, these pre-existing tensions were evident prior to the COVID-19 pandemic but became exacerbated under the relentless crisis and workforce degradation.[52,53,54]

Personal and relational integrity exists in an emerging, dynamic current of interconnection: both are needed to be true to what matters most in the various contexts where clinicians find themselves. These interconnected webs of personal morality and relational, collective ethical norms and values are constantly being appraised, discerned, and balanced or traded off in various ways. There will be times when clinicians must set aside their personal values so that those they serve can be true to their own. This does not suggest martyrdom or abandonment of one's values, but rather a temporary suspension of the priority given to one's point of view in the moment and under specific circumstances. Likewise, there will be circumstances in which adhering to the collective ethical values or norms would in fundamental ways undermine or violate our personal wholeness, harmony, or coherence with who we essentially are and our fundamental values and commitments. Acting with integrity does not imply that moral and ethical tensions will be eliminated or that the moral trade-offs will not carry weighty consequences or moral residue. Being able to discern these boundaries requires ongoing discipline, practice, and examination.

Relational integrity also means that the integrity or wholeness of one person resonates with the integrity or lack of integrity of others[55]. Consider a team of intensive care clinicians caring for a patient with complex autoimmune disease and multi-system organ failure. If the leader of the clinical team communicates through words and actions a tone of moral disregard for the concerns expressed by others on the team about the adequacy of disclosure of risks and the likelihood of benefits of an innovative therapy, it is likely that other team members will adopt the same tone and actions. The relational integrity of the leader can serve as a type of contagion, creating either a positive or negative resonance with the integrity of the rest of the team. It can either serve as an inspiration and a powerful fuel toward wholesome interpersonal, team, and community norms and behavior—or it can lead to normalizing ethically suspect behaviors that contribute to the overall degradation of ethical conduct and investment in serving the well-being of self and others.

Instead of fueling fear, anger, or disrespect, we can choose to shift our orientation toward basic goodness and kindness, leveraging our moral authority, however conferred, to serve as a role model for others and to coach and inspire them. If another ICU team member leverages her integrity by constructively offering an alternative view and models a robust notion of respectful engagement with the other members of the team, another path is possible. When we view integrity in this way, we are reminded of our interconnection, shared humanity, and requisite responsibility for our actions and their consequences for ourselves and others. The sphere of individual integrity is enlarged to include attention to honoring our own integrity and that of others, cultivating trustworthiness, and defining and honoring the boundaries and limits of relationships, roles, and authority.

Exercising cooperation and leveraging shared values and intentions protects our colleagues' integrity and our own, and it translates into preserving integrity for the whole. Consistent with this notion of our inherent interconnectedness, Kazuaki Tanahashi defines a broader notion of integrity as "whole oneness."[56] This broader notion of integrity opens the door to more closely uniting individual and interpersonal integrity with institutional and societal integrity—the organizational integrity reflected in social ecological resilience—that we hold to be the foundation of the cultural transformation we advocate in this book.

Conflicts of conscience arise in situations that call norms of conscientious judgment into question and can imperil both personal, professional, and relational integrity. Consider, for example, a patient who arrives in the emergency department in sickle cell crisis and requests a specific dose of analgesic. Although the typical response is to provide increasing doses of analgesia until pain is relieved, the treating clinician hesitates. Fearing substance abuse, she questions the patient's knowledge of the dosage, leading an observing clinician to view her behavior as violating norms of respect. Whether the witness remains silent or openly challenges his colleague, the individuals involved may be reluctant to uphold moral commitments now and in the future. These insidious patterns of responses impact not only the individuals involved but also the people we serve.

Claims of Conscience

The realization that one may be or has been propelled into acting against informed moral judgment—in effect, doing what one believes is morally wrong or at least morally tenuous—creates moral dissonance and tension and can imperil personal and relational integrity. Over time, if the call of conscience is not heeded, the signals generated in the body and psyche can become numbed, allowing more primitive instincts and preconscious processes to gain control.[37] Rationalization and self-protective patterns can diminish or extinguish the impact of conscience, leading to actions that are self-focused rather than altruistic[57] or to behaviors that are morally apathetic, lazy, or arrogant.[58] Patterns that are incongruent with our conscience and character can become normalized and no longer recognized as occasions for moral action. Similarly, we can deny our moral responsibility as a way to assuage our conscience.[34] Such a circumstance can lead to a state of moral impairment or moral disengagement. As is true of most processes, this state can be temporary or persistent; under the right circumstances, clinicians can choose to engage in rehabilitating activities designed to heal their suffering and restore their integrity.

A claim of conscience presumes that an individual has adopted core moral/ethical values and commitments that would be violated by engaging in a decision or action that fails to uphold them.[59] In healthcare, professional ethical standards establish the responsibility of clinicians to prioritize the integrity of the people they serve over their own.[59] However, this does not eliminate the need to consider the justification for and implications of asking caregivers to set aside their personal values when determining what weight to give to their claims.[60] Exercising a claim of conscience must also take into account the possibility for abuses that involve involuntary compliance or imposition of values in ways that cause harm or injustice to others.[37]

Appeals to conscience as a justification for one's action or inaction must be thoughtfully considered. Conscience violations that are asserted by clinicians may invoke personal sanctions ("I couldn't live with myself") as the motivation for their claim as a last resort to justify their actions or decisions.[34] In some cases this is coupled with an assertion that engaging in an act that fractures their integrity cannot be assuaged by any available justification. Claiming a violation of conscience that violates an important moral or ethical value or standard must be distinguished from situations where one must make a necessary and justified choice between two competing values that results in a moral residue or imperils integrity in some way.[34] Moreover, it is important to discern the motivation of such a claim to distinguish it from invidious discrimination.[60] When we fail to uphold an important moral/ethical value or commitment, we must be willing to retrospectively examine our patterns of responses, the justification for acting against an important moral/ethical value (especially if it causes harm to others), and whether amends or reparations to others who have been harmed are necessary.

A range of moral concessions and/or compromises may be considered or acted upon, each with the potential to restore or undermine integrity.[57] For example, Sandy, the neuro-critical care nurse described above, could protest what she considers prematurely limiting life-sustaining treatment and engage other physicians or nurse leaders to intervene in her particular case; alternatively, she could refuse to participate in the plan on grounds of a violation of her conscience. In either case, the integrity of relationships within the healthcare team would likely be temporarily or permanently imperiled, and Sandy's relationship with the patient compromised or terminated. She could also use the chain of command to escalate her concerns through organizational channels, utilize internal or external reporting mechanisms, or even consider whether this incident represents the final blow to her organizational commitment and resign.

Under conditions of moral adversity, when patient benefit and burdens are disproportionately imbalanced, alleviating suffering is thwarted or impossible, or treating patients with respect, dignity, and fairness is severely compromised, integrity may require taking principled action to uphold one's core values and commitments despite personal consequences. Exercising the "courage of one's convictions" may require action and fortitude to withstand internal turmoil, social rejection, malice, disregard, or overt or covert interpersonal violence, especially when the path of least resistance would be to succumb, compromise, or retreat into apathy or silence.[1] This does not imply that persons of integrity are meant to be martyrs or to engage in "heroic" courage;[61] rather, they are meant to discern the level of engagement needed to fulfill the voice of conscience and align with their commitments and character, regardless of the intended outcome, and act in a manner that reflects their personal and professional values and obligations.

Embedded in this is the acknowledgment that some aspects of our work are not easily amenable to modification, despite our most concerted and persistent efforts. As we note in Chapter 1, we will never extinguish suffering, death, moral and ethical disagreements, or conflicts in our clinical practice. They are an inherent part of the human condition, a reality with boundaries and responses that require ongoing inquiry, discernment, and action, not a predetermined prescription. There are also internal and external realities that may be resistant to our efforts to change. Clinicians may practice in environments that are increasingly antagonistic to their professional values and commitments; those at times erect insurmountable obstacles to providing care in alignment with their professional vows.[15]

Such instances require us to discern which moral harms and residue we are willing and able to live with and which we are not. More important, they are an invitation to determine whether constructive systemic reforms are possible and the degree to which our efforts are producing meaningful and sustainable results. Focusing on what is within our control to shift and the realistic opportunities to affect the broader systemic constraints requires the sober acknowledgment of the limits of our influence and power to bring about the results we desire.

Acknowledgement

Gratitude to Dr. Alisa Carse for her substantial contribution to the content related to integrity reflected in this chapter.

References

1. Calhoun C. Standing for something. J Philos. 1995;92:235–260.
2. Epstein EG, Hurst AR. Looking at the positive side of moral distress: why it's a problem. J Clin Ethics. 2017;28:37–41.
3. Juthberg C, Eriksson S, Norberg A, Sundin K. Perceptions of conscience in relation to stress of conscience. Nurs Ethics. 2007;14(3):329–343.
4. Laabs CA. Primary care nurse practitioners' integrity when faced with moral conflict. Nurs Ethics. 2007;14:795–809.
5. Halfon MS. Integrity: a philosophical inquiry. Philadelphia, PA: Temple University Press; 1989.
6. Halifax J. Standing at the edge: finding freedom where fear and courage meet. New York: Flatiron Books; 2018.
7. American Nurses Association. Code of ethics for nurses with interpretive statements. Silver Spring, MD: ANA; 2015.
8. American Medical Association. Code of medical ethics. Chicago, IL: AMA; 2017.
9. McFall L. Integrity. Ethics. 1987;98:5–20.
10. Carter SL. Integrity. New York: Basic Books; 1996.
11. Rodney P, Kadychuk S, Liaschenko J, Brown H, Musto L, Snyder N. Moral agency: relational connections and support. In Storch JL, Rodney P, Starzomski R, editors, Toward a moral horizon: nursing ethics for leadership and practice. Toronto, Canada: Pearson; 2013:160–187.
12. Mitchell C. Integrity in interprofessional relationships. In Agich GJ, editor, Responsibility in health care. The Netherlands: Springer; 1982:163–184.
13. Owens J, Singh G, Cribb, A. Austerity and professionalism: being a good healthcare professional in bad conditions. Health care analysis: HCA: journal of health philosophy and policy. 2019;27(3):157–170.

14. Irurita VF, Williams AM. Balancing and compromising: nurses and patients preserving integrity of self and each other. Int J Nurs Stud. 2001;38:579–589.
15. Carse A, Rushton CH. Harnessing the promise of moral distress: a call for re-orientation. J Clinical Ethics. 2017;28:15–29.
16. Thomas TA, McCullough LB. A philosophical taxonomy of ethically significant moral distress. J Med Philos. 2015;40:102–120.
17. Dyo M, Kalowes P, Devries J. Moral distress and intention to leave: a comparison of adult and paediatric nurses by hospital setting. Intensive Crit Care Nurs. 2016;36:42–46.
18. Trautmann J, Epstein E, Rovnyak V, Snyder A. Relationships among moral distress, level of practice independence, and intent to leave of nurse practitioners in emergency departments. Adv Emerg Nurs J. 2015;37:134–145.
19. Whitehead PB, Herbertson RK, Hamric AB, Epstein EG, Fisher JM. Moral distress among healthcare professionals: report of an institution-wide survey. J Nurs Scholarsh. 2015;47:117–125.
20. Whittaker, BA, Gillum, DG, Kelly, JM Burnout, moral distress, and job turnover in critical care nurses. International Journal of Nursing Studies. 2018;3(3):108–121.
21. Austin CL, Saylor R, Finley PJ. Moral distress in physicians and nurses: impact on professional quality of life and turnover. Psychological Trauma: Theory, Research, Practice, and Policy. 2017;9(4): 399–406.
22. Perlo J, Balik B, Swensen S, Kabcenell A, Landsman J, Feeley D. Institute for Healthcare Improvement white paper: framework for improving joy in work [Internet]. 2017. Available at http://www.ihi.org/resources/Pages/IHIWhitePapers/Framework-Improving-Joy-in-Work.aspx.
23. LeClaire M, Poplau S, Linzer M, Brown R, Sinsky C. Compromised integrity, burnout, and intent to leave the job in critical care nurses and physicians. Crit Care Explor. February 7, 2022;4(2):e0629.
24. Raso R, Fitzpatrick JJ, and Masick K. Nurses' intent to leave their position and the profession during the COVID-19 pandemic. JONA: The Journal of Nursing Administration. 2021;51(10): 488–494.
25. Falatah R. The impact of the coronavirus disease (COVID-19) pandemic on nurses' turnover intention: an integrative review. Nursing Reports, 2021;11(4):787–810.
26. https://www.ama-assn.org/practice-management/physician-health/pandemic-pushes-us-doctor-burnout-all-time-high-63.
27. Molinaro ML, Polzer, J, Rudman DL, Savundranayagam M. "I can't be the nurse I want to be": counter-stories of moral distress in nurses' narratives of pediatric oncology caregiving, Social Science & Medicine. 2023;320:4–8.
28. Lasater KB, Aiken LH, Sloane D, French R, Martin B, Alexander M, McHugh MD. Patient outcomes and cost savings associated with hospital safe

nurse staffing legislation: an observational study. BMJ Open. December 8, 2021;11(12):e052899.

29. Barnett SJ, Katz A. Patients as partners in innovation. Sem Pediatr Surg. 2015;24:141–144.
30. Schwartz JA. Innovation in pediatric surgery: the surgical innovation continuum and the ethical model. J Pediatr Surg. 2014;49:639–645.
31. Truog RD. The United Kingdom sets limits on experimental treatments: the case of Charlie Gard. JAMA. 2017;318:1001–1002.
32. Wilkinson D, Savulescu J. Hard lessons: learning from the Charlie Gard case. J Med Ethics. 2018 Jul;44(7):438–442.
33. Sulmasy DP. What is conscience and why is respect for it so important? Theor Med Bioeth. 2008;29:135–149.
34. Childress JF. Appeals to conscience. Ethics. 1979;89(4):315–335.
35. Vithoulkas G, Muresanu DF. Conscience and consciousness: a definition. J Med Life. 2014;7(1):104–108.
36. Kaszniak AW, Rushton CH, Halifax J. Leadership, morality and ethics: Developing a practical model for moral decision-making. MindRxiv. April 17, 2018. mindrxiv.org/8qby6. doi:10.17605/OSF.IO/8QBY6.
37. Vaiani CE. Personal conscience and the problem of moral certitude. Nurs Clin North Am. 2009;44(1):407–414.
38. Holtz H, Heinze K, Rushton C. Inter-professionals' definitions of moral resilience. J Clin Nurs. 2017; 27(3–4):e488–e494.
39. Solomon RC. Ethics and excellence: cooperation and integrity in business. New York: Oxford University Press; 1992.
40. A. L. Carse, personal communication, April 12, 2016. The content was adapted from previous non-published texts and were significantly influenced by her writings and collaboration.
41. American Nurses Association. Florence Nightingale pledge. www.nursingworld.org/FlorenceNightingalePledge-2017.
42. Pellegrino ED. Character, virtue and self-interest in the ethics of the professions. J Contemp Health Law Policy. 1989;5:53–73.
43. Eva KW. Trending in 2014: Hippocrates. Med Educ. 2014;48:1–3.
44. Halifax J. The precious necessity of compassion. J Pain Manag. 2011;41(1):146–153.
45. Halifax JS. G.R.A.C.E. for nurses: cultivating compassion in nurse/patient interactions. J Nurs Educ Pract. 2013;4:121.
46. Berwick DM. *Salve Lucrum:* the existential threat of greed in US health care. JAMA. 2023;329(8):629–630.
47. Fry-Bowers E, Rushton C. Reimagining nursing's social contract with the public. American Nurse Journal. 2023;18(9), 3-8.

48. Fry-Bowers E, Rushton C. Who will be there to care if there are no more nurses? Hastings Center Bioethics Forum. 2021:https://www.thehastingscenter.org/who-will-be-there-to-care-if-there-are-no-more-nurses/.
49. Kafle S, Paudel S, Thapaliya A, et al. Workplace violence against nurses: a narrative review. J Clin Transl Res. 2022;8(5):421–424.
50. Pagnucci N, Ottonello G, Capponi D, et al. Predictors of events of violence or aggression against nurses in the workplace: A scoping review. J Nurs Manag. 2022;30(6):1724–1749.
51. Henry LM, Rushton C, Beach MC, Faden R. Respect and dignity: a conceptual model for patients in the intensive care unit. Narrat Inq Bioeth. 2015;5: 5A–14A.
52. Swavely D, Romig B, Weissinger G, et al. The impact of traumatic stress, resilience, and threats to core values on nurses during a pandemic. J Nurs Adm. 2022;52(10): 525–535.
53. Hughes MT, Rushton CH. Ethics and well-being: the health professions and the COVID-19 pandemic. Academic Medicine: Journal of the Association of American Medical Colleges. 2022;97(3S): S98–S103.
54. Schlak AE, Rosa WE, Rushton CH, Poghosyan L, Root MC, McHugh MD. An expanded institutional and national-level blueprint to address nurse burnout and moral suffering. Nursing Management, 2022;53(1):16–27.
55. Rushton, C.H. Manbauman, C. Web of mutuality: Relational integrity in critical care nursing. AACN Advanced Critical Care, 2024;34(4), 381–390.
56. Personal communication, K. Tanahashi, December 9, 2014.
57. Rushton CH, Kaszniak AW, Halifax JS. A framework for understanding moral distress among palliative care clinicians. J Palliat Med. 2013;16:1074–1079.
58. Cribb A. Integrity at work: managing routine moral stress in professional roles. Nurs Philos. 2011;12(2):119–127.
59. Wiccliar MR. Conscientious objection in health care. Bioethics. 2000;14(3): 205–227.
60. Lewis-Newby M, Wicclair M, Pope T, Rushton C, Curlin F, Diekema D, et al. Managing conscientious objections in intensive care medicine: an official policy of the statement of the American Thoracic Society. Am J Respir Crit Care Med. 2015;191(2):219–227.
60. Hamric AB, Arras JD, Mohrmann ME. Must we be courageous? Hastings Cent Rep. 2015;45:33–40.

5

The Many Faces of Resilience

Cynda Hylton Rushton and Meredith Mealer

WHAT IS IT that allows some clinicians to navigate the inevitable ethical challenges and moral suffering they face without the despair and hopelessness that others experience?* What qualities and capacities do they possess? What helps them to find meaning in situations that appear senseless? How do they transform their clinical realities into integrity-preserving, growth-producing experiences? What practices do they employ that allow them to do so?[1] These questions point to the possibility that the negative consequences of moral suffering may be mitigated or transformed by leveraging our inherent resilient potential in the context of moral and ethical concerns. Instead of exclusively focusing on the detrimental effects of moral distress, it is important to examine what enables some clinicians to avoid them and to shift the paradigm to a strengths-based rather than a deficit-focused approach to addressing the sources and consequences of moral suffering in clinical practice.

In a narrative symposium calling for stories about moral distress that included examples of positive impact, only two of the twelve narratives highlighted these dimensions.[2] Embedded in the moral distress literature are understated or brief observations regarding the potential

* Portions of this chapter are excerpted or adapted from previous articles: (1) "Moral Resilience: A Capacity for Navigating Moral Distress in Critical Care," by C. H. Rushton, 2016, *AACN Advanced Critical Care*, 27, pp. 111–119. Copyright 2016 by the American Association of Critical-Care Nurses. Adapted with permission. (2) "Harnessing the Promise of Moral Distress," by A. Carse and C. H. Rushton, 2017, *Journal of Clinical Ethics*, 28, pp. 15–29. Copyright 2017 by Sage Publishing. Adapted with permission.

Cynda Hylton Rushton and Meredith Mealer, *The Many Faces of Resilience* In: *Moral Resilience*. Second Edition.
Edited by: Cynda Hylton Rushton, Oxford University Press. © Oxford University Press 2024.
DOI: 10.1093/oso/9780197667149.003.0006

for moral distress to be a catalyst for beneficial outcomes,[3,4] moral resilience[5,6,7,8,9,10,11,12] and growth.[13,14,15,16] Yet studies of moral action by nurses confronted with ethical challenges suggest there are methods of positive action and sense-making that can support integrity rather than imperil it.[17,18,19] Engaging the beneficial aspects of one's moral conscientiousness can offer an untapped resource when confronted with ethical challenges and moral distress.[6,12,20,21,22]

By definition, if one is morally resilient, it is possible to find ways of addressing moral suffering and distress that overcome their negative, debilitating aspects.[6] As spiritual, religious, and humanistic traditions hold, growth is possible, even after traumatic events. Yet, for those who are morally and emotionally depleted or dispirited, moral resilience may be inconceivable or even objectionable, provoking intense resistance to considering any constructive outcomes arising from moral distress. Clearly, the conditions for the possibility of moral resilience must be cultivated before some clinicians will be able to embrace the concept. For this reason, before we explore the contours of *moral* resilience and consider its application to the domain of clinical practice, we will first examine various threads of resilience found in practice and research in other domains. We will then define key concepts and relationships among them to explore how they may apply to the moral domain to address moral distress and other forms of moral suffering. This understanding will provide the framework—the strategies and the architecture—needed to support moral resilience among clinicians, enabling them to address moral suffering and distress in their many forms.[6]

The Concept of Resilience

The concept of resilience is a promising theoretical and empirical foundation that can be further specified to address threats to or violations of an individual's moral well-being and integrity. Resilience is a multifaceted construct that has been applied in various contexts, including neurobiology,[23] psychology,[24,25] social ecology,[26,27,28,29,30,31,32] and clinical practice.[33,34,35,36,37] While the concept has been applied to diverse disciplines and adverse events (e.g., war, natural disasters, business, climate change), there is no unifying definition. Resilience generally refers to the ability of an entity (an organism, person, or system) to withstand, adapt, or recover from adversity, stress, or trauma;[38,39] to be buoyant in adverse circumstances;[40] and to adapt flexibly to the changing contours of stress or adversity.[41] It presumes that humans have an innate resilient potential that evolves over time through the dynamic interplay of individual cellular, physiologic, and psychological factors as well as social, environmental, community, and societal conditions.[25] The normative self-righting tendencies of individuals can be leveraged and amplified in response to adversity.[42] Resilience can be understood as both a capacity that can be influenced and a process that unfolds in response to various forms of adversity. It is not a fixed state, and it dynamically matures and grows or declines depending on the characteristics of the individual and the ecosystem around them. People may be resilient at some times and not others depending on the circumstances they find themselves in and their personal profile and capabilities. Fundamentally, resilience focuses on strengths that foster patterns of positive adaptation rather than on sources of vulnerability that place individuals or groups at risk in adverse circumstances.[43]

Adversity is the primary antecedent to resilience.[44] Stressors that challenge or exceed one's capacity to adapt to challenging or disruptive life events, or various forms of suffering, are prerequisites for resilience.[45,46,47] Whether instigated by internal or external circumstances, adversity creates the conditions for individuals to access or develop their innate resilient potential, bolster their capacities for resilience, and achieve resilient reintegration.[32,33,48] However, the accumulation of adverse experiences can also increase the likelihood of traumatization.[33] The goal is to develop a "zone of resilience"[49,50,51] within which one can function without the detrimental consequences accompanying potentially stressful events or circumstances that are acute and time-limited or sustained and chronic. Within this zone there is the potential to face stressful events and to restore wholeness and, more positively, to attain higher-level functioning characterized by greater self-awareness, purpose, and growth.

Drawing from the literature on various dimensions of resilience, we highlight the threads that appear most relevant to the territory of moral resilience. They include neurobiological, psychological, and social ecological resilience and are summarized below. The content is illustrative, not comprehensive, and is offered to situate moral resilience within the field of resilience. Further research to validate these assumptions is needed.

Neurobiological Resilience

Human beings constantly adapt to survive. The body and brain are continuously adapting to moral, social, and ecological conditions. Adaptation, the capacity to withstand threats or restore stability, is a key feature of neurobiological resilience.[52] Research in the last ten years has identified several main neurobiological mechanisms implicated in individual variations of resilience levels. This chapter addresses primarily the central nervous system's role in stress; however, the neurobiology of resilience is a complex convergence of the central nervous system, genetics, epigenetics, the neuroendocrine system, the neuroimmune system, the enteric nervous system, and the gut microbiome.[53,54,55,56,57,58,59] Exploring these concepts with any level of detail is outside the scope of this chapter, but they offer an exciting and dynamic area of study that will continue to evolve.

The brain is the ultimate regulator and integrator of the process of allostasis that allows the human organism to withstand threats or challenges (stressors) to its homeostasis.[40] Physiologic and neural processes mediate the allostatic response and are activated in response to real or perceived threats. Both external threats, such as changes in the environment, and internal threats, such as patterns of blame, shame, or cognitive rumination,[60] can cause homeostasis to become imbalanced.

In humans, the stress response is hardwired, located in the most primitive parts of human brain. It is designed to detect threats and automatically signal the body to prepare for action through a predictable series of responses: fight, flight, or freeze.[61] Research has shown that resilience is associated with reduced activation of the brain regions responsible for threat appraisal, such as the amygdala, which is implicated in the fight, flight, or freeze response.[54] Instead, the prefrontal region of the brain is more engaged, allowing more efficient cognitive processing and reappraisal.[58,62,63] Threats to our biology, social ecosystem, and psychological well-being can take many forms, such as worry, emotional changes or upsets, or endangerment of personal goals, values, identity, and integrity, automatically activating the body's alarm system. When fear is present, consciously, or unconsciously, negative emotions are activated. Once the fight, flight, or freeze response is activated, the brain shifts to survival—narrowing the focus, preserving energy, and preparing for emergency responses.[61]

Current neuroscience documents this process. The amygdala and connected brain regions detect what is salient;[64,65] initiate multiple components of the fear response, including negative arousal;[66] narrow and bias attention to potential threats; [67,68] interfere with empathic concern and pro-social emotions;[59,69] and rely on automatic default patterns to guide responses.[67] In the short term, these responses are protective and necessary for survival, providing the stability for the body and brain to recover from or adapt to the threat and potentially the fuel for deliberate and constructive action.

Threats to homeostasis, activated by stressors that impact the biological system, can, over time, create chronic reliance on allostatic mechanisms that can contribute to myriad detrimental physical, emotional, behavioral, and spiritual consequences. Overuse and dysregulation of the allostatic response can deplete and disable homeostatic mechanisms and lead to disease or disability.[27] Cumulative strain on the stress-mediating systems of the brain, or allostatic load, is associated with enduring changes in self-regulation and coping.[70] Unlike positive or tolerable stress, toxic stress is characterized by its intensity, frequency, or prolonged duration that can overwhelm the body's stress response system and significantly alter neural pathways and brain structures.[70] Both short-term and longer-term neurobiological types of resilience are needed to regain homeostasis and minimize the detrimental effects of chronic, unrelieved stress.[40] Intentional efforts to shift the brain's "negativity bias" are needed to support neurobiological resilience.[71] In the context of clinicians who confront moral adversity, an awareness of the biological dimensions of resilience, the somatic manifestations of an activated stress response, and the skills to bring the body back into balance are vital to moral well-being and human flourishing. Neurobiological resilience is intertwined with the next category: psychological resilience.

Psychological Resilience

Psychological processes dynamically interact with human biology and the broader ecosystem to create the conditions for resilient potential to be realized. There are a variety of definitions of psychological resilience that encompass a dynamic, modifiable process [44] aimed at enabling an individual to regain stability in response to stress or adversity, "harness resources to sustain well-being,"[72(p1)] create meaning and live fully despite suffering,[73] and ultimately thrive despite acute or chronic stressors or adversity. This does not suggest that being resilient involves being "unscathed" by the experience of adversity and leaving the experience and its consequences behind.[74] Rather, a process of reintegration occurs. Resilient people not only return to their relative baseline but have the potential to use the experience to propel themselves forward in terms of growth, strength, and capability. This involves a "reintegration of self that includes a conscious effort to move forward in an insightful, integrated, positive manner as a result of lessons learned from an adverse experience" [32(p3)]—in effect, to "rise above" the adversity while harnessing and expanding one's repertoire of responses and resources.

There is no uniform response to adversity; people respond to it in unique and diverse ways.[75] Some people experience isolated stress or adversity that produces transient episodes that affect how they function but have little or no lasting impact. For others, chronic, stressful, and aversive events produce more enduring patterns of variability and lead to more sustained changes in a wide range of psychological and physiologic functions.[74] There may be predictable trajectories of responses to adversity that are particular to individuals while allowing for variations based on its intensity and circumstances.[32] Such variability is likely true when applied to the domain of moral resilience. It is conceivable that there is a wide range of responses to moral adversity. The specificity of these responses requires further investigation.

Psychological resilience is multi-faceted; it reflects a dynamic interaction between individual characteristics, risk, strengths, and protective factors.[43,74,76] One's resilient capacity may fluctuate depending on the particular circumstances, the environment, and the availability of resources.[75] Highly contextualized responses may change over time as a function of the risks posed,[77] experience, development, and the surrounding ecosystem.[76,78,79] This type of resilience may manifest in variable degrees across life domains,[80] suggesting, for example, that an individual may be resilient in the context of external engagement in the world but less resilient in more intimate contexts such as family.[81] Whatever the context, it is important to differentiate responses representing resistance characteristics that render one "impervious to the deleterious effects" of adversity from characteristics of recovery where one is able to "mend or restore psychological damage" or equilibrium.[82(p383)] Such distinctions may also be useful in understanding the various responses of clinicians to moral adversity.

How individuals see themselves and the world around them influences their resilient potential. The complex interplay among factors such as one's view of self, worldview, coping strategies, sense of purpose, safety and security, spirituality, gender, and race shapes one's response to adversity.[39,83] In particular, individual factors such as personal agency, self-efficacy, self-regulation, and positive emotionality all play important roles in the process of resilience.[74] While this is not an exhaustive list, it points to promising areas of psychological resilience research that are relevant to understanding moral resilience. Personal agency, which includes moral agency, generally refers to the freedom and capacity to responsibly initiate, control, and implement actions and embody behaviors in ways that are aligned with one's values and character. It includes the ability to influence one's thoughts, behaviors, and choices, and to have a sufficient internal locus of control to affect one's environment and experiences in response to adversity or stress.[76] Essentially, it means believing in and seeing oneself as capable and competent with enough sufficiency to confront whatever comes one's way.

Self-efficacy, a closely related concept, refers to believing one has the capability, fortitude, and agency to bring about one's desired goals or outcome; this belief has been associated with improved recovery after traumatic stress.[84,85] It involves the faith that one has the ability to manage a wide range of tasks, situations, and experiences. Perceived self-efficacy is cumulative; experiences of accomplishment resulting from goal attainment or mastery enhance perceived self-efficacy and encourage perseverance despite challenges.[86] Thus, both personal agency and self-efficacy influence people's ability to distinguish themselves from others and to be stable yet flexible amid adversity. The ability to distinguish oneself from others is a necessary element for emotion regulation and empathic engagement. According to Wright et al.,[74] a positive view of oneself includes self-confidence and self-esteem, additional factors that cluster together to enable resilience.

Self-regulatory abilities encompassing both biological and psychological mechanisms are vital in responding to and adapting to adversity.[87] Biological regulatory systems are constantly operating outside of conscious control to detect threats to homeostasis. In some instances, when biological stress responses are activated, emotional responses are also triggered. People learn to respond to the sensations and feelings that arise when the body's alarm system is activated. Psychological self-regulation includes the processes individuals use to modulate the incidence, intensity, and/or duration of their emotion reactivity and moderate their emotions and behavior.[88,89] It includes the capacity to attune to signals of distress in response to an emotional charge or unmet need, abide with them without detrimental reactivity, and choose to shift one's responses toward more wholesome and constructive outcomes. The ability to create a pause between the distress impulse and the response, correctly label the need or feeling, and discern and respond appropriately is foundational to self-regulation. Self-regulation of emotion and behavior affects the development of competence, which is related to both personal agency and self-efficacy.[90] Given the dynamic nature of emotion regulation, regulatory flexibility is critical.[75]

Insight into both positive and negative emotions can strengthen personal resilience.[41] Being resilient does not imply suppressing or disregarding the negative emotions that accompany threats to integrity or the causes of the threats; rather, it involves perceiving that negative emotions are present and inquiring into their significance. Such responses may be useful in the short term to mobilize in response to threats, but over time they may exhaust vital resources needed for adaptation or recovery. This awareness helps to orient oneself toward strategies that allocate energy in ways supportive of health and well-being. Likewise, positive emotions play a crucial role in enhancing coping resources and buffering stress or adverse events.[59,91,92] Positive emotions such as joy, gratitude, hope, serenity, awe, inspiration, pride, and love may be leveraged in response to adversity.[92] For example, hope, with its many dimensions, may be associated with a particular outcome or it may vacillate and change as one attempts to make sense of the circumstances or situation one finds oneself in. Hope can foster meaning and coherence amid adversity and can contribute to the development of a concordant narrative that links past, present, and future.[45]

Resilient people tend to be able to recognize the effects of adverse or stressful circumstances and to experience positive outcomes.[42] This does not mean they deny or overlook the adversity they confront; rather, they are able to experience positive emotions amid adversity, regardless of its source. Engaging positive emotions, choosing to shift one's focus away from the negative emotional arousal, contributes to the abilities of resilient people to physiologically regulate or recover from adversity.[41] In particular, positive appraisal of adversity as a challenge rather than a threat engages positive emotions that can help dissipate negative emotional experiences. Moreover, sustained engagement of positive emotions can help broaden the individual's repertoire of personal resources in response to adverse or negative circumstances.[93,94] Interventions such as meditations focusing on the cultivation of loving kindness or positive regard and kindness toward another have been effective in engaging positive emotions with impactful results on long-term behavioral change.[93,94] Applying these insights to situations arousing moral suffering is vital to efforts to engage their beneficial potential rather than focus on their debilitating and injurious aspects. These dimensions of psychological resilience have applicability to understanding the concept of moral resilience.

Social Ecological Resilience

Resilience is also understood as a multi-faceted construct that exists within a dynamic system of individuals and their environment. [95,96,97,98] Social ecological frameworks recognize that no single factor can explain or predict a particular phenomenon.[99] Hence, a broad definition of resilience as "the process of harnessing biological, psychosocial, structural, environmental and cultural resources to sustain well-being" reflects this complexity.[100(p1)] Consistent with an integrated theory of resilience,[39] individuals are embedded in a complex web of interrelated relationships, structures, and contexts. They are situated in families, organizations, communities, societies, and cultures that exert influence over their resilient potential and its expression in response to adversity. This ecosystem can enable or disable individual resilience and can itself be resilient or not. Ecosystem resilience has been defined as "the magnitude of disturbance that can be absorbed before the system changes its structure by changing the variables and processes that control behavior."[101(p2)] This suggests that shifts in one aspect of the ecosystem will have an impact on other, interrelated aspects. Such ecosystems are dependent on their natural resources for sustenance, developmental opportunities, and materials necessary for adaptation to adversity.[39] Extending this to healthcare, investments in health system resilience are a necessary component of creating healthy workplaces.[102,103] Features of the social ecosystem that have particular relevance to the response to moral adversity and cultivation of moral resilience focus on the interplay of factors at the level of individuals, the team, the organization, and broader community and society.[104] This complexity gives rise to a dynamic interplay among the dimensions that influence the broader culture, work environments, and intimate relationships when ethical issues arise.

Within the larger context of social ecological resilience, the relational or social context is vitally important in understanding how individuals leverage and foster their individual and collective resilience. "Social resilience is the capacity to foster, engage in, and sustain positive relationships and to endure and recover from life stressors and social isolation."[26(p44)] It leverages individual and group capacities to collaborate with others to transform adversity into "personal, relational, and collective growth."[26(p44)]

Social resilience reflects the dynamic interplay of relational characteristics and qualities with interpersonal and collective capacities. Self-regulation, for example, is necessary to avoid being excluded from one's social group, to gauge alignment with social norms, to detect threats, and to resolve conflicts.[105] Among the resources that foster social resilience are the capabilities to perceive, connect with, and communicate with others with respect and empathy; to honor oneself and others; to respond to and express social emotions; and to value trust, tolerance, and openness.[26] Social resilience also modulates and attenuates individual resilience. When groups can work together for their common benefit, their collective outcomes often exceed those attainable by individuals alone. This is applicable to clinical teams who work together to produce safe, quality outcomes for their patients.

Within interpersonal relationships, with family or professional colleagues, the individual's resilience depends upon the ability to cultivate social connections and positive relationships, avoid social isolation, and both give and receive social support.[27] These abilities are particularly important when interprofessional teams must interact in response to complex ethical issues. Cultivating positive relationships through respectful communication, emotional safety, and collaboration can support the resilience of individuals who come together to work toward a common goal. Broadly, social support is particularly important in fostering resilience across the lifespan.[52] Social support, which includes receiving informational or emotional support and various relationships from which support is received (e.g., family, friends, mentors, colleagues) is vital in responding to adversity with resilience. The sources and impact of social support are unique to the person, the circumstances, and the person's developmental stage.[52] This is important when considering interventions to address the needs of a diverse workforce, including those in training, those newly trained, and experienced practitioners. Nurses, for example, identify social support as a key element of their resilience.[35]

There is an often-unacknowledged interplay between the personal and professional lives of clinicians. Clinicians are dealing with the ethical challenges not only in their workplace but also in their families, communities, and broader society. The cumulative effects of multiple stressors, or cumulative risk, increase the likelihood of negative outcomes. [106,107,108] Risk becomes cumulative when the individual is exposed either to multiple different risk factors, multiple experiences of the same risk factor, or continuous adversity.[81] For example, a clinician may be involved in a morally distressing case at work while experiencing adversity at home. These realities came into sharp focus for clinicians during the COVID-19 pandemic as they attempted to respond to the rapidly changing healthcare landscape and disruptions to school, family, and societal life.

Social resilience and the impact of broader societal norms, culture, and structure are also important to consider in the context of clinical practice. Social resilience is reflected in a community's capacity to respond to adversity and challenges. Group bonds, trust, adaptability, and pro-social emotions amplify social resilience.[96] The effects of a specific type of adversity on a community depend on factors such as diversity, social capital, and the institutions within the community.[38] Communities are unique in the determinants of resilience; what works in one may not work in another. Thus, each community needs diverse methods for responding to various sources of adversity. This suggests that solutions to moral adversity will need to be designed at the local level and customized to the specific needs and culture of each.

Beyond the community level, a social ecological understanding of resilience acknowledges the interdependence of individuals and the ecosystems where they live and practice. When individuals and groups successfully navigate diverse sources of adversity, engage resources that support their respective resilient potentials, and address the systemic complexity of their ecosystem, they foster resilience.[44,109,110] A multi-tiered social ecological view can inform a deeper understanding of the processes that contribute to resilience. In the context of healthcare, it can guide clinicians and policymakers in the design and implementation of interventions effective for building individual and system resilience. Broadly defined, resilience is the capacity to "maintain its core purpose and integrity in the face of dramatically changed circumstances."[111(p126)] This has relevance when considering the application of social ecological frameworks to moral resilience. When individuals within teams and organizations can align their values and commitments with those of the organization where they practice and those of the broader societal and systemic systems, integrity and resilience can thrive.

Clinicians are most able to exert influence on the moral/ethical parameters of their work at the local level, the organizational ecosystem where they practice. This is where they experience the alignment or misalignment of their personal/professional values with those of the organization and where the infrastructure of the organization either enables or disables individual and collective resilience. So too, it is where their individual and

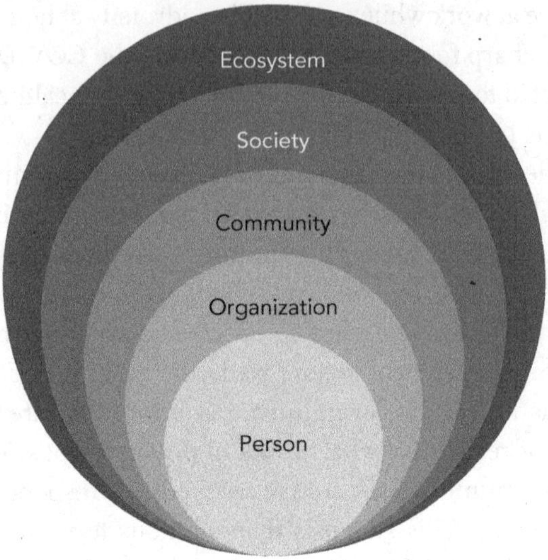

FIGURE 5.1. Social Ecological interdependence

collective resilience is fostered or undermined. These local environments within healthcare organizations are situated within a broader societal culture that exerts external influence on individual and collective resilience and integrity. This broader culture has wide-ranging influence in multiple arenas. Individuals are affected by social, political, legal, and economic issues regarding professional responsibility; the role of society and government in creating norms, policies, and incentives for healthcare professionals and organizations; and allocation schemes for distributing scarce resources. Embedded in societal, political, and economic understandings are also ethical and moral worldviews and values that shape the way ethical issues are identified, named, and dealt with. These worldviews influence what is deemed ethically salient, inform the range of options for addressing conflicts or uncertainty, and guide individual, interpersonal, social, and political behavior. As shown in Figure 5.1, the dynamic interplay among individual, organization, and community occurs within the context of society and culture, shaping and being shaped by the presence or absence of resilience.

Resilience in Clinicians

Resilience, broadly understood, has been studied in nurses and physicians utilizing qualitative and quantitative methods. These perspectives come from a variety of sources: literature reviews that have led to narrative synthesis, categorical analysis, and conceptual analysis;[33,34,48,112,113,114,115,116,117,118] interviews;[119,120,121,122,123,124] cross-sectional surveys;[35,125,126,127,128,129,130,131,132] and the development of conceptual models.[34] These investigations have focused on different populations representing the United States, United Kingdom, Europe, China, Australia, and New Zealand. Some studies interrogate resiliency in professions as a whole; others focus on specialties within each profession such as palliative care,[33,133,134,135,136,137] emergency medicine,[34,120,138,139,140,141] and primary care.[127] In addition, some explore the student perspective[113,142] or focus on using educational interventions to aid in the development of resilience.[143,144,145]

While these studies uncover many resilience-building themes, they show that possessing mindfulness skills, knowing core values, and having healthy relationships lead to resilient behaviors.[35,4,112,120,122,146,147,148,149,150,151,152,153,154,155,156] Having an open mind through cognitive reframing[112,140,150] and being present to think creatively and solve problems have aided in the ability to overcome difficult situation.[121,148] Lacking integrity or exhibiting feelings that are not in line with one's beliefs can lead to a sense of emptiness.[112] The opportunity for critical reflection can lead to abilities to adapt to the realities of current situations[150] and bring awareness to core values. Additionally, resilience is correlated with certain values, particularly honesty[148] and truthfulness;[121] these in turn lead to the second theme of trusting relationships. Having connections and support from family, friends, and others can create opportunities for values clarification and put challenges in perspective.[146,147,149] Close relationships also give clinicians an opportunity to cope with difficulties.[147] Interconnectedness, cooperation, and positive relations with colleagues in general are themes leading to resilient practices.[121,122,148] In testing a resilience model in operating room nurses, Gillespie et al. identified five explanatory variables: hope, self-efficacy, coping, control, and competence.[35] Hope is also a factor that can lead to increased levels of resilience in nurses.[157] Interestingly, in operating room nurses, personal characteristics such as age are not highly predictive of resilience, whereas years of experience is a significant contributor.[158]

Space for reflection and supportive relationships are not the only themes found in correlation with resilience. The environment a clinician works in and institutional practices can be a predictor of burnout[125,159] and resilience.[120,160] Clinician well-being is influenced by work demands,[33] especially if the occupation is challenging,[120] and a lack of work–life integration has led to burnout.[113] Job gratification seems to stem from self-demarcation, limitation of working hours, and making time for leisure activities.[121,146] Work environments where organizations act to curtail incidents that cause stress and to provide continuous professional development offer possibilities to foster resilience and work gratification.[121,122] Burnout ensues in scenarios with poor institutional support—for example, situations where there are poor resources for helping recent graduates make the transition into new positions. In contrast, by providing the resources (including equipment) that clinicians need to carry out their duties, institutions can help clinicians overcome difficult situations.[146,161,162,163,164]

What we can draw from these findings is an understanding that certain themes arise in resilient behaviors and certain aspects lead to an enhanced capacity to respond to adversity. If organizations want a resilient workforce, it is possible to create those opportunities and spaces. For example, interventions for improving mindfulness and addressing resilience can reduce burnout and workplace stress.[128,130,165] Interventions can help clinicians learn the skills to be resilient, potentially leading to higher retention.[113,165] Given that age, experience, and education are not shown to be predictors of resilience,[157] we can posit that such skills can be successfully taught to clinicians from all backgrounds and age groups. Fostering work culture and programming for resilience training can lead to greater worker satisfaction and competence[121] and can have direct effects on patient outcomes.[113,121,125,148]

Programs that provide spaces for mindfulness and values clarification, build relationships between colleagues, [165] and offer opportunities for employees to be mentally healthy through reflection, healthy eating, and exercise can go a long way in fostering healthy behaviors. What workers can gain from these interventions are strategies to develop mental, physical, and social resource pools that provide greater opportunities for effective decision-making.[121,158,166]

Several studies demonstrate the effects of using some of these interventions to promote resilience among nurses and physicians. West et al.[166] provided biweekly, protected time to seventy-four physicians to meet in small groups to practice mindfulness and reflection. Compared to a control group of physicians who had biweekly, protected time but received no intervention, physicians who received the mindfulness intervention showed significant increases in work engagement and significant decreases in burnout.[166] Mealer et al.[168] designed a two-day workshop, offered to twenty-nine critical care nurses, that allowed nurses to practice mindfulness skills, engaged them in psychological therapy, and encouraged them to exercise. The study suggested that such a forum could improve psychological health and increase resilience, although it was underpowered to determine whether these findings were statistically significant.[168] In other studies, interventions focusing on personal and environmental strategies have shown efficacy in treating and preventing burnout syndrome; [167,168,169] cognitive-behavioral interventions and relaxation activities have reduced occupational stress;[170] and positive psychology interventions focused on accomplishments and relationship development have led to values clarification, happiness, and higher levels of engagement.[171] Each of these studies points to the feasibility of implementing such programs and the willingness of participants to engage with curricula and interventions that may reduce psychological symptoms, moral distress, and burnout syndrome. These strategies and interventions are discussed in Chapters 7 and 8, following a more extensive examination of moral resilience in Chapter 6.

Future Direction in Clinician Resilience Research

Since the beginning of the COVID-19 pandemic, there has been a renewed focus on resilience and how building resilience at the system and individual level may improve the well-being of clinicians, which in turn may improve turnover rates and individual clinician satisfaction. There has also been an increase in intramural and extramural funding to support these efforts.

Despite a renewed focus and funding opportunities, there is not yet a robust body of evidence about the effectiveness of resilience interventions for clinician well-being. Two areas of concern are the measurement of resilience and the choice of outcome variables to determine the effectiveness of the intervention(s). There are several different instruments to measure resilience. [172,173,174,175] The Connor-Davidson Resilience Scale (CD-RISC-25 and CD-RISC-10)[174,176] are the instruments that have been the most used with nurses and other healthcare providers.[177]

In a recent systematic review and meta-analysis, a validated instrument to measure resilience in healthcare providers was used only 29% of the time[177] and there are questions as to whether these instruments are actually valid in a healthcare provider population. The CD-RISC was originally developed using a study sample of individuals from the general population, primary care outpatient setting, and a psychiatric outpatient setting and was conceptualized as a 5-factor model (personal competence, trust in one's instincts, positive acceptance of change, control and spiritual influences).[174] There is a paucity of evidence to support its factor structure as effective with healthcare providers, with one exploratory and confirmatory factor analysis supporting a 3-factor model in critical care nurses (personal competence, perseverance and leadership).[178] This may suggest that the concept of resilience in healthcare providers is different from that in the general population or other groups. In fact, concept analysis investigating resilience in nurses suggests entirely different defining attributes from those used in the general population, further highlighting the concerns with currently available measures.[179,180]

Outcome Variables

Resilience is not meant to "fix" everything nor does the absence of burnout signify resilience. Having more resilience does not exclude the need for evidence-based mental health treatment, in certain situations. Additionally, resilience has been heavily linked to burnout syndrome. The National Academy of Medicine launched the Action Collaborative on Clinician Well-Being and Resilience which has resulted in funding announcements and research geared toward reducing burnout syndrome in healthcare professionals.[181] However, before burnout syndrome is used as a primary outcome variable to determine the effectiveness of resilience interventions, it is important to understand how burnout syndrome was originally conceptualized. There are both subjective and objective criteria involved in the diagnosis of burnout syndrome. There is an abundance of evidence reported on subjective measures of burnout syndrome in healthcare professionals, primarily with the Maslach Burnout Inventory (MBI).[182,183,184,] These include emotional exhaustion, cynicism, and lack of personal accomplishment.[182] There is less information on the objective criteria. It is recommended that the symptoms associated with burnout <u>not</u> be related to (1) being a novice in your profession, (2) having symptoms or diagnoses of psychological disorders, or (3) experiencing non-work-related family problems[185] However, the prevalence of depression, anxiety, and posttraumatic stress disorder (PTSD) is high in healthcare professionals, which has been further exacerbated by the COVID-19 pandemic.[186,187,188] With this knowledge, there may be an overestimation of burnout syndrome among clinicians who commonly have coexisting contributors to their symptoms. As the field advances, more refined methods are needed to accurately diagnosis the underlying source and to better explicate and prioritize needs based on the findings. The authors of the MBI offer insights regarding the misuses and modifications of the scale and suggest ways to measure burnout accurately and ethically.[189] In the meantime, measuring well-being may be a more appropriate outcome measure for resilience interventions. The presence of resilience and well-being does not imply the absence of mental illness as these are related but distinct concepts that require targeted interventions to address them. Similarly, concepts such as moral distress and moral injury should not be conflated with burnout. While moral suffering may lead to burnout symptoms the concepts are distinct[190] and the types of resilience need to be differentiated and specified. Further conceptual and empirical work is needed to refine our understanding of the contributing mechanisms and measurement of relevant concepts.

Acknowledgment

Gratitude to Dr. Alford W. Kaszniak for his substantial contribution to the neuroscience section of this chapter.

References

1. Rushton CH. Moral resilience: a capacity for navigating moral distress in critical care. AACN Adv Crit Care. 2016;27:111–119.
2. Rushton CH, Boss R. The many faces of moral distress among clinicians: introduction. Narrat Inq Bioeth. 2013;3:89–93.
3. Lützén K, Kvist BE. Moral distress: a comparative analysis of theoretical understandings and inter-related concepts. HEC Forum. 2012;24:13–25.
4. Webster GC, Baylis FE. Moral residue. In Rubin SB, Zoloth L, editors, Margin of error: the ethics of mistakes in the practice of medicine. Hagerstown, MD: University Publishing; 2000:217–230.
5. Lützén K, Ewalds-Kvist B. Moral distress and its interconnection with moral sensitivity and moral resilience: viewed from the philosophy of Viktor E. Frankl. J Bioeth Inq. 2013;10:317–324.
6. Rushton, C. Transforming moral suffering by cultivating moral resilience and ethical practice. Amer Jour Crit Care. 2023;32 (4):238–248.
7. Wilson, MA. Analysis and evaluation of the moral distress theory. Nurs Forum. 2018;53:259– 266.

8. Holtz H, Heinze K, Rushton C. Interprofessionals' definitions of moral resilience. J ClinNurs. 2018; 27:e488– e49.4.
9. Silverman H, Kheirbek R, Moscou-Jackson G, Day J. Moral distress in nurses caring for patients with COVID-19. Nurs Eth. 2021;28:1137–1164.
10. Woods, M. Moral distress revisited: the viewpoints and responses of nurses. Inter Nurs Rev. 2020;67:68–75
11. Delgado J, Siow S, de Groot J, et al. Towards collective moral resilience: the potential of communities of practice during the COVID-19 pandemic and beyond. J Med Eth 2021;47:374–382.
12. Prentice TM, Gillam L, Davis PG, Janvier A. Always a burden? Healthcare providers' perspectives on moral distress. Arch Dis Child Fetal Neo Ed. 2018;103:F441–F445.
13. Rushton CH. Principled moral outrage: an antidote to moral distress? AACN Adv Crit Care. 2013;24:82–89.
14. Helmers A, Dryden Palmer K, Greenberg RA. Moral distress: Developing strategies from experience. Nurs Eth. 2020;27:1147–1156.
15. Tigard, DW. The positive value of moral distress. Bioethics. 2019;33:601–608.
16. Deschenes S, Kunyk D. Situating moral distress within relational ethics. Nurs Eth. 2020;27:767–777.
17. Goethals S, Gastmans C, de Casterlé BD. Nurses' ethical reasoning and behaviour: a literature review. Int J Nurs Stud. 2010;47:635–650.
18. Hanna DR. Moral distress: the state of the science. Res Theory Nurs Pract. 2004;18:73–93.
19. Traudt T, Liaschenko J, Peden-McAlpine C. Moral agency, moral imagination, and moral community: antidotes to moral distress. J Clin Ethics. 2016;27:201–213.
20. Carse A, Rushton CH. Harnessing the promise of moral distress: a call for reorientation. J Clin Ethics. 2017;28:15–29.
21. Guzys, D. Moral distress: A theorized model of influences to facilitate mitigation and resilience. Nurs Health Sci. 2021;23:658–664.
22. van Zuylen ML, de Snoo-Trimp JC, Metselaar S, Dongelmans DA, Molewijk B. Moral distress and positive experiences of ICU staff during the COVID-19 pandemic: lessons learned. BMC Med Ethics. 2023;24,40:1–17.
23. Szanton SL. Stress-resiliency model: bio behavioral pathways of risk and resilience. South Online J Nurs Res. 2009;9(2). http://www.resourcenter.net/images/snrs/files/sojnr_articles2/Vol09Num02S.html.
24. Bonanno GA. Loss, trauma, and human resilience: have we underestimated the human capacity to thrive after extremely aversive events? Am Psychol. 2004;59:20–28.
25. Bonanno GA. Meaning making, adversity, and regulatory flexibility. Memory. 2013;21:150–156.
26. Cacioppo JT, Reis HT, Zautra AJ. Social resilience: the value of social fitness with an application to the military. Am Psychol. 2011;66:43–51.

27. Karatsoreos IN, McEwen BS. Annual research review: the neurobiology and physiology of resilience and adaptation across the life course. J Child Psychol Psychiatry. 2013;54:337–347.
28. Luthar SS, Brown PJ. Maximizing resilience through diverse levels of inquiry: prevailing paradigms, possibilities, and priorities for the future. Dev Psychopathol. 2007;19:931–955.
29. Masten AS. Global perspectives on resilience in children and youth. Child Dev. 2014;85:6–20.
30. Masten AS. Invited commentary: resilience and positive youth development frameworks in developmental science. J Youth Adolesc. 2014;43:1018–1024.
31. Masten AS. Ordinary magic: resilience in development. New York: Guilford Press; 2014.
32. Southwick SM, Bonanno GA, Masten AS, Panter-Brick C, Yehuda, R. Resilience definitions, theory, and challenges: interdisciplinary perspectives. Eur J Psychotraumatol. 2014;5:1–14.
33. Back AL, Steinhauser KE, Kamal AH, Jackson VA. Building resilience for palliative care clinicians: an approach to burnout prevention based on individual skills and workplace factors. J Pain Symptom Manage. 2016;52:284–291.
34. Earvolino-Ramirez M. Resilience: A concept analysis. Nurs Forum. 2007;47:73–82.
35. Gillespie BM, Chaboyer W, Wallis M, Grimbeek P. Resilience in the operating room: developing and testing of a resilience model. J Adv Nurs. 2007;59:427–438.
36. Howe A, Smajdor A, Stöckl A. Towards an understanding of resilience and its relevance to medical training. Med Educ. 2012;46:349–356.
37. Finstad GL, Giorgi G, Lulli LG, Pandolfi C, Foti G, León-Perez JM, Cantero-Sánchez FJ, Mucci N. Resilience, coping strategies and posttraumatic growth in the workplace following COVID-19: a narrative review on the positive aspects of trauma. Inter J Environ Res and Public Health. 2021;18(18):9453.
38. Institute of Medicine. Building a resilient workforce: opportunities for the Department of Homeland Security: workshop summary. Washington, DC: National Academies Press; 2012.
39. Szanton SL, Gill JM. Facilitating resilience using a society-to-cells framework: a theory of nursing essentials applied to research and practice. ANS Adv Nurs Sci. 2010;33:329–343.
40. Carlson JL, Haffenden RA, Bassett GW, Buehring WA, Collins MJ, Folga S, et al. Resilience: theory and application. Argonne, IL: Argonne National Library; 2012.
41. Tugade MM, Fredrickson BL. Resilient individuals use positive emotions to bounce back from negative emotional experiences. J Pers Soc Psychol. 2004;86:320–333.
42. Masten AS. Ordinary magic: resilience processes in development. Am Psychol. 2001;56:227 238.

43. Masten AS, Wright MO. Resilience over the lifespan: developmental perspectives on resistance, recovery and transformation. In Reich JW, Zautra AJ, Hall JS, editors, Handbook of adult resilience. New York: Guilford Press; 2009:213–237.
44. Luthar SS, Cicchetti D, Becker B. The construct of resilience: a critical evaluation and guidelines for future work. Child Dev. 2000;71:543–562.
45. Panter-Brick C, Eggerman M. Understanding culture, resilience, and mental health: the production of hope. In Ungar M, editor, The social ecology of resilience: a handbook of theory and practice. New York: Springer-Verlag; 2012:369–386.
46. Richardson GE. The metatheory of resilience and resiliency. J Clin Psychol. 2002;58:307–321.
47. Richardson GE, Neiger BL, Jensen S, Kumpfer K. The resiliency model. Health Educ. 1990;21:33–39.
48. Young PD, Rushton CH. A concept analysis of moral resilience. Nurs Outlook, 2017;65:579–587.
49. Berkowitz SJ. Childhood trauma and adverse experience and forensic child psychiatry: the Penn Center for Youth and Family Trauma Response and Recovery. J Psychiat Law. 2012;40:5–22.
50. Leitch ML. Somatic experiencing treatment with tsunami survivors in Thailand: broadening the scope of early intervention. Traumatology. 2007;13:11–20.
51. Leitch L. Action steps using ACEs and trauma-informed care: a resilience model. Health & Justice. Apr. 28, 2017; 5(5):5.
52. Ozbay F, Fitterling H, Charney D, Southwick S. Social support and resilience to stress across the life span: a neurobiologic framework. Curr Psychiatry Rep. 2008;10:304–310.
53. Cathomas F, Murrough J, Nestler E, Han MH, Russo S. Neurobiology of resilience: interface between mind and body. Biological Psychiatry. 2019; 86:410–420.
54. Shi L, Sun J, Wei D, Qiu J. Recover from the adversity: functional connectivity basis of psychological resilience. Neuropsychologia. 2019;122:20–27.
55. Greydanus D, Calles J. Neurobiology of resilience: exciting research for practitioners of ephebiatrics. Int. J. Child Adolesc Health. 2021;14:219–222.
56. Rajkumar R. Harnessing the neurobiology of resilience to protect the mental well-being of healthcare workers during the COVID-19 pandemic. Frontiers in Psychology. 2021;12:doi: 10.3389/fpsyg.2021.621853.
57. Chichlowski M, Cutler J, Fawkes N, Pandey N. Feed your microbiome and improve sleep, stress resilience and cognition. Exploration of Medicine. 2022;3:331–344.
58. Kaye-Kauderer H, Feingold J, Feder A, Southwick S, Charney D. Resilience in the age of COVID-19. BJ Psych Advances. 2021;27:166–178.
59. Feldman R. What is resilience: an affiliative neuroscience approach. World Psychiatry. 2020;19:132–150.

60. Schulkin J, McEwen BS, Gold PW. Allostasis, amygdala, and anticipatory angst. Neurosci Biobehav Rev. 1994;18:385–396.
61. Thiel KJ, Dretsch MN. The basics of the stress response: a historical context and introduction. In Conrad CD, editor, The handbook of stress: neuropsychological effects on the brain. Oxford: Wiley-Blackwell; 2011:1–28.
62. Kong F, Ma X, You X, Xiang Y. The resilient brain: psychological resilience mediates the effect of amplitude of low-frequency fluctuations in orbitofrontal cortex on subjective well-being in young healthy adults. Soc Cogn Affect Neurosci. 2018;13:755–763.
63. Moreno-Lopez L, Ioannidis K, Askelund A, Smith A, Schueler K, van Harmelen, AL. The resilient emotional brain: a scoping review of the medial prefrontal cortex and limbic structure and function in resilient adults with a history of maltreatment. Biol Psych. 2019;5:392–402.
64. Cunningham WA, Brosch T. Motivational salience: amygdala tuning from traits, needs, values, and goals. Curr Dir Psychol Sci. 2012;21:54–59.
65. Santos A, Mier D, Kirsch P, Meyer-Lindenberg A. Evidence for a general face salience signal in human amygdala. Neuroimage. 2011;54:3111–3116.
66. Adolphs R. The biology of fear. Curr Biol. 2013;23:R79–R93.
67. Harrison LA, Hurlemann R, Adolphs R. An enhanced default approach bias following amygdala lesions in humans. Psychol Sci. 2015;26:1543–1555.
68. Todd RM, Talmi D, Schmitz TW, Susskind J, Anderson AK. Psychophysical and neural evidence for emotion-enhanced perceptual vividness. J Neurosci. 2012;32:11201–11212.
69. Cikara M, Van Bavel JJ. The neuroscience of intergroup relations: an integrative review. Perspect Psychol Sci. 2014;9:245–274.
70. Shonkoff JP, Garner AS, Committee on Psychosocial Aspects of Child and Family Health, Committee on Early Childhood, Adoption, and Dependent Care, Section on Developmental and Behavioral Pediatrics. The lifelong effects of early childhood adversity and toxic stress. Pediatrics. 2012;129:e232–e246.
71. Hanson R. Buddha's brain: the practical neuroscience of happiness, love and wisdom. Oakland, CA: New Harbinger; 2009.
72. Southwick SM, Pietrzak RH, Tsai J, Krystal JH, Charney D. Resilience: an update. PTSD Research Quarterly. 2015;25:1–10.
73. Bartone PT. Resilience under military operational stress: can leaders influence hardiness? Military Psychol. 2006;18:S131–S148.
74. Wright MO, Masten AS, Narayan AJ. Resilience processes in development: four waves of research on positive adaptation in the context of adversity. In Goldstein S, Brooks RB, editors, Handbook of resilience in children. Boston, MA: Springer; 2013:15–37.
75. Bonanno GA, Burton CL. Regulatory flexibility: an individual differences perspective on coping and emotion regulation. Perspect Psychol Sci. 2013;8:591–612.

76. Rutter M. Resilience in the face of adversity: protective factors and resistance to psychiatric disorder. Brit J Psychiatry. 1985;147:598–611.
77. Ungar M, Ghazinour M, Richter J. Annual research review: what is resilience within the social ecology of human development? J Child Psychol Psychiatry. 2013;54:348–366.
78. Kim-Cohen J, Turkewitz R. Resilience and measured gene-environment interactions. Dev Psychopathol. 2012;24:1297–1306.
79. Hofgaard LS, Nes RB, Røysamb E. Introducing two types of psychological resilience with partly unique genetic and environmental sources. Sci Rep. 2021;11:8624.
80. Pietrzak RH, Southwick SM. Psychological resilience in OEF–OIF veterans: application of a novel classification approach and examination of demographic and psychosocial correlates. J Affect Disord. 2011;133:560–568.
81. Wright MO, Masten AS. Resilience processes in development: fostering positive adaptation in the context of adversity. In Goldstein S, Brooks RB, editors, Handbook of resilience in children. New York: Springer; 2005:17–37.
82. Yehuda R, Flory JD, Southwick S, Charney DS. Developing an agenda for translational studies of resilience and vulnerability following trauma exposure. Ann NY Acad Sci. 2006;1071:379–396.
83. Rogers P, Bohland J, Lawrence J. Resilience and values: Global perspectives on the values and worldviews underpinning the resilience concept. Political Geography. 2020;83:1–9.
84. Bandura A. Self-efficacy: toward a unifying theory of behavioral change. Psychol Rev. 1977;84:191–215.
85. Benight CC, Bandura A. Social cognitive theory of posttraumatic recovery: the role of perceived self-efficacy. Behav Res Ther. 2004;42:1129–1148.
86. Bandura A. Self-efficacy: the exercise of control. New York: W. H. Freeman; 1997.
87. Masten AS. Competence, risk, and resilience in military families: conceptual commentary. Clin Child Fam Psychol Rev. 2013;16:278–281.
88. Eisenberg N. Empathy-related emotional responses, altruism, and their socialization. In Davidson RJ, Harrington A, editors, Visions of compassion. Oxford: Oxford University Press; 2002:131–164.
89. Rothbart MK, Derryberry D. Development of individual differences in temperament. In Lamb ME, Brown AL, editors, Advances in developmental psychology. Hillsdale, NJ: Erlbaum; 1981:37–86.
90. Masten AS, Coatsworth JD. The development of competence in favorable and unfavorable environments: lessons from research on successful children. Am Psychol. 1998;53:205–220.
91. Folkman S, Moskowitz JT. Positive affect and the other side of coping. Am Psychol. 2000;55:647–654.

92. Tugade MM, Fredrickson BL, Barrett LF. Psychological resilience and positive emotional granularity: examining the benefits of positive emotions on coping and health. J Pers. 2004;72:1161–1190.
93. Fredrickson BL. What good are positive emotions? Rev Gen Psychol. 1998;2:300–319.
94. Cohn MA, Fredrickson BL. Positive emotions. In Lopez SJ, Snyder CR, editors, Oxford handbook of positive psychology. Oxford: Oxford University Press; 2009:13–24.
95. Masten AS, Tellegen A. Resilience in developmental psychopathology: contributions of the project competence longitudinal study. Dev Psychopathol. 2012;24:345–361.
96. Adger WN. Social and ecological resilience—are they related? Prog Hum Geogr. 2000;24:347–364.
97. Elmqvist T, Folke C, Nyström M, Peterson G, Bengtsson J, Walker B, Norberg J. Response diversity, ecosystem change, and resilience. Front Ecol Environ. 2003;1:488–494.
98. Relman DA. The human microbiome: ecosystem resilience and health. Nutr Rev. 2012;70:S2–S9.
99. Baron SL, Beard S, Davis LK, Delp L, Forst L, Kidd-Taylor A, et al. Promoting integrated approaches to reducing health inequities among low income workers: applying a social ecological framework. Am J Ind Med. 2014;57:539–556.
100. Ager A, Annan J, Panter-Brick C. Resilience: from conceptualization to effective intervention. Policy brief for humanitarian and development agencies. New Haven, CT: MacMillan Center for International and Area Studies; 2013. http://crh.macmillan.yale.edu/sites/default/files/files/Resilience_Policy_Brief_Panter-Brick.pdf.
101. Gunderson LH, Holling CS, editors. Panarchy: understanding transformations in human and natural systems. Washington, DC: Island Press; 2002.
102. Forsgren L, Tediosi F, Blanchet K, Saulnier DD. Health systems resilience in practice: a scoping review to identify strategies for building resilience. BMC Health Serv Res. 2022;22:1173.
103. Biddle L, Wahedi K, Bozorgmeh, K. Health system resilience: a literature review of empirical research, Health Pol &Plan. 2020;35:1084–1109.
104. Davidson PM, Rushton CH, Kurtz M, Wise B, Jackson D, Beaman A, et al. A social-ecological framework: a model for addressing ethical practice in nursing. J Clin Nurs. 2018;00:1–9.
105. Heatherton TF. Neuroscience of self and self-regulation. Ann Rev Psychol. 2011;62:363–390.
106. Fergusson DM, Horwood LJ. Resilience to childhood adversity: results of a 21-year study. In Luthar SS, editor, Resilience and vulnerability: adaptation in the context of childhood adversities. Cambridge: Cambridge University Press; 2003:130–155.

107. Sameroff AJ, Fiese BH. Models of development and developmental risk. In Zeanah CH, editor, Handbook of infant mental health. New York: Guilford Press; 2000: 3–19.
108. Werner EE, Smith RS. Vulnerable but invincible: a longitudinal study of resilient children and youth. New York: McGraw Hill; 1982.
109. Gilligan R. Promoting resilience in young people in long-term care—the relevance of roles and relationships in the domains of recreation and work. J Soc Work Pract. 2008;22:37–50.
110. Rutter M. Resilience as a dynamic concept. Dev Psychopathol. 2012;24:335–e44.
111. Zolli A, Healy AM. Resilience: why things bounce back. New York: Free Press; 2012.
112. Gillespie BM, Chaboyer W, Wallis M. Development of a theoretically derived model of resilience through concept analysis. Contemp Nurse. 2007;25:124–135.
113. Hart PL, Brannan JD, Chesnay MD. Resilience in nurses: an integrative review. J Nurs Manage. 2014;22:720–734.
114. McGowan JE, Murray K. Exploring resilience in nursing and midwifery students: a literature review. J Adv Nurs. 2016;72:2272–2283.
115. Cooper AL, Brown JA, Rees CS, Leslie GD. Nurse resilience: a concept analysis. Int J Mental Health Nurs, 2020;29:553–575.
116. Wiig S, Aase K, Billett S, et al. Defining the boundaries and operational concepts of resilience in the resilience in healthcare research program. BMC Health Serv Res, 2020;20, 33.
117. Schwarz S. Resilience in psychology: a critical analysis of the concept. Theory & Psychology. 2018:28.4:528–541.
118. Brigham T et al. A journey to construct an all-encompassing conceptual model of factors affecting clinician well-being and resilience. NAM perspectives. 2018;8:201801b.
119. Russo G, Pires CA, Perelman J, Gonçalves L, Barros PP. Exploring public sector physicians' resilience, reactions and coping strategies in times of economic crisis; findings from a survey in Portugal's capital city area. BMC Health Serv Res. 2017;17:207.
120. Stevenson AD, Phillips CB, Anderson KJ. Resilience among doctors who work in challenging areas: a qualitative study. Br J Gen Pract. 2011;61:e404–410.
121. Tubbert SJ. Resiliency in emergency nurses. J Emerg Nurs. 2016;42:47–52.
122. Zwack J, Schweitzer J. If every fifth physician is affected by burnout, what about the other four? Resilience strategies of experienced physicians. Acad Med. 2013;88:382–389.
123. Aughterson H et al. Psychosocial impact on frontline health and social care professionals in the UK during the COVID-19 pandemic: a qualitative interview study. BMJ open. 2021;11;e047353.

124. Agarwal B, Brooks SK, Greenberg Neil. The role of peer support in managing occupational stress: A qualitative study of the sustaining resilience at work intervention. Workplace Health & Safety. 2020;68(2):57–64.
125. Eley DS, Cloninger CR, Walters L, Laurence C, Synnott R, Wilkinson D. The relationship between resilience and personality traits in doctors: implications for enhancing well-being. Peer J. 2013;1:e216.
126. Guo Y, Cross W, Plummer V, Lam L, Luo Y, Zhang J. Exploring resilience in Chinese nurses: a cross-sectional study. J Nurs Manage. 2017;25:223–230.
127. McCain RS, McKinley N, Dempster M, Campbell WJ, Kirk SJ. A study of the relationship between resilience, burnout and coping strategies in doctors. Postgrad Med J. Aug. 9, 2017 Published online: doi:10.1136/postgradmedj-2016-134683
128. Montero-Marin J, Tops M, Manzanera R, Piva Demarzo MM, Álvarez de Mon M, García-Campayo J. Mindfulness, resilience, and burnout subtypes in primary care physicians: the possible mediating role of positive and negative affect. Front Psychol. 2015;17:1895.
129. McKinley N et al. Resilience, burnout and coping mechanisms in UK doctors: a cross-sectional study. BMJ open. 2020;10.1: e031765.
130. Guo Yu-fang et al. Burnout and its association with resilience in nurses: A cross-sectional study. J Clin Nur. 2018;27(1–2):441–449.
131. Simpkin AL et al. Stress from uncertainty and resilience among depressed and burned out residents: a cross-sectional study. Acad Ped. 2018;18(6):698–704.
132. Barzilay R et al. Resilience, COVID-19-related stress, anxiety and depression during the pandemic in a large population enriched for healthcare providers. Transl psyc. 2020;10(1):291.
133. Zanatta F, Maffoni M, Giardini A. Resilience in palliative healthcare professionals: a systematic review. Supp Care in Cancer. 2020;28:971–978.
134. Powell MJ, Froggatt K, Giga S. Resilience in inpatient palliative care nursing: a qualitative systematic review. BMJ Suppor & Pallia Care. 2020;10(1):79–90.
135. Grauerholz, KR et al. Fostering vicarious resilience for perinatal palliative care professionals. Front in Peds. 2020;8:572933.
136. McKinley N et al. Resilience in medical doctors: a systematic review." Postgr Med J. 2019; 95(1121):140–147.
137. Venegas CL et al. Interventions to improve resilience in physicians who have completed training: a systematic review. PLoS One. 2020;14(1):e0210512.
138. Musso M et al. The relationship between grit and resilience in emergency medical service personnel. 2019;19(3):199–203.
139. Son C et al. Investigating resilience in emergency management: an integrative review of literature. Applied Ergonomics. 2020;87:103114.
140. Azizoddin DR et al. Bolstering clinician resilience through an interprofessional, web-based nightly debriefing program for emergency departments during the COVID-19 pandemic. Journal of Interpro Care 3. 2020;4(5):711–715.

141. Kelker H et al. Prospective study of emergency medicine provider wellness across ten academic and community hospitals during the initial surge of the COVID-19 pandemic. BMC Emerg Med. 2021;21:1–12.
142. Hughes V, Cologer S, Swoboda S, Rushton, C. Strengthening internal resources to promote resilience among pre-licensure nursing students. J Prof Nursing. 2021;37(4):777–783.
143. McAllister M, McKinnon J. The importance of teaching and learning resilience in the health disciplines: a critical review of the literature. Nur Educ Today. 2009;29:371–379.
144. McDonald G, Jackson D, Wilkes L, Vickers MH. A work-based educational intervention to support the development of personal resilience in nurses and midwives. Nurse Educ Today. 2012;32:378–384.
145. Pines EW, Rauschhuber ML, Cook JD, Norgan GH, Canchola L, Richardson C, et al. Enhancing resilience, empowerment and conflict management among baccalaureate students: outcomes of a pilot study. J Adv Nurs. 2014;68:1482–1493.
146. Ablett JR, Jones RS. Resilience and well-being in palliative care staff: a qualitative study of hospice nurses' experience of work. Psycho-oncology. 2007;16:733–740.
147. Burge F, McIntyre P, Twohig P, Cummings I, Kaufman D, Frager G, et al. Palliative care by family physicians in the 1990s. Can Fam Phys. 2001;47:1989–1995.
148. Everly GS, McCormack DK, Strouse DA. Seven characteristics of highly resilient people: insights from Navy SEALs to the "greatest generation." Int J Emerg Ment Health. 2012;14:87–93.
149. Glass N. An investigation of nurses' and midwives' academic/clinical workplaces. Holistic Nurs Pract. 2009;23:158–170.
150. Hodges HF, Keeley AC, Troyan PJ. Professional resilience in baccalaureate-prepared acute care nurses: first steps. Nurs Educ Perspect. 2008;29:80–89.
151. Kornhaber RA, Wilson A. Building resilience in burns nurses: a descriptive phenomenological inquiry. J Burn Care Res. 2011;32:481–488.
152. Vos LMW et al. Optimism, mindfulness, and resilience as potential protective factors for the mental health consequences of fear of the coronavirus. Psych Res. 2021;300:113927.
153. Joyce S et al. Road to resilience: a systematic review and meta-analysis of resilience training programmes and interventions. BMJ Open. 2018;8*6):e017858.
154. Labrague LJ. Psychological resilience, coping behaviours and social support among health care workers during the COVID-19 pandemic: A systematic review of quantitative studies. J Nurs Manag. 2021; 29(7):1893–1905.
155. Schierberl Scherr AE, Ayotte BJ, Kellogg MB. Moderating roles of resilience and social support on psychiatric and practice outcomes in nurses working during the COVID-19 pandemic. SAGE Open Nursing. 2021;7:23779608211024213.

156. Labrague LJ, De los Santos JAA. COVID-19 anxiety among front-line nurses: predictive role of organisational support, personal resilience and social support. Nurs Manag. 2020;28(7):1653–1661.
157. Rushton CH, Batcheller J, Schroeder K, Donohue P. Burnout and resilience among nurses practicing in high-intensity settings. Am J Crit Care. 2015;24:412–420.
158. Gillespie BM, Chaboyer W, Wallis M. The influence of personal characteristics on the resilience of operating room nurses: a predictor study. Int J Nurs Stud. 2009;46:968–976.
159. Dordunoo D et al. The impact of practice environment and resilience on burnout among clinical nurses in a tertiary hospital setting. Inter J Envir Res and Pub Heal. 2021;18(5): 2500.
160. Lowe LD. Creating a caring work environment and fostering nurse resilience. Int J Human Caring. 2013;17:52–59.
161. Xu Z, Yang F. The impact of perceived organizational support on the relationship between job stress and burnout: a mediating or moderating role? Curr Psych. 2021;40:402–413.
162. Srivastava S, Agrawal S. Resistance to change and turnover intention: a moderated mediation model of burnout and perceived organizational support. J Org Change Manag. 2020;33(7):1431–1447.
163. Wang Q, Wang C. Reducing turnover intention: perceived organizational support for frontline employees. Front Res in China. 2020;14(1):1–16.
164. West CP, Dyrbye LN, Shanafelt TD. Physician burnout: contributors, consequences and solutions. J Int Med. 2018;283(6):516–529.
165. Rushton C, Swoboda S, Reimer T, Boyce D, Hansen G. The Mindful Ethical Practice & Resilience Academy (MEPRA): Sustainability of impact. Amer Jour Critl Care. 2023;32(3):184–194.
166. West CP, Dyrbye LN, Rabatin JT, Call TG, Davidson JH, Multari A, et al. Intervention to promote physician well-being, job satisfaction, and professionalism: a randomized clinical trial. JAMA Intern Med. 2014;174:527–533.
167. Wong AV, Olusanya O. Burnout and resilience in anaesthesia and intensive care medicine. BJA Educ. 2017;17:334–340.
168. Mealer M, Hodapp R, Conrad D, Dimidjian S, Rothbaum BO, Moss M. Designing a resilience program for critical care nurses. AACN Adv Crit Care. Winter 2017;28(4):359–365.
169. Holliday R, Ricke DJ, Ricklefs C, Mealer M. Brief narrative writing program implemented in a neurosurgical intensive care unit during the COVID-19 pandemic. Am J Crit Care. Mar 1, 2023;32(2):131–135.
170. Ruotsalainen JH, Verbeek JH, Mariné A, Serra C. Preventing occupational stress in healthcare workers. Cochrane Database Syst Rev. 2015;4:CD002892.
171. Gander F, Proyer RT, Ruch W. Positive psychology interventions addressing pleasure, engagement, meaning, positive relationships, and accomplishment

increase well-being and ameliorate depressive symptoms: a randomized, placebo-controlled online study. Front Psychol. 2016;7:686.

172. Sinclair VG, Wallston KA, The development and psychometric evaluation of the Brief Resilient Coping Scale. Assessment. 2004;11: 94–101.
173. Smith BW, Dalen J, Wiggins K, Tooley E, Christopher P, Bernard J. The brief resilience scale: Assessing the ability to bounce back. Inter J Behav Med. 2008;15(3);194–200.
174. Connor KM, Davidson JRT. Development of a new resilience scale: The Connor-Davidson Resilience Scale (CD-RISC). Depres & Anx. 2003;18(2):76–82.
175. Block J, Kremen AM. IQ and ego-resiliency: Conceptual and empirical connections and separateness. J Pers and Soc Psych. 1996;70(2):349–361.
176. Campbell-Sills, L., Stein, MB. Psychometric Analysis and Refinement of the Connor-Davidson Resilience Scale (CD-RISC): validation of a 10-Item Measure of Resilience. J Trau Stress; 2007: 20, 1019–1028.
177. Cheng C, Chua J, Cheng L, Ang W, Lau Y. Global prevalence of resilience in health care professionals: A systematic review, meta-analysis and meta-regression. J Nurs Manag.2022: 30:795–816.
178. Mealer M, Schmiege S, Meek P. The Connor-Davidson Resilience Scale in critical care nurses: a psychometric analysis. J of Nurs Meas. 2016;24:28–39.
179. Turner SB. The resilient nurse: An emerging concept. Nurse Leader. 2014;12(6):71–90.
180. Fisher D, Law R. How to choose a measure of resilience: an organizing framework for resilience measurement. Appl Psych. 2021;70:643–673.
181. National Academies of Medicine Action Collaborative on Clinical Wellbeing and Resilience. https://nam.edu/action-collaborative-on-clinician-well-being-and-resilience-network-organizations/.
182. Maslach C, Jackson SE, Leiter MP. Maslach Burnout Inventory. Palo Alto, CA: Consulting Psychologists Press; 1996.
183. Dyrbye LN, West CP, Satele D, et al. Burnout among US medical students, residents, and early career physicians relative to the general US population. Acad Med. 2014;89(3):443–451.
184. Maslach C, Jackson SE. MBI: Human Services Survey for Medical Personnel. https://www.mindgarden.com/315-mbi-human-services-survey-medical-personnel.
185. Bibeau G, Dussault G, Larouche LM, Lippel K, Saucier JF, Vezina M, Vidal JM. Certains aspects culturels, diagnostiques et juridiques de burnout [Some cultural diagnostic and juridical aspects of burnout]. Montreal: Confederation des Syndicats Nationaux; 1989.
186. Varghese A, George G, Kondagul S, Naser A, Khakha D, Chatterji R. Decline in mental health of nurses across the globe during COVID-19: a systematic review and meta-analysis. J Glob Health. 2021;11:05009..

187. Chutiyami M, Cheong A, Salihu D, Bello V, Ndwiga D, Muharaj R, Naidoo K, Kolo M, Jacob P, Chhina N, Ku T, Devar L, Pratitho P, Kannan P. COVID-19 pandemic and overall mental health of healthcare professionals globally: a meta-review of systematic reviews. Front in Psych. 2022;12:
188. Hill J, Harris C, Christian D, Buland P, Doherty A, Benedetto V, Bhutani G, Clegg A. The prevalence of mental health conditions in healthcare workers during and after a pandemic: system review and meta-analysis. J of Adv Nurs. 2022;78:1551–1573.
189. Maslach C, Leiter M. How to measure burnout accurately and ethically, Harvard Bus Rev. 2021, https://hbr.org/2021/03/how-to-measure-burnout-accurately-and-ethically.
190. Antonsdottir I, Rushton CH, Nelson KE, Heinze KE, Swoboda SM, Hanson GC. Burnout and moral resilience in interdisciplinary healthcare professionals. J Clin Nurs. 2021;00:1–13.

6

Conceptualizing Moral Resilience

Cynda Hylton Rushton

CONCEPTUALIZING RESILIENCE WITHIN the moral domain in healthcare encompasses both normative and descriptive dimensions of individual and collective intentions, decisions, behaviors, and actions.* Clinicians are responsible for upholding professional standards, ethical norms, and policies in myriad ethical issues within the healthcare environment. They are also responsible for making sure that their actions and behaviors are congruent with their values, commitments, and conscience. This requires an understanding of moral resilience that is grounded in a robust notion of integrity rather than more narrowly in terms of moral distress and moral residue[1,2,3] and further applies the body of resilience scholarship outlined in Chapter 5.

To arrive at this understanding, we synthesized findings from two studies that form the basis of our conceptualization. The first study, a literature search using eleven databases, identified 192 occurrences of the term in seventeen sources; concept analysis yielded five definitions

---

* Portions of this chapter are excerpted or adapted from previous articles: "Moral Resilience: A Capacity for Navigating Moral Distress in Critical Care," by C. H. Rushton. *AACN Advanced Critical Care*. 2016; 27: 11–119. Copyright 2016 by the American Association of Critical-Care Nurses. Adapted with permission; "Harnessing the Promise of Moral Distress," by A. Carse and C. H. Rushton. *Journal of Clinical* Ethics. 2017; 28: 15–29. Copyright 2017 by Sage. Adapted with permission; "'Inter-professionals' Definitions of Moral Resilience," by H. Holtz, K. Heinze, and C. Rushton. *Journal of Clinical Nursing*. 2017;1–7. Copyright 2017 by John Wiley & Sons. Adapted with permission; and C. H. Rushton. "Transforming Moral Suffering by Cultivating Moral Resilience and Ethical Practice," by C. H. Rushton. *American Journal of Critical Care*. 2023; 32(4): 238–248. Adapted with permission.

Cynda Hylton Rushton, *Conceptualizing Moral Resilience* In: *Moral Resilience*. Second Edition.
Edited by: Cynda Hylton Rushton, Oxford University Press. © Oxford University Press 2024.
DOI: 10.1093/oso/9780197667149.003.0007

through 2015 and added two from 2016.[4] Since then others have added their interpretations to the literature. These are summarized in Table 6.1. The implications of this evolving body of scholarship are explored later in Chapter 9.

We discuss the second study here and, later in the chapter, offer insights from it and the raw data upon which it is based. The researchers asked 184 interprofessional clinicians and twenty-three non-clinician healthcare workers the open-ended question, "How do you define moral resilience?" and then conducted a formal content analysis of their answers.[5] The key attributes of moral resilience they identified—personal and relational integrity, buoyancy, moral efficacy, self-regulation, and self-stewardship—inform our definition.

The hallmark of our definition of moral resilience is "the capacity of an individual to sustain or restore their integrity in response to moral adversity."[6(p112)] As Chapter 3 documents, moral adversity can take many forms. It can begin insidiously as unrelieved moral stress; it can consist of moral challenges punctuated by dissonance, confusion, uncertainty, or conflict; it can be experienced as a result of setbacks and disruptions that constrain one's moral agency; or it can arise in the *anticipation* of moral threat, especially when the moral stakes are weighty.[1,6] Morally resilient clinicians draw upon their inner strength and fortitude when they encounter or realistically anticipate moral threat. Indeed, some clinicians report being more engaged in morally distressing situations, igniting compassion and signaling their moral conscientiousness.[7,8,9,10,11]

While moral resilience can be viewed as a signal of moral conscientiousness, we are not suggesting that moral suffering in and of itself is desirable or necessarily positive. Rather, we are proposing that moral suffering to some degree is inevitable in the context of human existence—particularly in the context of clinical practice. By leveraging our self-efficacy and moral agency we can determine our responses to it. With intention and the development of preventive and proactive skills and capacities, we can shift our relationship to it in ways that can reduce its detrimental impact and protect or restore our integrity when it is imperiled. Instead of seeing ourselves as broken and permanently damaged, it is possible to restore ourselves to wholeness, not by denying our moral suffering but by intentionally and constructively engaging in a process of moral repair that weaves together both the suffering and our basic goodness in a new way. In so doing we can strengthen our integrity and capacity to learn and

Table 6.1. Contemporary Definitions of Moral Resilience in the Academic Literature

Author	Definition of Moral Resilience
Oser and Reichenbach Oser, F. K., and Reichenbach, R. (2005). Moral resilience—the unhappy moralist. In W. Edelstein and G. Nunner-Winkler (Eds.), Morality in context (pp. 203–224). Amsterdam, The Netherlands: Elsevier.	Moral resilience means to be good (and prove one's integrity and character) under conditions of risk.
Swierstra Swierstra, T. (2013). Nanotechnology and technomoral change. Etica e Politica: Rivista De Filosofia on-Line, 15(1), 200–219.	Moral resilience is "an attitude that is simultaneously robust and flexible."
Lützén and Ewalds-Kvist Lützén, K., and Ewalds-Kvist, B. (2013). Moral distress and its interconnection with moral sensitivity and moral resilience: Viewed from the philosophy of Viktor E. Frankl. *Journal of Bioethical Inquiry*, 10(3), 317–324.	Moral resilience is defined as a "distinctive sense that life is meaningful under every condition."
Monteverde Monteverde, S. (2014a). Caring for tomorrow's workforce: Moral resilience and healthcare ethics education. Nursing Ethics, 23(1), 104–116. Monteverde, S. (2014b). Undergraduate healthcare ethics education, moral resilience, and the role of ethical theories. *Nursing Ethics*, 21(4), 385–401.	Moral resilience is defined operationally as "a reduction of moral distress in a given axis of time measured by a validated tool." It can also be "understood as the capability to 'name' and 'frame' ethical issues."
Baratz Baratz, L. (2015). Israeli teacher trainees' perceptions of the term moral resilience. *Journal for Multicultural Education*, 9(3), 193–206.	Moral resilience is "the ability to cope with crisis situations and particularly, crises related to moral principles."
Rushton Rushton, C. H. (2016). Moral resilience: A capacity for navigating moral distress in critical care. *AACN Advanced Critical Care*, 27(1), 111–119.	Moral resilience is "the capacity of an individual to sustain or restore their integrity in response to moral complexity, confusion, distress or setbacks."

Table 6.1. Continued

Author	Definition of Moral Resilience
Holtz, H.K., Weissinger, G.M., and Swavely, D., et al. (2023). The long tail of COVID-19: Implications for the future of emergency nursing. *Journal of Emergency Nursing*, 49(2), 198–209.	
Swavely, D., Romig, B., and Weissinger, G., et al. (2022). The impact of traumatic stress, resilience, and threats to core values on nurses during a pandemic. *Journal of Nursing Administration*, 52(10), 525–535.	
Albaqawi, H., and Alrashidi, M.S. (2022). Perceived stress and its relationship to moral resilience among nurses in the Hail Region, Saudi Arabia. *Makara Journal of Health Research*, 26(3), 159–164.	
Kovanci, M.S., and Ozbas, A.A. (2023). Examining the effect of moral resilience on moral distress. *Nursing Ethics*. Online ahead of print.	
Lachman	Moral resilience is "the ability and willingness to speak and take right and good action in the face of an adversity that is moral/ethical in nature."
Lachman, V. D. (2016). Ethics, law, and policy. Moral resilience: Managing and preventing moral distress and moral residue. *MEDSURG Nursing*, 25(2), 121–124.	
Defilippis	Moral resilience is "a character trait (virtue) that allows people to remain open to compromises without compromising themselves."
Defilippis, T.M.L.S., Curtis, K., and Gallagher, (2019) A. Conceptualising moral resilience for nursing practice. *Nursing Inquiry*, 26.	
Quigg	Moral resilience is "the ability to effectively navigate through moral adversity."
Quigg L. *Evaluating a brief mindfulness-based self-care intervention on critical care nurses' resilience and well-being during the COVID-19 pandemic*. [Doctoral dissertation]. Los Angeles: University of California–Los Angeles; 2022.	

Source: "A Concept Analysis of Moral Resilience," by P. D. Young and C. H. Rushton, 2017, *Nursing Outlook*, 65, p. 581. Copyright 2017 by Elsevier. Used with permission and adapted.

grow in response to moral adversity. For individual moral resilience to thrive, clinicians must practice in a moral ecosystem that supports this resilience rather than contributing to moral adversity and moral suffering. Chapter 10 and Chapter 11 take up these issues in detail.

Key Attributes of Moral Resilience

The content analysis of definitions of moral resilience upon which we ground our understanding identifies essential themes.[5] The primary or overarching one—integrity, both personal and relational—is viewed as foundational to our understanding of moral resilience. The concept of buoyancy emerged as a prominent theme, exceeding the remainder of the themes in frequency of occurrence. Three secondary themes that support *moral* resilience and integrity are moral efficacy, self-regulation, and self-stewardship. More global qualities and skills that enable one to be more morally resilient emerge from these themes. None of these concepts is discrete; they are interrelated and synergistically aligned. While progress has been made in understanding these relationships, further research is needed to fully explicate the dimensions and contours of each theme and to determine the relationship of each one to other concepts such as moral distress or other forms of moral suffering.[**]

Integrity

Integrity, a state of being whole and undiminished, is foundational to human flourishing and ethically grounded clinical practice. It can be nurtured over a lifetime in ways that are generative and constructive and that reflect one's personal and professional standards, values, and commitments. Based on our analysis, integrity can be further classified into personal and relational integrity. Aspects of each concept are highlighted here and elaborated in Chapter 4.

** The following sections quote definitions of moral resilience provided by clinicians in the study conducted by Holtz et al. (2017). Comments quoted in this chapter that come from the published article are cited with page numbers; comments drawn from the raw data gathered as part of the study are cited with the reference number but no page number.

Personal and Professional Integrity

Broadly, integrity points to a state of moral wholeness and as such is a primary attribute of moral resilience for clinicians. It is a state of being integrated in terms of all aspects of one's being and the ecosystem that one is embedded within. This state of harmony aligns one's inner values, intentions, and commitments so that one can authentically embody them in one's choices, spoken and unspoken communications, motives, and actions. The act of embodying one's highest values reflects honesty, sincerity, and integration of moral character. Embodying integrity requires intimate self-knowledge, including the contours of one's own conscience along with the core commitments that make up one's personal moral compass and professional code of ethics.

Moral integrity is secured when one's thoughts, intentions, words, and actions align and one is faithful to one's moral and ethical norms, values, and commitments. It is not merely doing what is ethically justified but doing so with the properly nuanced knowledge, intention, and attitude. In moments of integrity, fear is balanced with self-awareness, insight, and principled action, and these encourage self-respect, calm, and peacefulness. As outlined in Chapter 4, clinicians may experience conflicting responsibilities and commitments within their professional roles. For example, when patient benefit and burden are disproportionately imbalanced, the ability to alleviate suffering is thwarted or impossible and the ability to treat patients with respect, dignity, and fairness is severely compromised. Under conditions of adversity such as these, integrity may require one to take principled action despite the risk of personal consequences to uphold one's fundamental values and commitments. Integrity goes beyond acting for the sake of duty or the apparent justification of an action when doing so is contradictory to one's moral inclinations, intentions, or cognitive appraisal.

Integrity "fundamentally entails conscientiousness—the diligent, resolute, and thoughtful ongoing effort to live in alignment with one's own principles and value commitments," despite countervailing forces such as conflicting views or values, resistance, or defensiveness.[1(p22)] As one clinician stated, "A person of integrity is able to distinguish one's values and commitments from those of others and to be accountable for upholding them and strives to protect and preserve the integrity of relational systems."[5]

Relational Integrity

Personal and professional integrity is reciprocally intertwined with relational integrity—a communal stance that embraces one's interconnection with others who share a common humanity and the broader ecosystem one resides within. In the context of clinical practice, it is the ability to be grounded in one's own moral principles and commitments while interfacing with others in ways that do not impose those values on others or discredit or disable the integrity of others. A clinician framed relational integrity this way: "Being able to act compassionately in the best interest of the patient regardless of personal thoughts, feelings or beliefs and not feeling conflicted in doing so."[5] Oriented to serve the interests of others, clinicians are called upon to suspend or subordinate their own interests in service of the interests of others while preserving their moral wholeness within their role constraints. This requires the ability to honor diverse and at times conflicting points of view, emotional attunement (empathy), and cognitive attunement (perspective-taking). It also involves acting in the best interests of others, even when doing so is contrary to one's personal point of view, and doing so without abandoning one's values, commitments, responsibilities, or sense of wholeness. One clinician reflected that being morally resilient involves "maintain[ing] my own morals but be[ing] respectful and accepting of other people's morals."[5] Other clinicians distinguished their ability to stay true to their values "despite what you may *do* to respect what others believe."[5] Relational integrity does not require individuals to abandon their values, beliefs, or commitments. Rather, it suggests that maintaining personal integrity is possible while fulfilling one's professional role—even when one must carry out decisions requiring actions that may on the surface imply abandonment or disregard for personal values or be contrary to one's conscience. Respecting or honoring another's moral or ethical point of view does not suggest that one is agreeing with or endorsing it. This distinction is particularly important when considering current definitions of moral distress that rely on one's appraisal of what is "right" in a situation without the ability to act upon it.[12,13] Relational integrity considers the diverse moral perspectives reflected in different notions of what is morally justified by the people we serve and among clinicians themselves.

Congruent with the concept of relational integrity, sustaining it must "involve more than a single-minded focus on one's own moral agency."[14(p86)] In the inherently collaborative clinical context, "[being] ethical . . . involves perpetual responsiveness to others," a "recognition of the messy . . . interdependence of decisions, interests, and persons."[11(p84)] Exercising moral agency in these contexts is not primarily a "matter of independent, individual effort, but of collaborative engagement in forging paths that are walked together, and shaped in ongoing ways through shared, collective effort."[1(p22)]

The topic of relational integrity is elaborated in Chapter 4.

Buoyancy

Another primary theme in moral resilience is buoyancy. Morally resilient individuals do not succumb to adversity or fear; "they are buoyant, able to recover, recall their commitments, and reorient in ways that work constructively with possibilities available, and in some instances to grow and learn from adversity."[1(p22)] One clinician describes moral resilience as the "capacity to recover to a healthy state, mentally and physically from crisis or lack of ability to respond to a situation in an ideal manner."[5] Being morally resilient does not imply that such individuals escape adversity or its consequences; they suffer and struggle with unexpected and uncontrollable threats and moral complexity but are nonetheless able to restore, maintain, or in some instances even enhance their moral well-being. They may forge enduring strengths amid adversity and constructively work with it rather than give in to its negative effects. Moral resilience implies the capacity to recover from tension and pressures, to restore wholeness or integrity, and to re-integrate or transform forces of adversity—in effect, to recognize and shift their responses while marshaling resources before becoming impaired in some way or unable to recover or grow.

Buoyancy also includes the ability to interpret moral adversity in a way that leverages a constructive or positive mindset rather than a detrimental or negative one. In studies involving children, it is possible to interrupt negative interpretations of adverse events and positively impact outcomes following the event.[15,16] Extending this to clinicians, when our mindsets are fixed, rigid, or judgmental, we are more likely to focus on the negative aspects of the situation. In cases involving threats to integrity, we can attune to the distress and despair of the situation and disable our ability to perceive the more promising or less harmful moral choices. This kind of mental and emotional buoyancy allows clinicians to acknowledge the difficulties and threats and to shift their focus to finding principled solutions rather than succumbing to the negative appraisal and narrative.

When one is buoyant, moral adversity may displace integrity but does not destroy it. Buoyancy—the ability to recover from moral setbacks with optimism and a hopeful, positive, but realistic mindset—unleashes the energy to regain or sustain moral agency and wholeness, to restore one's moral values when they have been compromised in some way.[5] Instead of being permanently depleted, dispirited, or disengaged, morally resilient clinicians are able to rebound, reorient, and continue to serve. They recover their essence in the face of disturbance without recreating the past; they create a new future that integrates the experience into their current reality. They are able to harness "wise" hope[17] to support their efforts to make sense or meaning of dissonant, confusing, or uncertain circumstances and to support their efforts to restore coherence and wholeness.[18] Hope has been identified as a key feature of resilience in nurses.[19,20,21] Being buoyant may also engage one's foresight to recognize and honor one's limits by discerning when sufficient effort has been exerted, especially if doing so protects one's fundamental values and/or well-being.

Embedded in buoyancy are flexibility and adaptability to the changing stream of experience and situations without compromising what matters most—to be willing and able to begin again while still understanding the degree of moral adversity one can withstand and still renew or grow. Buoyancy is the ability to adapt to changed circumstances while fulfilling one's core purpose and commitments. One aspect of buoyancy is the ability to re-integrate moral adversity by gaining a new perspective or outlook. As one clinician stated, buoyance is being able to "look at a situation with new eyes—taking time to process each morally distressing experience so that the residue does not taint future experiences and allows fresh eyes for each situation."[5] A fresh view can enable clinicians to release the effects of the situation, including moral suffering, and to thrive despite a negative experience. When accommodating various levels of disturbance that imperil integrity, buoyancy involves learning—"building a new skill set for the next encounter."[5] Flexibility and adaptability of mind and emotion fuel buoyancy by cultivating openness, non-attachment to one's position, and a robust repertoire of strategies responsive to the demands of the situation. Being able to adhere to one's moral commitments without rigidity is key to remaining open without being personally wounded or diminished.

A characteristic of buoyancy includes a growth orientation that allows individuals experiencing moral suffering to deepen their commitment and connection to their intentions, values, and commitments, and thus learn and grow in ways that are wholesome and constructive. This reflective capacity is vital if clinicians are to realize the full potential of their moral agency and efficacy; it involves the ability to discern appropriate levels of moral responsibility in morally complex or conflicting situations. While moral resilience requires fortitude and perseverance, it is not simply a matter of individual discipline, willpower, or resoluteness, which are of limited value at best in navigating the kinds of integrity-challenging pressures that often generate moral suffering. Nor does it imply a stance of complacency, disregard, or suppression of the adversity that leads to moral suffering or distress. Rather, it represents the cultivation of skills and practices such as mindfulness that support clinicians as they strive to navigate ethically complex situations without disabling costs to themselves and the people they serve.[1(p22)] It requires them to be cognizant of their own individual breaking points, beyond which they cannot withstand or transform the pressure or tension of their moral adversity without detriment to themselves. Buoyancy is fundamentally supported by a culture of ethical practice that creates the infrastructure for limits to be honored and provides sufficient resources to preserve and restore integrity.

Moral Efficacy

Integrity is closely tied to a cluster of attributes, a related constellation of concepts that includes self-respect, self-efficacy or agency, self-perception, and self-esteem. While each concept is slightly different, they overlap and generally refer to a proper sense of respect for one's place and value in the world. Building on this orientation, moral efficacy is the belief in one's ability to bring about desired and beneficial results through one's efforts and the exercise of one's moral agency individually and collectively.[22] As clinicians, the contours of moral agency are informed by norms and values reflected in their profession's codes of ethics. Possessing moral agency involves viewing oneself as capable of recognizing, deliberating about, embodying, and acting upon moral commitments and responsibilities.[23,24,25] This includes an individual's moral identities and self-conception; it acknowledges social, historical, political, cultural, and organizational contexts; and it recognizes the boundaries of authority and freedom to act autonomously within one's roles and social ecology.[21] Within this context are influences of power and structures that can enable or disable moral efficacy. These issues are vital when considering situations that constrain moral agency and contribute to moral suffering in any form.[21,26]

Having moral efficacy involves possessing the capability, fortitude, and repertoire of skills needed to enable integrity-preserving action. It presumes the requisite degree of moral and ethical competence to recognize the moral contours of a challenging situation, to discern and analyze the ethically permissible or justified options, and to be motivated and committed to skillfully carry out the action that, all things considered, best serves those involved. The foundation of moral/ethical competence must be adequately developed for moral efficacy to be realized.[27] It is closely tied to having a clear and articulate voice that arises from one's moral core rather than from reaction or projection. Being morally efficacious empowers clinicians to leverage their knowledge and skills in situations where advocacy or principled action is needed. The capacity to articulate one's beliefs, defend them, when necessary, provide sound reasons for one's choices and actions, and speak up even when the result is not what one hoped for is vital to moral efficacy. Championing one's values or commitments for oneself or on behalf of others, even when meeting with resistance or rejection, is a core element of personal integrity and is reflected in one's moral efficacy. Self-regulatory capacities support the ability to encounter moral ambiguity and remain principled and grounded in what matters most. It includes having confidence in one's capability to achieve one's moral purpose and the courage to respond in the face of moral adversity and persevere through challenges reflecting "moral potency."[28]

It must be acknowledged, however, that people's moral efficacy is not solely determined by their individual capacities. Individuals are socially and relationally situated, making them dependent upon and vulnerable to the moral ecosystem they reside in.[21] This is why, for example, moral efficacy is diminished when the norms of an institution effectively silence the voices of its members. It can also be diminished when one must make incommensurate choices between personal and professional values and commitments that produce weighty consequences and imperil personal integrity to uphold organizational mandates. There may also be circumstances where moral agency is justifiably constrained.[29] Clinicians during a pandemic, for example, may have experienced legitimate constraints on resources because of scarcity created by disproportionate numbers of people who need healthcare services. Though these circumstances are no fault of individual clinicians, their ability to determine responses was largely determined by local, state, or governmental policies.

Further elaboration of the interplay between individual, collective, and organizational dynamics is included in Chapter 10 and Chapter 11.

Self-Regulation

Broadly, self-regulation refers to the ability to mindfully recognize what is happening in the moment (body, heart, and mind) and to employ influence over one's intentions, motivations, affective or emotional states, thought processes, behavioral patterns, and actions. Adjustments arise through internal processes involved in self-monitoring that allow individuals to recognize and honor their experience, choose their responses, change, or overcome habitual patterns or unconstructive responses, and align with their values, commitments, responsibilities, and priorities.[30,31] It is the capacity to be spiritually, emotionally, somatically, and cognitively grounded amid a threat to integrity or ethical challenge. Essentially, it is the ability to achieve a state of balance that allows one to perceive things clearly and act in accordance with one's values, commitments, and responsibilities.

Self-regulation is a person's capacity for self-monitoring and subsequent internal efforts to accept, adjust, or release feelings, thoughts, or actions in response to self-sanctions, standards, or goals. Together with mindfulness, it can lead to the mental and emotional stability and the composure and equanimity that prove especially useful when difficult, ethically challenging circumstances arise. Like the ballast of a ship amid strong winds, self-regulatory capacities allow individuals to remain centered during whatever is happening by not denying their experience and by leveraging their inner stability and strength. Such capacities are cultivated with mindful, diligent practice and bolster the ability to act in alignment with one's deepest values and commitments, thereby supporting integrity. One must have the capacity to direct one's behavior and modulate one's impulses to adhere to relevant standards, achieve goals, or attain ideals. It is particularly important when seeking to align intentions, values, behaviors, and actions in the context of ethically challenging situations.

In a psychological context, self-regulation helps a person to modulate positive and negative affective states and to be emotionally agile.[32,33] This includes the processes used to modulate the incidence, intensity, and/or duration of emotional reactivity and to moderate emotions and behavior.[34,35] It includes the capacity to attune to signals of distress in response to an unmet need or threat, to abide with them without detrimental reactivity, and, when necessary, to release them. Emotional inhibition is related to emotion regulation and positively related to resilience.[28] Being able to create a pause between the distress impulse and the response, correctly label the need or feeling, discern the contours of the situation, and respond constructively is foundational to self-regulation. Emotions are important for discerning the morally relevant aspects of the situation; they are not ends in themselves but rather a means of directing attention and garnering motivation to act.[36] Focusing solely on the emotional content of morally challenging situations has the potential to amplify, magnify, or distort their meaning and importance. Accounting for the emotional dimension can help to shift the focus to the values that underlie and inform deliberations, decision-making, and moral action. Self-regulation of emotion and behavior of children has been shown to affect children's development of competence.[37] Applying this to the context of moral resilience, moral/ethical competence is related to both moral agency and moral efficacy.

When faced with adversity, skillful self-regulators are able to experience the full range of both positive and negative feelings, let go of what does not serve them, focus their attention on achieving their goal, persist with properly balanced engagement when challenges arise, and flexibly use a variety of skills while maintaining confidence that their efforts will result in desired outcomes.[38] In contrast, individuals who lack self-regulation skills may become overwhelmed with the overstimulation of their nervous system, lapse into victimhood, and focus on the actions of others while narrowing their perspective toward their own interests. Sympathy from others may intensify their struggles and keep them stuck in an unchanging cycle of powerlessness and despair. People who are self-regulated can work constructively with negative reactions and self-defeating patterns, form positive attributions about their situation, leverage their potential to intensify their properly bounded resolve and effort, and apply diverse strategies when confronted with subsequent challenges, fatigue, or frustration.[39,40]

Self-regulation enables people to be receptive to circumstances without forming rigid attachments to the experience that block any release from its grip to create space for insight and learning. As one clinician wrote self regulation is manifest when:, "In the midst of the seemingly impossible situation of being confronted with conflicting views, values, and information from others and experiencing a resolution different from how you see it or a deeply unsatisfactory outcome and being able to go into the next room and being fresh with space for something new and not getting damaged by what came up."[5] The ability to recognize that a situation is beyond one's control and then to adopt a new perspective or release expectations or emotions that no longer serve a useful purpose is a byproduct of skillful self-regulation and robust humility.[41] Some clinicians cited the wisdom of the Serenity Prayer as a symbol of this aspect of their moral resilience.

Self-Stewardship

Moral resilience requires clinicians to invest in their own well-being as an acknowledgment of their inherent dignity and worthiness as human beings and secondarily enables them to manifest their service to others. Many clinicians risk abandoning their own health and well-being when they deny signals indicative of their basic needs. In some professions such as nursing, self-stewardship is considered a moral imperative that is necessary to fulfill professional commitments.[42] It demands a stance of self-respect and positive regard to honor one's wholeness and that of others. Investing in their own well-being enables clinicians to honor their uniqueness and their commonality with others, without fear of becoming self-centered or self-indulgent. Self-stewardship includes the attitudes, behaviors, and actions that one takes to maintain or improve one's health and well-being. It can include an array of strategies aimed at nurturing the body, mind, and spirit. When we are balanced in all aspects of ourselves, body, mind, and spirit are in harmony. One clinician repeated Jack Kornfield's assertion: "We can feel this possibility of balance in our hearts in the midst of life when we recognize that life is not in our control. We are a small part of a great dance."[43(p331)]

Self-stewardship embodies a commitment to know oneself, to manage one's personal resources responsibly and mindfully, to recognize and compassionately respect one's limitations, and to choose actions that are wholesome and life-affirming. It includes being able to humbly accept the situation and the circumstances as they are and to shift the focus to what can be done rather than what is not possible or ineffective. This entails adopting "intentional strategies to foster [one's] sustainability when participating in situations that are counter to one's own moral compass" when confronted with morally complex or distressing situations.[5]

Clinicians must use their energy in a mindful, principled manner. Self-stewardship is grounded in respect and generosity toward oneself, not selfishness. It includes a "clear, proper and appropriate assessment of honoring [one]self."[5] As Parker Palmer states: "Self-care is never a selfish act—it is simply good stewardship of the only gift I have, the gift I was put on earth to offer others."[44(p30)] Investing in one's wholeness and well-being is not optional. This ethical mandate, reflected in the American Nurses Association Code of Ethics for Nurses,[36] provision 5 and the "quadruple aim," suggests that both individuals and the institutions where they practice are obliged to honor the inherent dignity of the people providing care.[45] This ethos is reflected in the Beryl Institute's pledge to create enabling healthcare environments that honor the humanity of everyone.[46] These powerful mandates for investing in self-stewardship are situated in a complex "paradoxical coexistence" of individuals within the settings where they practice and the broader healthcare ecosystem.[47] Depending on the meaning and interpretation assigned to these mandates is the potential to harness them as support for cultivating self-stewardship; or for weaponizing them as an evaluation of clinician deficiency and outsized responsibility for enacting them.

In situations that drain our vital energy, especially when we may be expending disproportionate effort to bring about a particular result, we look to evidence of our depletion in our thoughts, emotions, and bodies. As self-stewards, we must continuously calibrate clear, but not rigid, boundaries to help us resist being pushed past critical thresholds while we simultaneously expand the range of ways we can adapt if pushed beyond the critical point. With the sustained high levels of burnout among clinicians,[48,49,50,51,52,53,54,55] awareness of its symptoms is vital. As self-stewards, we must acknowledge the evidence that our ability to respond to burnout or moral adversity is associated with resilience[17] and that moral distress is a factor that contributes to burnout syndrome.[44,56,57] Associations between moral distress, moral injury, burnout, turnover intention, and moral resilience have demonstrated that moral resilience serves as a protective resource and moderator of the impact of potentially morally injurious circumstances[9,10,58] (see Chapter 9 for research).

When we allocate our gifts, talents, time, and energy to the highest and best use, we nourish our purpose and sense of fulfillment. Self-stewardship includes being able to derive meaning from our work despite the challenges we confront. Moral resilience enables us to make sense out of adversity and find a place of coherence by crafting a narrative about the situation we can live with and creating a more balanced post hoc account of our experiences.[59] The ability to reinterpret morally distressing experiences is an essential element of moral repair, as moral distress and its residue have the potential to reshape the architecture of one's integrity. Chapter 7 and Chapter 8 offer strategies for cultivating these skills and practices.

Qualities and Skills to Support Moral Resilience

These attributes of moral resilience are supported by a variety of related qualities and skills. The responses of interprofessional clinicians expanded the contours of moral resilience to include qualities of courage, empathy, humility, and compassion as instrumental in responding to moral adversity.[5] Several participants acknowledged the importance of "standing up for what you believe in without fear" and engaging in action despite resistance; this quality of courage is understood as a vital driver of integrity.[5] One participant described moral resilience as the ability to "put yourself in their shoes and offer only kindness and compassion." This response brings together empathy (the ability to attune to the affective experience of others and to take their perspective) and compassion (the ability to engage in and take action in response to another's suffering).[60,61,62] Both qualities are present in the definitions offered by a number of those surveyed, consistent with the view of empathy as a critical precursor of compassion.[63] Another quality that emerged in the analysis was humility, the stance of not knowing all the answers, being open to discovering what will work best in the particular situation, and accepting things as they are, without judgment. According to one participant, this quality involves "having the willingness and courage to accept when a decision was, in hindsight, the wrong one and to be willing to adjust course without a need to blame or self-criticize." It involves having realistic expectations of one's own performance, including the ability to take responsibility and to take action "to begin again."

These qualities of courage, empathy, compassion, and humility are augmented by the resilience skills of being mindful—that is "pausing," "stepping back," "taking a breath," and taking time to recheck one's thoughts, ideas, and feelings. Mindfulness skills also require being grounded in one's values, intentions, and current reality, or in the words of one participant, "being stable and non-reactive in the midst of changing or uncertain circumstances."[5(p5)]

Other skills that participants use to foster moral resilience included developing self-awareness, including the capacity for introspection and inquiry; practicing listening skills; and using various reflective practices. While these may not be an exhaustive list of qualities and skills, they are key dimensions that provide fertile ground for moral resilience to arise. Many of these skills can be learned, strengthened, and refined to proactively build one's "moral resilience muscle." They may also serve as protective factors that enable clinicians to act with integrity and to be buoyant in response to moral adversity. Moral distress and its residue become only two of many possible responses to sources of moral adversity; clinicians may also leverage their moral agency and moral imagination to foster positive relationships, manage conflict, and empower effective communication within a moral community.[64] Further exploration of these qualities and skills is warranted.

Insights from Neuroscience

Attributes such as buoyancy, self-regulation, self-awareness, and the qualities and skills that support moral resilience described above provide an opportunity to explore how contemporary neuroscience may provide an additional dimension. In understanding the mechanisms of moral suffering and self-regulatory capacities and their relevance to moral resilience, it can be helpful to consider the results of relevant experiments from the rapidly developing new field of social neuroscience. Understanding the brain processes involved in complex social phenomena can provide us with insights into new ways of conceptualizing and responding to difficulties that arise in social situations, including moral suffering and moral distress, and how we might leverage them to amplify moral resilience.

Although there is an absence of neuroscientific research specifically focused on moral suffering or moral distress, there are several studies on the related construct of empathic distress. For clinicians, empathic distress (feeling distress when seeing another's suffering) and empathic over-arousal (unpleasantly high physical arousal when witnessing another's suffering) are common. Both can lead one to act in ways focused on reducing one's own over-arousal,[65] including ways that ignore the patient's needs and thus potentially interfere with morally congruent decision-making. Moral distress, as already noted, can similarly be accompanied by high emotional arousal, potentially decreasing the ability to make good decisions. Research has demonstrated that states of high emotional arousal, including anxiety, fear, and anger, bias attention[66] and prevent clinicians from apprehending the various dimensions of a situation that are important for making sound decisions. The emotional arousal of moral distress has also been associated with long-term psychological consequences and burnout. For these reasons, it is helpful to examine the psychological and neural processes by which empathic distress, and by extension moral distress, may occur.

Experiments have shown that humans attune to and spontaneously mimic the emotional arousal, distress, and expression of others, beginning as young as six months of age[67] and continuing into adulthood.[68] Spontaneous mimicry and emotional contagion appear to involve brain systems referred to as "mirror neurons."[69] When one observes another in pain or distress, brain systems responsible for the emotional distress that accompanies one's own pain experience and expression are activated.[70] These mirror neuron processes are considered by a number of neuroscientists to be a core component of empathy.[71]

Empathy can lead to compassion or "empathic concern," where empathy is accompanied by the intent to decrease another's suffering,[72] often leading to helpful behavior.[73] However, empathy can also sometimes lead to empathic distress, especially when the physiologic arousal of empathy is very high. This empathic over-arousal often results in failure to attend to or come to the aid of a distressed person; instead, one focuses on strategies to reduce one's own distress.[74]

However, if the emotional arousal of empathy is modulated by executive brain systems that direct attention, inhibit impulsive action, and plan alternative responses, then empathic concern is more likely than empathic distress.[75] Burnout in helping professionals may reflect "empathy fatigue" (from repeated empathic distress) rather than "compassion fatigue." Some have argued that empathic concern/compassion, wherein there is emotional balance and the intention to help another who is suffering, tends to be associated with positive emotional experience and does not fatigue the person.[76,77,78]

Experiments have shown that empathic distress is more likely than empathic concern/compassion when a person is taking a self-focused perspective rather than the perspective of the person who is distressed.[54] This often reflects difficulty in disengaging from a self-focused perspective and shifting perspective to that of the other person.[79] Overall, self-centered psychological functioning has been found to be related to greater degrees of unhappiness.[80] Thus, the ability to shift perspective is an important skill that leads to empathic concern/compassion rather than empathic distress.[81,82]

People who experience empathic over-arousal and distress are likely to engage in various ways of reducing their distress. In addition to shifting attention away from the suffering of another person, they may try to suppress their emotions. Emotional suppression is considered a "consequent-focused" emotion-regulation strategy (i.e., employed after the emotion has been aroused). It is often ineffective in reducing unpleasant emotional arousal and may increase measured physiologic arousal. In contrast, "antecedent-focused" emotion regulation strategies (i.e., focused on events and their interpretations that initiate emotional responses) are often more effective in reducing emotional arousal, including empathic over-arousal. The antecedent-focused strategy of reappraisal (seeing a different meaning of the event) can be particularly effective.[83]

In a clinically relevant example of neuroscientific research on emotion regulation in empathic emotional arousal,[84] persons without specific training who viewed a patient undergoing a potentially painful clinical procedure (acupuncture) were likely to themselves experience emotional distress and showed activation (by functional magnetic resonance imaging) in those brain systems related to the emotional aspects of one's own pain experience. However, clinicians trained in acupuncture were able to shift perspective, appraising the situation differently (as a treatment to reduce suffering), and showed activation of those brain systems associated with perspective-shifting and the modulation of emotional arousal. Reappraising the situation and incorporating awareness of other perspectives are also arguably relevant in situations of moral distress and other forms of moral suffering.[1,85]

Taken together, social neuroscience experiments on empathic distress (should similar results be found in future studies of moral suffering, including moral distress) suggest several ways in which moral suffering might be reduced and moral resilience enhanced. These include approaches to facilitate flexibility in perspective-taking, to decrease self-focus, and to develop skills in antecedent-focused emotion regulation strategies such as reappraisal. Augmenting existing neuroscientific evidence with further empirical investigation into the context of moral resilience offers a promising direction for designing and testing interventions.

A Way Forward

Central to our definition of moral resilience is a robust understanding of integrity that encompasses personal, professional, and relational integrity. In our definition, moral resilience is not defined by external circumstances but rather invites individuals to return to the fundamental state of wholeness as the basis for determining their responses, choices, and actions.

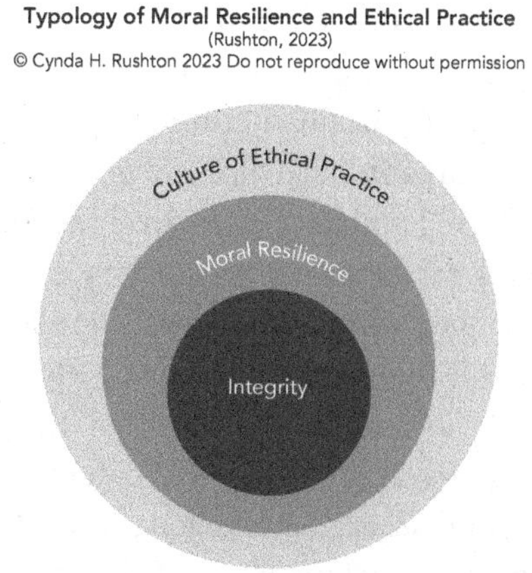

FIGURE 6.1. Typology of Moral Resilience and Ethical Practice

Moral resilience thrives in a practice environment where the modifiable factors that cause moral adversity and moral suffering are systematically addressed. Figure 6.1 reflects our typology of moral resilience and ethical practice. With integrity as the core, moral resilience enables personal and relational integrity in response to moral adversity within a culture of ethical practice.

Amid moral suffering and ethical challenges, the current paradigm tends to overlook the potential for growth, meaning, and integrity-preserving moral agency. Largely absent from narratives of moral distress are examples of integrity-preserving action that allowed individuals to navigate ethically troubling situations without accumulating moral residue or experiencing burnout or despair. Notably, the most used measure of moral distress does not include questions regarding how people who do not report detrimental levels of moral distress (when exposed to the same situations that cause higher levels in others) avoid the same degree of distress or suffering.[86] This has led some authors to question what the scale is measuring.[87,88] Other areas of inquiry (e.g., the post-traumatic growth literature observing psychological growth in response to traumatic or stressful events)[89,90] may be applicable to experiences of moral suffering. While not all clinicians can transform their suffering, taking proactive steps to create conditions that strengthen their inherent resilient potential offers hope for those confronted by ethical complexity and suffering.

We believe it is possible to grow and learn in the wake of morally distressing or injurious experiences—to find meaning, to reconnect to one's commitments and aspirations, and to release the destructive residue fueled by frustration, anger, despair, and shame.[91(p351)] Doing so unleashes the constructive energy and engagement to mitigate the destructive consequences of repeated and sustained attunement to the negative aspects of moral distress. Such an approach also provides an opportunity to turn toward our moral suffering and to constructively and intentionally engage in a process of moral repair that incorporates elements of the entire experience into a stronger whole.[92] However, transforming these possibilities into realities will require us to reorient the ways we understand and work with moral adversity and suffering.[1] In clinical practice, we must more fully recognize and harness the potential of moral resilience while acknowledging and accepting that some aspects of our practice are unlikely to be modified, regardless of our efforts. As clinicians, our work includes confronting disease, injury, suffering, and death in its most raw and intimate expressions. We must work with human vulnerability, injustices, tragedies, and the complexities that accompany the people we serve.[1] Moral resilience is a necessary protective resource that helps clinicians confront these realities in ways that preserve their own integrity and do not disproportionately undermine their own well-being. Rather than denying their moral suffering, it makes the consequences visible and therefore amenable to constructive, integrity preserving repair. Cultivating the wisdom to discern what can and cannot be changed is a vital element of moral resilience.

Clinicians may view moral suffering as an inevitable reality in healthcare today that they are powerless to change or a condition that should be extinguished altogether since suffering serves no purpose. This view animates despair and a victim narrative that is devoid of moral agency or power to change one's responses or the circumstances. It breeds cynicism to believe that nothing can change or there is nothing an individual can do, further incapacitating and disempowering them. Such attitudes and beliefs have been exacerbated during the COVID-19 pandemic and have intensified cynicism and despair. Repeating these disempowering narratives only solidifies the despair rather than transforming it and intensifies suffering rather than relieving it. Such characterizations overlook the power of individuals to choose in accordance with their values and denies their inherent capacities for integrity and resilience that are not defined by external circumstances but can be influenced or degraded by them. Moral resilience is fundamentally about restoring agency and empowering individuals to choose integrity-preserving responses rather than become victims of the realities they find themselves in.

Being morally resilient does not imply a spineless acquiescence to the very real and complex challenges that are present in healthcare. Nor does it imply putting a positive spin on unethical behaviors or practices.[93] It does not suggest a state of oblivion or complacency that allows avoidance of enacting immoral acts.[94,95] Moral resilience does not place a disproportionate burden on individuals to address the moral adversity and thereby "blame" the victim.[90,91,96,97] Rather, moral resilience reflects a realistic appraisal of the situation, acknowledges its contours and constraints, and provides a foundation for principled action, including constructive moral outrage.[98] Our recognition and response to moral adversity is an important signal of moral conscientious rather than moral weakness.[1,99] Without moral resilience, we risk making ungrounded, disrespectful, and potentially harmful responses that ultimately undermine our personal and relational integrity.[100] When we remain entrenched in our negativity, we put at risk the effectiveness of our efforts and our own health. Moral resilience orients us toward our basic goodness and that of others. To do otherwise denies the essential nature of human beings and their power to adapt, grow, and learn amid moral adversity. Under the right circumstances, morally resilient people can make sense out of their adversity, create a more balanced post hoc account of their experiences, and find meaning despite the challenges. This ability to reinterpret experiences, release the negative, and re-construct our experience into a new whole is a vital part of moral repair.

Crucially, from our perspective, moral suffering itself is not the enemy. If properly worked with, it can heighten awareness that an occasion calls for careful moral consideration, prompt fruitful reflection and insight, and lead to effective and compassionate moral action. The ability to cultivate mental and emotional stability and foster resilience is crucial to sustaining conscientious integrity in the face of moral adversity in clinical practice that too often leads to reactivity and outrage, numbness, or withdrawal (see Chapter 3). It is essential to find ways of supporting clinicians' suffering in response to moral adversity to help them regain their sense of moral efficacy and voice and sustain the resilience they need to navigate the turbulent waters of clinical work.[101] Absent this, moral suffering will remain a recalcitrant pattern that continues to undermine compassion, erode clinician wellbeing, and imperil clinicians' ability to sustain a sense of moral efficacy and integrity in their work.

By confronting adversity from a place of wisdom rather than reaction, we have the potential to shift from powerlessness and despair to empowered moral agency and moral efficacy. Leaders who foster cultures that are intentionally designed to enable the integrity of all stakeholders—including patients, families, clinicians, staff, and the leaders themselves—must also invest in and support efforts to foster the resilient potential of everyone. Individual moral resilience is unlikely to flourish unless the organization meets its ethical responsibility to create environments that support a culture of ethical practice.[102] Throughout this book, we call attention to the influence of the systems in which clinicians practice on their integrity and the potential resource moral resilience offers. Pivoting toward the possibility of a more life-affirming possibility does not overlook or minimize the adversity that is present in healthcare. Doing so does not imply that the goal is to fortify people to tolerate unacceptable conditions. Considering the neurobiological, psychological, and social ecological elements of resilience as discrete yet interactive and intertwined forces can be useful in understanding what it means to be morally resilient individually and collectively.

We must confront the reality that clinicians work in imperfect systems that include both modifiable and non-modifiable elements.[103] Systems of communication, modes of decision-making, resource allocation, and budgets, for example, are largely modifiable with leadership, discipline, and systematic solutions. Conceivably, morally resilient clinicians will be better able to engage in efforts to devise solutions when they are less burdened by their distress about things they cannot change and are able to engage their creativity, sustain their energy, and adopt collaborative solutions. But other elements of the work environment are not easily or immediately modifiable. Electronic medical records, malpractice laws, prescription drug regulations, and reimbursement methods, for instance, have a significant impact on day-to-day clinical practice but are not immediately or easily modified.[104] While the impact of these systemic factors must be addressed, moral resilience can be a resource for addressing these realities in ways that reduce the negative impact on clinicians as larger-scale reforms are undertaken.

Clearly, we should not be complacent in addressing those aspects of our practice that need modification. On the contrary, moral resilience involves being able to discern which aspects of our clinical practice are amenable to change and which reflect an immutable reality. Reorienting our approach requires practical recognition of the embedded nature of individual moral agency, its limitations, and the beneficial potential it represents.[1] We must seek to empower individual moral efficacy and support individual integrity through creative innovation within clinical organizations and systems of practice.[3] Some have asserted that focusing on individual moral resilience will undermine systems change,[79] but we believe that framing the options as either focusing on individuals or the system creates an unnecessary and binary choice. Well-intentioned efforts to separate individual agency from the cultures in which clinicians practice creates an unbalanced polarity.[105] Individuals are members of systems by choice or circumstance and are embedded in systems that support or degrade their integrity. While it is unquestionable that keeping the pressure on the system to change is vital, it is not the only way to make progress. Exclusively focusing on the system can inadvertently leave those in the system feeling abandoned waiting for large-scale changes to be implemented. Instead, we advocate an inclusive "both/and" approach that leverages both individual capacities of moral resilience and intentional systemic design that creates and sustains cultures that support ethical practice (see Chapters 10 and 11). Whether one engages in integrity-preserving actions or what Morley and colleagues have termed "critical resilience" to address systemic issues of austerity,[106] change requires that the people who engage in these efforts have the requisite skills, capabilities, and structures that enable effective action and "wise hope" rather than despair.[16] The foundation for both types of resilience begin with a robust notion of integrity and must include concurrent investments to create a culture that enables ethical practice. Focusing on moral resilience in no way suggests that we should abandon the excellent scholarship on moral distress to date; rather, we propose building upon it to shift the orientation toward solutions and possibility rather than despair and depletion.[90] Aligning the polarities of the individual and the system is needed to avoid over-emphasis on either component or to avoid strengthening unintended consequences.[102]

Terms like resilience and moral resilience have the potential to be applied in ways that are incongruent with their meaning. How they are interpreted depends on the intention and tone of their communication—either as a demand that conveys a sense of deficiency or as an invitation to harness the basic goodness and inherent resilient potential everyone possesses. As is true in some institutions, the moral distress narrative can be misapplied in some contexts—used as a threat to others' authority or decision-making; so too can terms like moral resilience be corrupted.[107] These insidious patterns can cause leaders to view addressing moral adversity and moral suffering solely as an individual responsibility that requires more education or training to withstand the workplace pressures, ignoring the broader systemic factors that contribute to moral suffering and erode well-being. In both cases, it is vital to understand the danger of creating and repeating a narrative that animates fear and resentment rather than engagement. When we continually activate the threat system in our nervous system we undermine our flexibility, creativity, and collaboration. By aligning individual and system interventions we amplify the impact by taking a social ecological approach.[108] Changes in one area impact the whole; designing interventions that account for these interrelationships has the greatest potential for lasting and meaningful change.

Currently no established evidence-base for specific strategies for cultivating moral resilience exists. However, borrowing from the literature on resilience in various contexts offers several promising possibilities that can be applied to moral resilience. We take up the capacities for moral resilience in Chapters 7 and 8 and the design of system-level interventions in Chapters 10 and 11.

Acknowledgment

Gratitude to Dr. Alford W. Kaszniak for his substantial contribution to the neuroscience section of this chapter. Portions of the chapter were excerpted in a subsequent article summarizing our work.[92] The concepts of relational integrity[109] and self stewardship[110] are further elaborated in later articles.

References

1. Carse A, Rushton CH. Harnessing the promise of moral distress: a call for reorientation. J Clin Ethics. 2017;28:15–29.
2. Lachman VD. Ethics, law, and policy. Moral resilience: managing and preventing moral distress and moral residue. MedSurg Nurs. 2016;25:121–124.
3. Thomas TA, McCullough LB. A philosophical taxonomy of ethically significant moral distress. J Med Philos. 2015;40:102–120.
4. Young PD, Rushton CH. A concept analysis of moral resilience. Nurs Outlook. 2017;65:579–587.
5. Holtz H, Heinze K, Rushton C. Inter-professionals' definitions of moral resilience. J Clin Nurs. 2017;27(3–4):e488–e494.
6. Rushton CH. Moral resilience: a capacity for navigating moral distress in critical care. AACN Adv Crit Care. 2016;27:111–119.
7. Garros D, Austin W, Carnevale FA. Moral distress in pediatric intensive care. JAMA Pediatr. 2015;169:885–886.

8. Henrich NJ, Dodek PM, Gladstone E, et al. Consequences of moral distress in the intensive care unit: a qualitative study. Am J Crit Care. 2017;26:e48–e57.
9. Rushton CH, Thomas TA, Antonsdottir IM, et al. Moral injury and moral resilience in health care workers during COVID-19 pandemic. J Palliat Med. 2022;25(5):712–719.
10. Prentice TM, Gillam L, Davis PG, Janvier A. The use and misuse of moral distress in neonatology. Semin Fetal Neonatal Med. 2018;23(1):39–43.
11. Spilg E, Rushton CH, Phillips J, et al. The new frontline: exploring the links between moral distress, moral resilience, and mental health in healthcare workers during the COVID-19 pandemic. BMC Psychiat. 2022;22(19):1–12.
12. Jameton A. Nursing practice: the ethical issues. Englewood Cliffs, NJ: Prentice-Hall; 1984.
13. Johnstone M, Hutchinson A. "Moral distress"—time to abandon a flawed nursing construct? Nurs Ethics. 2015;22:5–14.
14. Austin W. The ethics of everyday practice: healthcare environments as moral communities. Adv Nurs Sci. 2007;30:81–88.
15. Dweck CS. Mindset. New York: Random House; 2006.
16. Yeager DS, Dweck CS. Mindsets that promote resilience: when students believe that personal characteristics can be developed. Educ Psychol. 2012;47:302–314.
17. Halifax RJ. Wise hope in the time of the pandemic. Upaya Zen Center. Published April 14, 2020. Accessed February 12, 2023. https://www.upaya.org/2020/04/wise-hope-in-the-time-of-the-pandemic-by-roshi-joan-halifax/.
18. Bonanno GA. Meaning making, adversity, and regulatory flexibility. Memory. 2013;21:150–156.
19. Gillespie BM, Chaboyer W, Wallis M. Development of a theoretically derived model of resilience through concept analysis. Contemp Nurse. 2007;25:124–135.
20. Gillespie BM, Chaboyer W, Wallis M, Grimbeek P. Resilience in the operating room: developing and testing of a resilience model. J Adv Nurs. 2007;59:427–438.
21. Rushton CH, Batcheller J, Schroeder K, Donohue P. Burnout and resilience among nurses practicing in high-intensity settings. Am J Crit Care. 2015;24:412–420.
22. Rathert C, May DR, Chung HS. Nurse moral distress: a survey identifying predictors and potential interventions. Int J Nurs Stud. 2016;53:39–40.
23. Hannah ST, Avolio BJ, Walumbwa FO. Relationships between authentic leadership, moral courage, and ethical and pro-social behaviors. Bus Ethics Q. 2011;21:555–578.
24. Peter E, Liaschenko J. Perils of proximity: a spatiotemporal analysis of moral distress and moral ambiguity. Nurs Inq. 2004;4:218–225.
25. Rodney P, Kadychuk S, Liaschenko J, et al. Moral agency: relational connections and support. In Storch JL, Rodney P, Starzomski R, editors, Toward a moral horizon: nursing ethics for leadership and practice. Toronto, ON: Pearson; 2013:160–187.

26. Morley G, Sankary LR. Re-examining the relationship between moral distress and moral agency in nursing. Nurs Philosophy. 2024;25(1):e12419.
27. Cannaerts N, Gastmans C, Dierckx de Casterlé B. Contribution of ethics education to the ethical competence of nursing students: educators' and students' perceptions. Nurs Ethics. 2014;21:861–878.
28. Hannah ST, Avolio BJ. Moral potency: building the capacity for character-based leadership. Consult Psychol J Pract Res. 2010;62:291–310.
29. Morley G, Sankary LR. Moral distress and justifiable constraints on moral agency. AJOB. 2023;23(4):77–79.
30. Baumeister RF, Heatherton TF. Self-regulation failure: an overview. Psychol Inq. 1996;7:1–15.
31. Carver CS, Scheier MF. On the self-regulation of behavior. Cambridge: Cambridge University Press; 1998.
32. Cortes L, Buchanan MJ. The experience of Columbian child soldiers from a resilience perspective. Int J Adv Counsel. 2007;29:43–55.
33. Davidson RJ. Affective style, psychopathology, and resilience: brain mechanisms and plasticity. Am Psychol. 2000;55:1196–1212.
34. Eisenberg N, Spinrad TL, Morris AS. Regulation, resiliency, and quality of social functioning. Self Identity. 2002;1:121–128.
35. Rothbart MK, Derryberry D. Development of individual differences in temperament. In Lamb ME, Brown AL, editors. Advances in developmental psychology. Hillsdale, NJ: Erlbaum; 1981:37–86.
36. Beauchamp TL, Childress JF. Principles of biomedical ethics. New York: Oxford University Press; 2013.
37. Masten AS, Coatsworth JD. The development of competence in favorable and unfavorable environments: lessons from research on successful children. Am Psychol. 1998;53:205–220.
38. Schunk DH. Self-regulated learning: the educational legacy of Paul R. Pintrich. Educ Psychol. 2005;40:85–94.
39. Weiner B. An attributional theory of achievement motivation and emotion. Psychol Rev. 1985;92:548–573.
40. Zimmerman BJ. Becoming a self-regulated learner: an overview. Theory Pract. 2002;41:64–70.
41. Walsh A. Pulling the heartstrings, arguing the case: a narrative response to the issue of moral agency in moral distress. J Med Ethics. 2010;36:746–749.
42. American Nurses Association. Code of ethics for nurses with interpretive statements. Silver Spring, MD: ANA; 2015.
43. Kornfield J. A path with heart. New York: Bantam Books; 1993.
44. Palmer PJ. Let your life speak: listening for the voice of vocation. San Francisco, CA: Jossey-Bass; 2000.
45. Bodenheimer T, Sinsky C. From triple to quadruple aim: care of the patient requires care of the provider. Ann Fam Med. 2014;12:573–576.

46. The Beryl Institute. About us. Updated 2023. Accessed February 12, 2023. https://theberylinstitute.org/about-us/.
47. Christofield M, Moon P, Allotey P. Navigating paradox in self-care. BMJ Global Health. 2021;6:e005994.
48. Busis NA, Shanafelt TD, Keran CM, et al. Burnout, career satisfaction, and well-being among US neurologists in 2016. Neurology. 2017;88:797–808.
49. Gómez-Urquiza JL, Aneas-López AB, Fuente-Solana EI, et al. Prevalence, risk factors, and levels of burnout among oncology nurses: a systematic review. Oncol Nurs Forum. 2016;43:E104–E120.
50. Gómez-Urquiza JL, De la Fuente-Solana EI, Albendín-García L, et al. Prevalence of burnout syndrome in emergency nurses: a meta-analysis. Crit Care Nurse. 2017;37:e1–e9.
51. Lebares CC, Guvva EV, Ascher NL, et al. Burnout and stress among US surgery residents: psychological distress and resilience. J Am Coll Physicians. 2018;226:80–90.
52. Moss M, Good VS, Gozal D, et al. An official Critical Care Societies collaborative statement: burnout syndrome in critical care health care professionals: a call for action. Am J Crit Care. 2016;25:368–376.
53. Shenoi AN, Kalyanaraman M, Pillai A, et al. Burnout and psychological distress among pediatric critical care physicians in the United States. Crit Care Med. 2018;46:116–122.
54. Kim Y, Lee E, Lee H. Association between workplace bullying and burnout, professional quality of life, and turnover intention among clinical nurses. PLOS ONE. 2020;15(1):e0228124.
55. Dordunoo D, An M, Chu MS, et al. The impact of practice environment and resilience on burnout among clinical nurses in a tertiary hospital setting. Int J Environ Res Public Health. 2021;18(5):2500.
56. Fumis RR, Amarante GA, de Fátima Nascimento A, Junior JV. Moral distress and its contribution to the development of burnout syndrome among critical care providers. Ann Intensive Care. 2016;7:71.
57. Johnson-Coyle L, Opgenorth D, Bellows M, et al. Moral distress and burnout among cardiovascular surgery intensive care unit healthcare professionals: a prospective cross-sectional survey. Can J Crit Care Nurs. 2016;27:27–36.
58. Antonsdottir I, Rushton CH, Nelson KE, et al. Burnout and moral resilience in interprofessional healthcare professionals. J Clin Nurs. 2021;31(1–2):196–208.
59. Lützén K, Ewalds-Kvist B. Moral distress and its interconnection with moral sensitivity and moral resilience: viewed from the philosophy of Viktor E. Frankl. J Bioeth Inq. 2013;10:317–324.
60. Halifax J. A heuristic model of enactive compassion. Curr Opin Support Palliat Care. 2012;6:228–235.
61. Hein G, Singer T. I feel how you feel but not always: the empathic brain and its modulation. Curr Opin Neurobiol. 2008;18:153–158.

62. Singer T, Claus L. The social neuroscience of empathy. Ann NY Acad Sci. 2009;1156:81–96.
63. Singer T, Klimecki OM. Empathy and compassion. Curr Biol. 2014;24:R875–878.
64. Traudt T, Liaschenko J, Peden-McAlpine C. Moral agency, moral imagination, and moral community: antidotes to moral distress. J Clin Ethics. 2016;27:201–213.
65. Batson CD, Early S, Salvarani G. Perspective taking: imagining how another feels versus imagining how you would feel. Pers Soc Psychol Bull. 1997;23: 751–758.
66. Yiend J. The effects of emotion on attention: a review of attentional processing of emotional information. Cogn Emot. 2009;24:43–47.
67. Fawcett C, Wesevich V, Gredeback G. Pupillary contagion in infancy: evidence for spontaneous transfer of arousal. Psychol Sci. 2016;27:997–1003.
68. Dimberg U, Thunberg M, Elmehed K. Unconscious facial reactions to emotional facial expressions. Psychol Sci. 2000;11:86–89.
69. Rizzolatti G, Sinigaglia C. Mirrors in the brain: how our minds share actions and emotions. Oxford: Oxford University Press; 2008.
70. Lamm C, Batson CD, Decety J. The neural substrate of human empathy: effects of perspective-taking and cognitive appraisal. J Cogn Neurosci. 2007;19:42–58.
71. Decety J. A social cognitive neuroscience model of human empathy. In Harmon-Jones E, Winkielman P, editors. Social neuroscience: integrating biological and psychological explanations of social behavior. New York: Guilford; 2007:246–270.
72. De Waal FB. Putting the altruism back in altruism: the evolution of empathy. Ann Rev Psychol. 2008;59:279–300.
73. Winczewski LA, Bowen JD, Collins NL. Is empathic accuracy enough to facilitate responsive behavior in dyadic interaction? Distinguishing ability from motivation. Psychol Sci. 2016;27:394–404.
74. Eisenberg N. Empathy-related emotional responses, altruism, and their socialization. In Davidson RJ, Harrington A, Visions of compassion. Oxford: Oxford University Press; 2002:131–164.
75. Eisenberg N, Eggum ND. Empathic responding: sympathy and personal distress. In Decety J, Ickes W, editors. The social psychology of empathy. Cambridge, MA: MIT Press; 2009:71–83.
76. Ricard M. Altruism. New York: Little, Brown, 2015.
77. Preckel K, Kanske P, Singer T. (2018). On the interaction of social affect and cognition: Empathy, compassion and theory of mind. Curr Opin Behav Sci. 2018;19:1–6.
78. Hofmeyer A, Kennedy K, Taylor R. Contesting the term "compassion fatigue": Integrating findings from social neuroscience and self-care research. Collegian. 2020;27(2):232–237.
79. Royzman EB, Cassidy KW, Baron J. I know you know: epistemic egocentrism in children and adults. Rev Gen Psychol. 2003;7:38–65.

80. Dambrun M, Ricard M. Self-centeredness and selflessness: a theory of self-based psychological functioning and its consequences for happiness. Rev Gen Psychol. 2011;15:138–157.
81. Batson CD. The empathy-altruism hypothesis: issues and implications. In Decety J, editor. Empathy: from bench to bedside. Cambridge, MA: MIT Press; 2013:41–54.
82. Zaki J, Ochsner K. The cognitive neuroscience of sharing and understanding others' emotions. In Decety J, Empathy: from bench to bedside. Cambridge, MA: MIT Press; 2013:207–226.
83. Gross JJ, Thompson RA. Emotion regulation: conceptual foundations. In Gross JJ, editor, Handbook of emotion regulation. New York: Guilford Press; 2007:3–24.
84. Cheng Y, Lin CP, Liu HL, et al. Expertise modulates the perception of pain in others. Curr Biol. 2007;17:1708–1717.
85. Rushton CH, Kaszniak AW, Halifax JS. A framework for understanding moral distress among palliative care clinicians. J Palliat Med. 2013;16:1074–1079.
86. Hamric AB, Borchers CT, Epstein EG. Development and testing of an instrument to measure moral distress in healthcare professionals. AJOB Prim Res. 2012;3:1–9.
87. Kolbe L, de Melo-Martin I. Moral distress: what are we measuring? Am J Bioeth. 2023;23(4):46–58.
88. Morley G, Bena JF, Morrison SL, Albert NM. Sub-categories of moral distress among nurses: a descriptive longitudinal study. Nurs Ethics. 2023; 30(6):885-903.
89. Tedeschi RG, Calhoun LG. A clinical approach to posttraumatic growth. In Linley PA, Joseph S, editors. Positive psychology in practice. Hoboken, NJ: John Wiley; 2004:405–419.
90. Cunningham T, Pfeiffer K. Posttraumatic growth as a model to measure and guide implementation of COVID-19 recovery and resiliency. Nurs Add Q. 2022;46(1):81–87.
91. Pike AW. Moral outrage and moral discourse in nurse-physician collaboration. J Prof Nurs. 1991;7:351–362.
92. Rushton, C. Transforming moral suffering by cultivating moral resilience and ethical practice. American Journal of Critical Care. 2023;32(4):238–248.
93. Epstein EG, Hurst AR. Looking at the positive side of moral distress: why it's a problem. J Clin Ethics. 2017;28:37–41.
94. Sala Defilippis TML, Curtis K, Gallagher A. Conceptualising moral resilience for nursing practice. Nurs Inq. 2019;26(3):e12291.
95. Wocial LD. Resilience as an incomplete strategy for coping with moral distress in critical care nurses. Crit Care Nurse. 2020;40(6), 62–66.
96. Traynor, M. Critical resilience for nurses: An evidence-based guide to survival and change in the modern NHS. Oxford: Routledge; 2017.

97. Traynor M. Guest editorial: What's wrong with resilience? J Res Nurs. 2018;23: 5–8.
98. Rushton CH. Principled moral outrage: an antidote to moral distress? AACN Adv Crit Care. 2013;24:82–89.
99. Thomas TA, McCullough LB. A philosophical taxonomy of ethically significant moral distress. J Med Philos. 2015;40:102–120.
100. Rushton C, Thompson L. Moral outrage: promise or peril. Nurs Outlook. 2020;68(5):P536–538.
101. Browning A. Moral distress and psychological empowerment in critical care nurses caring for adults at end of life, Am J Crit Care. 2013;22(2):143–152.
102. Musto LC, Rodney PA. Moving from conceptual ambiguity to knowledgeable action: using a critical realist approach to studying moral distress. Nurs Philosophy. 2016;17:75–87.
103. National Academies of Medicine. Keynote address Q&A: psychological distress in critical care health care professionals (Marc Moss). July 17, 2017. https://www.youtube.com/watch?v=YRARouBzi74.
104. Berwick DM. *Salve lucrum*: The existential threat of greed in US health care. JAMA. 2023;329(8):629–630.
105. Johnson, B. Polarity management: identifying and managing unsolvable problems. Amherst, MA: HRD Press; 1996.
106. Morley G, Ives J, Bradbury-Jones C. Moral distress and austerity: an avoidable ethical challenge in healthcare. Health Care Anal. 2019;27(3):185–201.
107. Prentice TM, Gillam L, Davis PG, Janvier A. The use and misuse of moral distress in neonatology. Semin Fetal Neonatal Med. 2018;23(1):39–43.
108. Davidson PM, Rushton CH, Kurtz M, et al. A social-ecological framework: a model for addressing ethical practice in nursing. J Clin Nurs. 2018;27(56): e1233–e1241.
109. Rushton, C.H. Manbauman, C. Web of mutuality: relational integrity in critical care nursing. AACN Adv Crit Care.2023; 34(4), 381–390.
110. Rushton, C. Self stewardship: an ethical imperative for nurses. AACN Adv Crit Care; 35(2), 280–291.

7

Cultivating Essential Capacities for Moral Resilience

Cynda Hylton Rushton, Alfred W. Kaszniak, and Roshi Joan S. Halifax

EVERYONE POSSESSES THE seeds of moral resilience, but like other human capacities, there is wide variability in how that resilience evolves over a lifetime.* Because each person's experience of suffering is unique, their suffering is not amenable to strict characterization or interpretation of its meaning, purpose, or consequences. It requires that we embrace each other's reality and commit to bearing witness, while resisting our inclinations to fix or change the other or prescribe how to understand it.[1,2] Our connection to another's suffering can ignite a connection with our own suffering and help shape our responses to and relationships with ourselves and others.

Our approach to moral resilience holds that it is possible to cultivate the innate resilient potential we all possess by developing the capacities that help us recognize moral adversity and suffering in daily life and particularly in clinical settings. If diligently developed, these capacities will support us as we work to design and practice strategies that protect the

* Portions of this chapter are from: C. H. Rushton, A. Kaszniak, and J. Halifax (2013). "Addressing moral distress: Application of a framework to palliative care practice," *Journal of Palliative Medicine*, 16(9), pp. 1080–88. Adapted with permission.

Cynda Hylton Rushton, Alfred W. Kaszniak, and Roshi Joan S. Halifax, *Cultivating Essential Capacities for Moral Resilience* In: *Moral Resilience*. Second Edition. Edited by: Cynda Hylton Rushton, Oxford University Press.
 DOI: 10.1093/oso/9780197667149.003.0008

integrity at the heart of clinical practice. This is the topic of this chapter and the one that follows. For us to be successful, these capacities need to be integrated with and supported by the interpersonal and system-focused strategies that create a culture of ethical practice (discussed in Chapters 10 and 11).[3]

Know Our Fundamental Values

A foundational capacity for moral resilience is the reflective and intentional adoption of values and behavior for realizing good, for self and others, and for the social and material world. Values, consciously chosen, provide the anchor for integrity. They serve as our moral compass to help us navigate situations that engage our fundamental understandings of moral and ethical behavior, our intentions, and our commitments. They are reflected in our character and our decision-making, in what we as individuals stand for. When a situation or choice under conditions of risk, danger, and uncertainty calls upon us to act with integrity, our moral compass guides and grounds our actions. Like any sensitive navigational instrument, our compass requires careful, ongoing calibration with our core values. For each of us, this means determining and embodying our core values, asking, and answering key questions, such as "What matters most to you in life and work? What rules, principles, spiritual/religious traditions, norms, or beliefs guide decisions and behavior? How is your character reflected in your choices and behavior? When confronted with an opportunity to choose or act in alignment with your values, what guides you?" Our moral compass invites us to choose the direction of our path, determine the course to get there, and continually recalibrate as we journey toward our destination.

Attune to Intentions and Motivations

Detecting, clarifying, and evaluating our own intentions can fuel conscientiousness to act ethically and in accordance with our fundamental values. Admittedly, our intentions and motivations are rarely pure; indeed, they are often quite complex.[4] Mindfully connecting to who we fundamentally are and why we chose our profession helps to bring that awareness into our "working memory," that cognitive capacity for briefly holding limited amounts of information in conscious awareness, making it available to interact with other cognitive contents and processes.[5,6] By doing so, we have greater connection with associated insights and can summon the energy to prevail despite challenges or adversity. Alignment with our intentions and motivations can help to focus problem-solving and cognitive processes that draw upon values, goals, expectations, and spiritual or religious beliefs that can be instrumental in appraising or reassessing challenges in the context of moral complexity. Tuning into and clarifying how we intend to be as a person and within our professional roles requires awareness and connection to our core values and goals and a process for appraising congruence with them.[7] Pausing to reflect upon our fundamental motivations for being a clinician can illuminate a pathway for ethically sound action. So too can appreciating how our intentions and motivations align with our character and ethical values. Discerning the answers to key questions—"Why *am* I doing this? What makes it matter? Are my actions in tune with the person I want to be? What kind of person will I be if I engage in a particular manner in this circumstance?—helps intensify alignment or illuminate areas of malalignment. For example, a critical care nurse's perception that the treatments she is implementing prolong dying can undermine her intention to relieve her critically ill patient's suffering and threaten her image of herself as a "good" nurse; advocating for the interests of the patient may have the effect of compromising her personal or professional values. Noticing the physical, emotional, and behavioral manifestations of this tension can provide insight for investigating its meaning and significance.

Stand for What Matters Most

Above all, we must stand for what matters most. Preserving or restoring integrity requires an intimate understanding of the foundation of who we are, our character, and what matters most, both when our values are threatened and when they are aligned. We may assume as clinicians that our moral foundation is clear until we are challenged to articulate and defend it. Self-awareness includes ongoing, disciplined self-exploration; it depends upon a robust capacity for reflection, introspection, and self-effacement. Discerning which values we will protect or defend above all others helps create our moral compass and ground our actions in integrity. Distinguishing what we stand *for* as opposed to what we stand *against* can shift the tenor of our response to challenges and threats to our integrity. Within this process, it is vital to acknowledge the subjectivity embedded in the clinical encounter and to be aware of our stance toward ourselves,

Table 7.1. Questions to Evaluate Alignment© 2018

- What will it take for me to do what I say? What will it take for me to deliver on what I plan to accomplish?
- What do I see when I inquire into the congruence between my actions and strategies and my values/commitments/purpose? Is there something I need to modify?
- On which occasions did I speak out for the values I stand for?
- When did I manifest the values/commitments I cherish and honor in myself?
- When did I stretch and take a risk and manifest my courage to create something important?

other persons, and the clinical environment. Intentionally connecting to our inner landscape and noticing the quality of our own inner resonance with our purpose and values is a precondition for appraising alignment with or threats to integrity. This grounding is essential to discerning the impact of our values and character on our actions, especially when confusion, dissonance, and uncertainty arise. Table 7.1 offers questions to guide discernment regarding alignment of values, commitments, and behavior.

Cultivate Mindful Awareness and Self-Attunement

Among the capacities for moral resilience and the foundation for all those that follow, mindful awareness means paying attention in the moment openheartedly without reaction or judgment.[8,9] It is the ongoing practice of humbly bringing one's attention back into the present each time it wanders into the past or future or is put off balance. A core skill, mindfulness involves noticing, tracking, and training the mind to remain non-judgmentally aware in the present and stable amid distractions, emotional arousal, and proliferation of thoughts. Thus, it allows for self-attunement to bodily signals and emotions that offer insights into the ethical contours of the situation, relevant perspectives, and possible courses of action.

Practitioners of mindfulness appear to be more emotionally regulated than non-practitioners,[10,11,12] and highly experienced meditation practitioners have been shown to have enhanced compassion-related brain responses to the distress of others.[13,14] Mindfulness seems an unattainable skill for some people, but even brief periods of mindfulness practice can be beneficial, as evidenced by assessments of altered brain physiology and by behavioral measurement of increased emotion regulation.[10,15] Although mindfulness without emotional intelligence renders its benefits less effective,[16] just a few weeks of mindfulness meditation training has been shown to increase altruistic responding to another's distress[17] and to enhance activation of the brain systems related to emotion regulation, correlated with evidence of greater compassionate behavior.[18] A growing body of research suggests that mindfulness can enhance self-awareness of internal states and allow different meaning to be made of adversity, shifting emotion in a more positive direction.[19,23] Importantly, research has found that mindfulness is a skill that clinicians can learn and use for self-regulation, stress management, and well-being.[20,21,22,23,25]

Mindfulness involves self-attunement that encompasses being aware of somatic cues,[24,25,26] emotional tone and tenor, thought patterns, intention, and motivation.[18,27] Below we discuss strategies that can help us to identify and define what we are experiencing so that we can activate integrity-preserving responses.

Acknowledge What Our Bodies Tell Us

Our bodies are instrumental in perceiving the intricacies of a situation, our responsiveness to others, and the implications of ethical nuances on our own integrity; the dynamic interplay among these elements informs the process of enacting ethical actions. Somatic modes of awareness help us locate what is of value and awaken our concern. They are especially important related to reactions, threats to integrity, or activation of conscience. Paying attention to the signals that indicate either alignment with our intentions and motivations or discontent, confusion, or potential conflict is necessary for robust ethical attunement.

Consider, for example, a clinician who connects with a patient in a moment of crisis and can communicate, using presence, words, and actions, deep respect, and reverence for the magnitude of the situation without fear or anxiety. The embodied experience is free of tension or confusion; words flow without effort. The clinician's parasympathetic nervous system (PNS) is activated; decreased heart rate, respiration, blood pressure, and muscle tension and general relaxation of the nervous system are accompanied by contentment or ease.

In contrast, imagine a clinician who perceives that his actions to uphold a patient's preference for life-sustaining treatment despite evidence of its limited effectiveness conflict with their professional duty to "do no harm." Before they become consciously aware of the threat to their well-being or integrity, they may feel a heaviness around the heart or a knot in the gut, muscle tension, or increased heart rate, respiration, or blood pressure—all signals of sympathetic nervous system (SNS) arousal as the body prepares for "fight, flight, or freeze." Or they may turn to increased nurturing, protective, and supportive behaviors (tending) and seek out connections to other people (befriending) in a pattern known as "tend and befriend."[28,29]

Awareness of typical patterns of physiologic and somatic responses to stressors (which may include behavioral and gender differences) can help us navigate difficult clinical situations.[23,29,30,31] This is particularly important when our basic physiologic needs are not met; this can shift us from a place of balance and wholeness to dysregulation and fractured integrity. Low blood sugar levels can mimic symptoms of panic or anxiety. Fatigue and exhaustion can lead to foggy thinking, delayed reaction time, and errors. Over-reliance on self-protective patterns and adverse responses can lead to exhaustion, negative health outcomes, and compromised integrity. Self-attunement to responses such as these may give us clues about the alignment of our intentions, values, and actions. These clues, in turn, can help us discern the contours of ethical issues, understand our emotional responses, and calibrate our ethical responses.

Our bodies hold vast knowledge that includes a reservoir of memories and experiences. According to Nancy Eisenberg,[32] one of the preconditions of empathic arousal, a necessary element for attunement to self and other, is the memory that resides not only in our mind but also in our bodies. Shards of our experiences become integrated into our muscles, internal organs, impulses, and bodily movements. Typically, bodily sensations precede feeling and thought. Our minds are aware of our experiences and can construct the narrative surrounding them. Verbally telling the story about a troubling case, for example, may trigger "somatic remembering"[33,34,35] that manifests as physical sensations, numbing, dysregulated arousal, and involuntary movements; it may also activate emotions such as dread, helplessness, hopelessness, shame, or responses such as moral outrage. The moral residue of experiences when a clinician chooses not to address an ethical issue or participates in moral wrongdoing is likely imprinted consciously or unconsciously in the body.[36,37] Although often pre-reflective and easily overlooked, these sensory and somatic aspects can inform how we interpret and assign an emotional valence to a situation—a precondition for moral discernment.[13]

Respect and Respond to Our Emotions

Normally we experience a range of emotions every day. When we use them constructively, they can help us locate what matters and motivate us to action. We have preferences for the kinds of emotions we embrace and those we tend to push away. With mindfulness we acknowledge them all,[18] but we do not invite all of them to remain where they can create distraction or cause harm. Often, we try to repress, ignore, or reject strong emotions such as anger, fear, frustration, or sadness. Rather than pushing an emotion away, however, we can use the experience of the emotion arising to pause and invite reflection and insight: "Where in my body am I experiencing this feeling? What is the intensity of this feeling? Mild? Moderate? Strong? Am I appraising it as positive, negative, or neutral?" When we pause, we can use our full repertoire of input and choose whether an emotion needs to be fueled, witnessed, or released. Through our bodies we begin to interpret the particularities of a situation and assign it an emotional valence that can anchor our understanding of its moral significance.[38,39]

Positive or negative emotions can be a part of sensory and somatic perceptions and nervous system activation. In cases of flight, fright, or freeze, SNS activation is an aspect of negative emotions, for example, when a nurse perceives that treatment plans being implemented are contrary to the patient's expressed or written preferences for life-sustaining therapy. Fear is an ingredient that intensifies the likelihood of lapses of integrity. When expectations for performance are heightened, when the requirements of the situation exceed one's competence or confidence, or when one experiences situations that do not turn out as desired or expected, fear may be more likely to arise. Situations where there are abuses of power at some level of the team or hierarchy can destabilize individuals to the point that they will behave in ways incongruent with their moral core and integrity. For example, when a superior insists that subordinates lie or cover up another's lapse, fear can cause them to act in ways contrary to their personal and professional moral commitments and norms. Strong emotions such as anger, while a normal human response, can lead to reactionary responses, unregulated venting, or outbursts.[40] Similarly, feeling lonely, misunderstood, or rejected can lead to withdrawal or self-imposed isolation, which can override our need for social connection.[41] Humans, who are hardwired for negative emotions to be rapidly triggered, can begin to resonate with each other's negative emotional energy, creating a "stress contagion effect" that can affect individual perception and responsiveness and influence the ways that people resonate with each other.[42,43] Seeing another person experience distress can reinforce and exacerbate our own negative emotions.

In contrast, positive emotions may arise in conjunction with PNS activation—for instance, in response to actions where interventions are implemented in a way that fosters respect, relieves suffering, or creates meaning amid crisis. Consistent with PNS activation, focus and attention tend to broaden and become more flexible.[44] The clinician's claims of futility and moral distress may be transformed from negative emotions into evidence of commitment, moral character, and intention to "do the right thing," lightening the clinician's burden and offering the opportunity to leverage what was distress into principled, integrity-preserving, compassionate action. This requires internal spaciousness, stability, and focus both to neutralize the negative impact of physiologic and emotional activation and to garner additional internal and external resources that support resilience rather than depletion.[18] Most likely, shifting the response pattern will require strong, intentional efforts to overcome the human tendency to focus on the negative aspects of situations, appraisals, and responses.[45,46] Yet, when people co-experience positive emotions, they begin to experience "positivity resonance" that can create biobehavioral synchrony, broaden collective mindsets, and build collective resources.[47,48]

Thus, both positive and negative signals invite further investigation to discern their relevance, offer more nuanced interpretation, or identify gaps in our knowledge or understanding. Detecting and responding to signals of imperiled integrity and situations that make one vulnerable to them is a first step in taking corrective action.

Monitor Our Thought Patterns

Recognizing and tracking thought patterns that are often overlooked makes them available for further examination. Frequently, the mind organizes itself to preserve what is appraised to be of value, instigating thought patterns that preserve the status quo. We may seek justification for conscious or unconscious biases or what we have already determined we want to do to allay the uncomfortable sensations associated with confronting the arising dissonance.[49] The mind is likely to release its grip only reluctantly on what is familiar or to defend what may threaten its stability. When arousal is not regulated and emotions escalate, cues from various sources are misinterpreted and attention is dispersed, sabotaging the ability to appraise the situation accurately. This is why, in situations associated with moral suffering, especially moral distress or injury, assumptions about the decisions, outcomes, and ethical valence of issues can become distorted. For example, after experiencing negative emotion with SNS activation in a series of situations, a clinician may interpret a new situation to be similar, despite insufficient information or data. Negative thought patterns such as "This family doesn't get it" or "This is futile" may set off a cascade of responses that constrain possibilities, undermine relationships, and fuel feelings of self-doubt, shame, self-loathing, or anger at being powerless to escape from or successfully resolve the situation.[50] In such cases, a clinician's thought patterns can become stuck in an endless cycle of rumination, replaying the events over and over without new insight or action. Alternatively, thought patterns arising from positive emotions with PNS activation can stimulate a spaciousness and curiosity about other possibilities, and potentially emotions such as compassion and altruism. Witnessing the suffering of a patient and her family can arouse empathy and lead the clinician to openness and perspective-taking in service of greater understanding, alignment, and harmony.

When our minds and emotions overwhelm our awareness, we begin to lose connection with somatic and physiologic information. Attentional balance helps to perceive the contours of the situation clearly and contributes to stability of the nervous system. Attunement to somatic signals, noticing the valence of the emotional response and thought patterns, expands the repertoire of information that can be leveraged toward appraising the situation more calmly and discerning ethically grounded options. When we notice what is happening within and around us, we can choose to shift our responses and options to align with our values, beliefs, roles, and worldviews. This in turn can impact our stance in the situation, its dynamics, and ultimately how it unfolds.

Likewise, we need to learn about and notice our thought patterns. The brain is a thought generator, constantly producing thoughts and predictions. Often our mind is focused on the past or the future and not what is happening right now. Recent evidence suggests that a wandering mind tends to be less caring toward oneself and others.[51] Given clinicians' constant exposure to myriad distractions, it stands to reason that they are at high risk for depletion of their disposition toward caring and compassion. It takes practice to notice when our mind has wandered and to bring our attention back to the present. Thoughts are not necessarily reality; like other sources of information, they require discernment to verify their veracity and relevance. When we are unable to distinguish our thought patterns, we may begin to believe a whole range of thoughts that may or may not be true. For example, if we begin to question our ethical competence, we may listen to the background conversation in our mind that says, "I'm not good enough. I'm not smart enough. I'll look stupid if I speak up. No one cares what I have to say. Why *are* we doing this?" Believing these messages can make us feel powerless, distracting us from what matters most. Monitoring the stream of our thoughts creates an opportunity to recognize patterns that enable or disable our integrity and to choose to shift or release them.[52] A continuous repeat of the same narrative can lead to rumination and "sticky" attachment to the content of the thought pattern. Enhancing cognitive control enables us to guide our thoughts and behaviors in accord with our intentions, to be more flexible, to "down-regulate" our nervous system, and potentially to override habitual responses that no longer serve a useful role in the situation.[53]

Adopt Mindfulness Practices

A range of mindfulness practices can support awareness of body, heart, and mind, focused attention, mental and emotional balance, and self-regulatory skills. Sensing into the body—the viscera, body structures, and physiology—is a helpful tool to stabilize or ground the mind.[23] Being aware of patterns of breathing, areas of constriction or comfort, and how we navigate through our day cultivates focused attention and offers insight into our physical experience. It is often said that the status of the body reflects the quality of the mind. Somatic attunement—the ability to recognize what is happening in our own bodies—uses the same neurological circuits as empathy, which is necessary to attune to others.[54,55] We can also become aware of our emotional states and begin to notice and sit with both pleasant and unpleasant sensations such as joy or contentment, or sadness, fear, anxiety, or distress. Being able to identify and locate where these feelings live in our bodies expands our repertoire of awareness. Similarly, being able to notice and track patterns of awareness, thoughts, attitudes, and beliefs creates greater attunement to our repetitive and often preconscious patterns. Tracking our attentiveness or distractedness, the cognitive processes we use in reflection or decision-making, and where we hold on to ideas and where we can release them offers insights and data from which to discern the path of integrity in the complex situations where we find ourselves.[56]

But first we must become intimately familiar with our own inner processes and response patterns, and most of us need guidance and practice to be able to cultivate a robust awareness and language of bodily sensations, emotional tenor, and the content and meaning of our thought patterns. In our over-stimulated lives, we rarely carve out time for stillness or solitude. As Dan Siegel notes, "Each of us needs periods in which our minds can focus inwardly. Solitude is an essential experience for the mind to organize its own processes and create an internal state of resonance. In such a state, the self is able to alter its constraints by directly reducing the input from interactions with others."[32(p235)] Using practices that invite stillness such as meditation, biofeedback, visualization, insight practices, or movement practices such as yoga or tai chi can support the development of new patterns of awareness.[23,26]

To build a foundation for moral resilience, clinicians can benefit from learning basic mindfulness techniques to support them when ethical challenges arise. There are many ways that mindfulness practices can support moral resilience and help to down-regulate the nervous system and reduce reactivity; examples are learning to be aware of the breath, intentionally extending the inhale and exhale and noticing the differences, and practicing bringing awareness to the soles of one's feet on the floor to focus attention during stressful or adverse events. Practices such as a mindful body scan can help clinicians to become more aware of their body sensations and patterns of responses. A variety of resources are available to develop a regular mindfulness practice. Programs such as Mindfulness-Based Stress Reduction (MBSR) or other guided programs can be effective.[26,57]

Committing to technology breaks and periods of stillness throughout the day enables us to take advantage of our capacities for insight, reflection, and non-reactive responses. Intentionally employing ways to create pauses in the workflow, decision-making process, and communication can create more spaciousness for insight and reflection. Taking an in-breath and remembering one's intentions before entering a patient's room or responding to a colleague can enhance our clarity and focus.

Cultivate Reflection and Insight

Reflection and insight are vital elements of moral resilience; without them we risk repeating autopilot patterns, inadequate or ineffective discernment, and potential harm to others and ourselves. Intentionally creating pauses in the process of ethical discernment to enhance clarity, insight, and accurate perception of the situation can support ethically grounded action. Pausing creates space to notice what is present; it allows us to gather our attention and attune to our bodily signals. Emotions and thought patterns can offer useful insights regarding the ethical contours of clinical situations. Noticing what is happening in our bodies can free us from being caught up in the speed and importance of our thoughts. Pausing to notice with intention allows us to acknowledge the presence of our biases, judgments, internal conflict, and painful feelings. It helps relax our fear and resistance and creates space to let things be as they are—and space for us to choose a next step. When we can create more spaciousness, we have the opportunity to empower our moral agency to take principled action rather than to acquiesce, shut down, or become complacent. According to an observation often attributed to Victor Frankl, "Between stimulus and response, there is a space. In that space is our power to choose our response. In our response lies our growth and our freedom."[58] Inviting spaciousness enables us to connect more deeply with our own being, which in turn awakens our compassion and caring and supports us in making wiser choices. When we pause, we are able to notice what is happening; we have the space to choose whether we need to adjust our attention and our perspective, and the space to rest in the midst of whatever is happening.

Maintain an Open Mindset

Embedded in creating space for insight is an opportunity to monitor our own mindset and that of others. Our mindsets can be open or closed, porous or rigid. When our mindset is closed, we are more likely to be defensive, critical, narrow-minded, and judgmental. We are more likely to be reactive, to give way to primitive autopilot reactions based in fear and survival. We become more negative or blame-focused and adopt "either/or" thinking that frames the problem as win–lose and leads to scarcity thinking—the perception that there is a lack of possibilities, competence, personal agency, time, and so on. Alternatively, when we are open and curious, we can choose and use our higher brain function to be more flexible, non-reactive, and responsibility oriented. We engage pro-social qualities such as generosity, kindness, and altruism. Instead of focusing only on the problem, we become more solution-focused, creating win–win situations by considering new possibilities and ways of being.

Our mindsets can also be reflected in narratives of the confusion and conflict that surround ethically troubling situations. Telling and retelling stories of moral adversity has the potential to project our experiences and memories or to retraumatize us to the unprocessed suffering associated with them into the current situation, or they can serve to illuminate our moral conscientiousness, values, and commitments.[59] Without a disciplined process, these stories can solidify a narrative that may or may not be accurate and that may unintentionally undermine the individual and collective moral agency of clinicians and clinical teams. Typical compensatory mechanisms and patterns of responses to situations that cause moral suffering may involve moralistic narratives that make others wrong or deny our contribution to the situation. With an imperfect understanding of the other and perceiving that we are the ones who are acting rationally, social incentives derived from role, gender, race, and so on can lead us to make unsafe or marginally ethically robust decisions. Over time the narrative becomes solidified into "truth," and clinicians rally around it to justify their actions, behaviors, and choices. This can begin to marginalize voices that are not consistent with the collective narrative. People who raise alternatives are silenced or discredited; consultants who are not likely to agree are marginalized, all in service of maintaining the status quo. But this marginalization often insidiously erodes individual and collective integrity, with consequences such as burnout,[60] turnover, medical errors, reduced employee engagement, and low patient and family satisfaction. Unaware of their cause, we may blame patients and their families, other clinicians, the organization, and society for "making us do things we do not want to do." This kind of mindset can be corrosive and ultimately can threaten the very core of our work as clinicians and our relational integrity. It can also point to moral disengagement as a response to our individual and systemic adversity.[61,62]

Noticing the threads of these narratives and engaging in a disciplined process of inquiry—being willing to ask and consider new questions—can lead to greater insights that preserve or restore integrity. Inquiry and curiosity are key elements of ethical competence; they allow us to engage our whole being, not just our immediate reactivity. With the intention to be constructive—not to intimidate, prove that we are right, or demonstrate how much we know—we can gain clarity and use questions to serve the highest good. Discerning the purpose of our questions—whether to focus attention, gather information, clarify facts or assumptions, discover solutions, or negotiate or resolve conflicts—informs our communication and decision-making. It can help us discover what new questions we should ask to understand the situation, options, or solutions more fully. In difficult cases, we also need to ask, "What is the tone surrounding the conversation? Is it collaborative, angry, defensive, or judgmental? What is the cost of remaining in this tone?" Discerning the consequences of our behaviors and decisions (action or inaction) and being responsible for them are fundamental to integrity.

Learn to Pause

Being able to pause, notice, and reflect to gain perspective—about others and ourselves—is an important dimension of both personal and relational integrity. Pausing, even for one breath, creates space for us to refocus our attention, to allow our mind and body to relax, and to perceive more clearly what is true in the moment. This allows us to expand our awareness to include the feelings and experiences of others; sensing and empathizing with their experiences and their situations and listening allows us to distinguish the contours of our own experience, validate our assumptions, and monitor our mindset and biases. By so doing, we can foster "the Art of Pause"[63] and enhance clarity, insight, and accurate perception of the situation (Table 7.2).[63]

Pausing in this way gives others the space to express their views, especially if they differ from our own. When we are clear about where each

Table 7.2. Developing Skills in Pausing

- Anchor yourself in your breath.
- Create spaciousness.
- Be transparent.
- Monitor your mindset.
- Explore personal responses.
- Ask questions.
- Get clarification.
- Be open to new possibilities.
- Let go of outcome.
- Become a witness rather than an actor.

Source: Rushton CH. Ethical discernment and action: the art of pause. AACN Adv Crit Care. 2009;20:108–111

person in the situation stands, we are better able to transform difficult situations in effective and compassionate ways. Asking "What's actually going on here?" and listening to the answers that come back will help to cultivate curiosity and humility. This helps us to weigh and decipher the importance of different opinions, values, rights, and decisions to determine if some are more important than others, with integrity and without bias or assumptions. Being open to new information also can help us to revise or reinforce the discernment process.

Embedded in the discernment process is a commitment to transparency from the very beginning of the dialogue or decision-making process. This includes shared responsibility for the quality of the decisions made and their consequences as they are occurring and after they have been implemented. The goal is not to focus on criticism or punishment for those viewed as unjustified but rather to encourage self-corrective action and improvements before unreflective or harmful decisions have been enacted.

Practice the Art of Listening

Listening is a foundational skill for insight and reflection. Like mindfulness, it takes a combination of intention and attention. Intention involves having a genuine interest in the other person's experiences, views, feelings, and needs. Attention requires us to focus and to stay present, open, and unbiased to the other person's verbal, non-verbal, and energetic responses, even when they don't align with our own ideas, views, or desires. It means asking ourselves, "What is alive in my body, heart, and mind right now? Is there anything that is getting in the way of being present for the other person? If something is getting in the way, does it need to be addressed now or can it wait until another time?" Pausing in this way and bringing your awareness to sensations in your body (sensing into our own experience) before we extend our attention to the other person helps us connect to our intention to listen fully and openly. Also embedded in the skill of listening is a collateral skill of inviting and holding silence. Cultivating a quality of silence as a way of being[64] can help to create more spaciousness in the discernment process.[65] Silence can allow us the spaciousness to notice our own responses as they arise within an encounter, and to release those thoughts, feelings, judgments, and memories of them so we can return our full attention to the speaker.

Practice Empathy

A necessary element of insight, empathy is commonly understood as including two dimensions: affective and cognitive. Affective empathy occurs when a person "perceives someone else's affect . . . and this triggers a response such that the observer partially feels what the [other person] is feeling."[66(p82),67] It expands our awareness to include the somatic and affective experience of another in an embodied manner without being consumed or overwhelmed by it. Our ability to do this is in part based on emotional contagion or being affected by another person's affective state. Because we are hardwired to resonate with others, an important element of affective empathy is the ability to distinguish our own affective state from another's and to acknowledge when our affective arousal is arising from the experience of the other.[53] This requires self-awareness, focused attention, contextual appraisal, and conscious choice to adapt our response to amplify or to inhibit our feeling state in response to the circumstances and our personal resources.

Cognitive empathy or perspective-taking involves using cognitive reasoning to bring awareness to and seek to understand another person's intentions, values, beliefs, or point of view. Like affective empathy, it helps us to differentiate our own mental processes from those of another person.[68] When we are attuned to the affective experience of another, we can explore that perspective with openness and curiosity.[69] As clinicians, we distinguish ourselves from others when we acknowledge that we are not our patients, although we are able to attune to their experience. Over-identification can cause a loss of boundaries, and this can have an adverse effect on us. When we cannot distinguish the experience of another from our own, we are more vulnerable to empathic over-arousal.[13] Cultivating a stance of equanimity by embodying a healing presence with awareness of the present moment supports stability. When signs of negative arousal arise, it is useful to pause to recalibrate attention and intentionally make the distinction between self and other. Alternatively, clinicians may notice that they are unable to resonate with the experience of the people they serve, leading to feelings of disconnection or numbness. Some clinicians report "going through the motions" without being able to attune to the suffering, confusion, or despair of patients or their families. Both extremes can undermine empathy. Mindfulness practices that cultivate awareness of bodily experience help decrease a tendency to get caught up in self-relevant narratives or imagery that blurs the distinction between one's own experience and that of others.[70] Developing peer support systems can help clinicians to recognize when their responses are disproportionate to the situation or reflect disconnection and can create a zone of stability that maintains clear boundaries of responsibility for both the process and the outcomes of their actions.[13]

Develop Moral Efficacy

Moral efficacy, the belief in our ability to bring about desired and beneficial results though our efforts and the exercise of our moral agency both individually and collectively,[71] is essential to moral resilience. When we develop moral efficacy, we can bring our values and principles into alignment with the actions we take in response to ethically challenging situations.[49] The foundation of moral efficacy involves well-developed ethical awareness, sensitivity, and attunement as antecedents for discernment and action.[72,73] It includes cultivating a rich moral vocabulary, moral imagination, coherent character, and openness to understanding the values, motivations, and hopes and fears of others. Clinicians need cognitive skills to appraise and respond to ethically challenging situations,[74,75] but they also need mindful awareness and stability to address the complicated, intertwined issues that shape interdisciplinary clinical practice, with its diverse power relationships, communication patterns, and other ongoing matters.[49,73,76,77] In the context of clinical practice the moral and ethical domains are often overlapping but at times are distinct. Moral/ethical efficacy requires knowledge and cognitive capabilities; it also requires moral/ethical embodiment, perception/attunement, reflection/discernment, analysis, and behavior or action,[78] along with skills to mitigate the detrimental impact of moral adversity and suffering.

Embodiment of our values and commitments is a foundation for ethically grounded action. When we embody our moral conscientiousness, our diligent, intentional, and thoughtful efforts are reflected in how we live in alignment with our values and commitments despite obstacles or challenges.[49] Margaret Walker writes, "Human beings have prodigious resources of imagination, invention, insight, and resistance that can open spaces of possibility and images of agency even under desperate conditions."[79(p64)] Moral imagination engages our curiosity, which allows us to simultaneously hold paradoxically different views and envision possibilities beyond our current perception that may produce alternative outcomes.[80] Imagining beyond what is present in the moment carries the inherent risk of stepping into unknown or unfamiliar territory.[78] Mental and emotional stability and spaciousness in thinking and responding enhance the opportunity for intuition and imagination to operate. Because we resonate with what captures our attention, we need to rebalance our nervous system when it becomes activated so we can discern the relevance of its signals. If we fail to do so, it is more likely that default responses, linked to our prewired experience and patterns, will automatically take over without conscious thought.

Develop Moral Sensitivity

Moral perception and attunement are vital elements of moral efficacy. An expanded concept of moral sensitivity[71,81,82] refers to an acute perception of the morally salient features of the situation—the interests and values of the people involved and the possible choices and courses of action relevant to an ethical question, conflict, or dilemma—and a state of self-awareness in which one is attuned to the wisdom of the body, emotions, and mind. It requires us to perceive and respond to the nuances and hidden meanings of a situation's moral/ethical dimensions while we also maintain a state of awareness, openness, and inquiry. As such, moral sensitivity and attunement are foundational to principled, compassionate action that retains our own integrity while being responsive to and respectful of the integrity of others. It is the ability to locate and name the source of moral confusion, dissonance, uncertainty, disagreement, or conflict and to perceive the situation and its meanings without projection, bias, or misinterpretation. This requires the awareness of one's moral and ethical values, intentions, and dispositions toward oneself and others, and the capacity to notice the aspects of a situation that activate responses that foster alignment or alienation with one's character and conscience or cause one to quicken in response to a real or perceived threat to one's ethical values and commitments. This requires the ability to mentally "self-distance"[83] to inquire about the interpretation and implications for others.

"If one's moral sensitivity is not well developed, one may not accurately identify an occasion for moral action and may inappropriately tolerate ethically objectionable acts."[71(p325)] Without recognizing and being clear about what the ethical problem is, it is impossible to determine what to do about it, or to be motivated to act once an obligation or commitment to do so is identified. Moral apathy, frustration, disagreement, and confusion can arise as a function of ambiguity about defining the ethical problem or the morally contoured response. Likewise, the negative impact of ethical violations on patients, families, clinicians, or leaders can be overlooked and can lead to tolerating inappropriate behaviors or decisions.

Without a stable mental and emotional continuum and refined moral sensitivity, salient features of the situation may be overlooked, overemphasized, or disregarded, and ethical actions are more likely to be guided by unconscious projections, unexamined assumptions, and faulty reasoning. This can lead to actions that lack sufficient ethical justification or are unethical. The foundation of moral sensitivity is the cultivation of a variety of personal strategies aimed at supporting mental stability, reducing reactivity, and enhancing awareness of the somatic, emotional, and behavioral signals that are relevant to ethical decision-making.[61] This awareness, coupled with systems that support ethical practice, is needed for integrity to be preserved. See Chapters 10 and 11 for details.

Cultivate Moral Attunement

Being attuned to the moral/ethical dimensions of clinical cases helps to illuminate the relevant contours of the situation, focus attention, clarify the justification for different perspectives, and inform ethically grounded and integrity-preserving actions. Being true to one's own convictions while attuning to the particularities of the situation of the other person is a rigorous and demanding balancing effort that requires principled processes and disciplined awareness. Moral sensitivity and attunement anchor us to the ethically relevant aspects of the situation so that our moral judgments can be fully informed. It is essential to engage curiosity to uncover the hidden meanings of the situation and the values of the persons involved, to challenge one's assumptions, and to notice evidence of bias or misinterpretation. This kind of awareness invites a robust, dynamic process of inquiry.

At the same time, we must be aware of the ways that attuning with others might distract or displace our attention and understanding. Conscious safeguards and intentional pauses are needed to avoid misunderstanding or misinterpreting the meanings of various aspects of the situation, the options under consideration, and their alignment with important ethical values and principles. Misinterpretation, in our attempted attunement, may be a particular risk when we strongly identify with another, potentially leading to over-arousal and personal distress rather than empathic responding.[84]

Being morally attuned is an invitation to see what we do not yet perceive and to consciously resist drawing conclusions prematurely. It guides clinicians to focus on the special circumstances and context of the specific situation, not merely the isolated ethical theories and principles involved. It invites consideration of other aspects of the moral life, such as care, harmony, compassion, and responsibility for self and others, to reduce the adversarial tensions that often occur when people take hard, immutable stances. Moral sensitivity and attunement allow for a more comprehensive appreciation of the attitudes, values, and ethical commitments of all who are affected—patients, families, professionals, and others. Holding the space to perceive and non-judgmentally investigate the ethically salient features of a challenging clinical situation by attuning to oneself and others is also crucial to acknowledging unwanted thoughts, feelings, and sensations and resisting the urge to run away from them, deny their existence, or discount or push them away.

Moral attunement calls for exquisite attentiveness and genuine respect for ethical values and perspectives that are aligned with or are different from one's own. Given the diversity of moral and ethical perspectives, reaching consensus in situations where there are contentious ethical issues, or wide-ranging but dissonant justifications may not always be possible. Responsiveness to others and their claims, requests, and actions reflects the dynamic process of enacting ethically grounded actions and upholding relational integrity. Alignment of values and commitments often diffuses conflict and distress. In the clinical setting when values and actions are in harmony, there is often greater ease, generosity, creativity, and flexibility. When there is disagreement or conflict about values, commitments, or responsibilities (e.g., if the patient or family request treatments that the members of the treating team believe are ineffective), malalignment results, creating dissonance and mobilizing the conditions where unconscious processes can take over and allow moral indifference or disregard to occur.[85] Awareness of cultural, religious, gender, or other biases that may be present is vital; without attunement, they can provide the fuel for disconnection, projection, and deepening conflict. Investment in individual and systemic processes that foster robust relational integrity can support greater moral attunement.

Engage in Moral/Ethical Analysis

A foundation of moral sensitivity and attunement informs the cognitive processes that follow from our awareness of an ethical issue and invites more nuanced moral analysis. This dialectic process of appraisal and discernment flows from locating the elements that create or undermine harmony. What we are aware of and resonate with informs the range of choices we consider when we deliberate what actions to take and how to implement them. Being responsive and flexible in complex ethical situations without compromising our core moral values and principles is vital to our integrity and leverages our moral conscientiousness—the resolute and thoughtful ongoing effort to live in alignment with our principles and values, even in the face of challenges and obstacles.

Appraisal and discernment are primed by robust moral sensitivity and attunement to the morally salient dimensions that support various courses of action. Resonating with and responding in accord with one's values preserves integrity and is often accompanied by a sense of clarity and peaceful emotions such as empathy, positive regard, kindness, or love. In contrast, when one's values are misaligned because of a perceived violation of an ethical principle, the feelings that arise can range from discomfort and anxiety to anger and outrage. In some situations, these negative emotions may instigate a process of ethical appraisal and discernment to determine the ethically justified response.

When the need for moral discernment is recognized, cognitive processes are activated to identify the morally relevant aspects of the situation, understand the conflicting perspectives, explore the nature of the value conflicts, identify the range of morally permissible actions, and determine the best course of action (all things considered). This iterative process involves an appraisal of how one's actions affect oneself and others and how the actions taken or not taken promote or undermine integrity and/or result in one's participation in a spectrum of moral wrongdoing.[86] The preconditions of empathy and perspective-taking, moral sensitivity, and attunement support or undermine the capacity to respond in an emotionally balanced, ethically grounded, and compassionate manner.[53] The ultimate goal is to embody our moral commitments in each moment and every encounter, to be coherent with our choices and behaviors.

Weigh Competing Moral/Ethical Claims

Throughout this process, we must weigh all relevant evidence and subject our own views to the same rigorous examination that we give to competing perspectives. Our openness to criticism and to reassessment of all views involved, including our own, can create the conceptual clarity we need to make justifiable moral modifications that support both individual and relational integrity.[87] In some situations, various members of the clinical team, or the patient or family, may hold different assumptions or worldviews, or perceive the same information differently. In others, conflicts or disagreements may occur about the proper course of action or which ethical principles apply. Reasonable people do disagree, and dilemmas can reflect conflicting principles or actions that result in different outcomes, none of them clearly preferable from a moral/ethical point of view. In situations where options are highly constrained, it is possible that none of the options created will be viewed as morally desirable. Often the facts may be disputed, uncertainty is likely, and there may or may not be a clearly preferable moral action that leaves all stakeholders satisfied. Even if there is, moral residue may occur for at least some of the stakeholders. In situations involving irreconcilable conflicts or impossible and non-negotiable moral requirements, doubt and moral suffering are common features. Even when one has done what is least harmful, moral residue may be unavoidable.[88] In these situations, the integrity-preserving path may be obscured by the depth of moral suffering and the constraints that limit the exercise of moral agency.

Ongoing application of ethical decision-making processes can help to illuminate important moral/ethical claims, various courses of action, and their justifications.[72,89] Discerning how best to fulfill one's moral ideal or goal involves clarifying factual, conceptual, and ethical issues to determine what course of action can be justified. For example, when a critically ill patient is dying, it is important to understand the diagnosis and prognosis and to clarify any factual issues related to medical care. Conceptual issues such as the patient's view of what constitutes an adequate quality of life or a life worth living may also need discussion. In addition, clinicians need to consider their fundamental ethical obligations and commitments to do good, avoid harm, respect the autonomy of patients and their surrogates, treat persons fairly, tell the truth, maintain privacy, and so forth. This effort requires making reasoned judgments about the quality of arguments that a particular course of action preserves a moral value or standard essential to personal and relational integrity.

In making moral/ethical judgments, clinicians appeal to ethical theories and principles to avoid making decisions solely based on individual viewpoints.[54] Within a theoretical framework, they must pay meticulous attention to the contextual features of the case they are appraising—the personal characteristics and relationships of everyone involved in the situation. Values, life history, and commitments that may be related to race, gender, education, or social status all help to shape the ongoing narrative of a person's life and preferences. Discerning these factors helps establish the range of permissible responses and their impact on oneself and others, which in turn informs the intention and way decisions are implemented.[71] Determining whether an action upholds or violates important moral/ethical values or commitments demands reflection to differentiate one's position or desired outcome from what is ethically unjustified. For example, one may perceive that securing a do-not-resuscitate order for a patient in multi-system organ failure is the best outcome because the cumulative burdens outweigh the possible benefits. Being morally attuned invites a non-judgmental evaluation to determine whether a particular action falls within a morally permissible range of options, regardless of our own endorsement. If it is morally permissible, our moral suffering may not be grounded in an ethical violation but rather a cognitive, emotional, or spiritual conflict or dissonance. If it falls outside that permissible range, acting in alignment with our intentions, values, and character may require us to resist by conscientiously objecting or requesting not to participate. Such distinctions require careful discernment to resist exerting unacknowledged biases or assumptions.

Exercise Moral Agency

The ability of clinicians to maintain their integrity or, when the situation requires, to engage successfully in moral repair depends upon their sense of moral agency. In ethically difficult cases especially, clinicians may find themselves vulnerable to asymmetries of power and authority within the practice environment as they struggle to protect their moral values.[39] In such circumstances and in routine care as well, clinicians exercise their moral agency by actively considering the perspectives of others while potentially reevaluating their own considering new information or insights. They neither abdicate their moral authority nor abandon their values, but intentionally balance and attune their own moral stance to the complexities of the situation and the positions taken by others involved in it.[39] In ethically challenging cases, where life and death may be at stake, decisions must be made when outcomes are uncertain, and the path of integrity is unclear. At such times, the exercise of moral agency demands the objectivity, insight, and courage to resolve any confusion or dissonance that may occur.

Determining the ethically justified path means discerning whether action or inaction is required. There are myriad instances where one must carefully consider what will serve those involved or the situation itself. This requires us to hold lightly to our opinions and viewpoints to discover the path of least harm and greatest benefit. In some instances, the path involves taking conscientious action; in others, bearing witness to the reality of the situation or remaining silent or *not* acting is the most ethically responsible action. Attention to the consequences of action or inaction is necessary to discern whether certain paths will cause more suffering for those involved in the situation (e.g., patient, family, clinicians, or others) or relieve it. Awareness of professional obligations may in some cases re-orient clinicians to prioritize the interests of those they serve above their own.

Discerning the wise and compassionate path may include examining a range of possible actions, such as seeking an integrity-preserving compromise, speaking up to bring awareness to the situation or advocate for an alternative, and engaging others, including leaders. In some instances, it may require requesting relief from or refusing to participate on grounds of imperiled integrity or choosing not to act. In egregious situations, it may involve considering acts such as bringing the issue to public attention by "blowing the whistle" or choosing to remove oneself from the situation or organization. In all cases, *how* one enacts one's decision must be as carefully considered as the decision itself. (See Chapter 8 for further details).

Take, Defer, or Decline Action

The resolution of ethical quandaries requires wisdom and skillful means. At times action is required; other times the wise path is to wait or not act. How one ultimately implements a decision is as important as the decision itself. Discerning what will serve the stakeholders involved in the situation—including oneself—requires leveraging all the elements of moral efficacy to bring about the conditions for integrity-preserving action. Grounded in a state of mental and emotional stability in which anger and distress are modulated and action is compassionate, principled action seeks to reestablish a moral value or standard. It requires discernment, inquiry, and self-effacement to determine the right and best response to these situations. It is *not* ungrounded tolerance of unacceptable conditions or passive inaction. Embedded in this discernment process is awareness of the degree to which the person is embodying their values with the actions they take and whether their essence as a person is shining through in their behaviors and actions.

Decisions about how to proceed in morally/ethically challenging situations require realistic expectations of ourselves and others. Being morally resilient in such situations is an invitation to accept things as they currently are, to acknowledge the boundaries of power and influence, and to recognize that the evidence of effective moral agency is reflected both in one's conscientious efforts and in the outcomes produced.[90] Accepting things as they are does not imply agreeing with or endorsing the decisions, circumstances, or causes of the conflict or distress, or being complacent. Rather, it suggests recognizing the situation with all its complexity as it is—not how we prefer it would be or the outcome we prefer. Consider how often clinician suffering arises from wanting the patient or the family to "get it" and see the situation in same way we do, or from wanting the surgeon to agree that the continued treatment is causing more harm than benefit. Continually using the same approaches to change what is currently solidified often exacerbates our own suffering and may cause further recalcitrance. We are not suggesting giving up; rather, we should consider how well our current approaches are working and whether a new approach is possible if we view the situation without our agenda being prominent. Sometimes letting go of the grip of our own agenda creates the space for other possibilities to emerge.

In other situations, the patterns of decisions and actions within the practice environment may accumulate to the point where one must consider whether continuing in one's role or profession is justified. Discernment is necessary to determine the proper threshold of effort to justify a decision to leave a position or the profession. Individual awareness and action are necessary to begin the process of restoring personal integrity but alone are insufficient if the root causes of the sources of moral suffering are not also addressed. Sometimes leaving an institution reflects reaching one's threshold of effort to change the systemic patterns and culture that contribute to erosion of integrity. See Chapters 10 and 11.

Engage in Activities that Support Self-Stewardship

Self-stewardship arises from the fundamental moral obligation to honor and safeguard our health and well-being to serve others. It is neither a static formula of behaviors and activities nor a whimsical, self-indulgent means of escapism. It is an ever-changing component of a responsible approach to health and to living our lives as fully as possible within the context of our own circumstances. As clinicians, we unconsciously transmit to each other an unspoken attitude of self-sacrifice, delayed gratification, and a demanding work ethic that denies even basic physiologic needs for nourishment, sleep, or hydration.[91,92,93] Many clinicians report that they rarely take their full meal break or take care of their needs for hydration or elimination during their shifts; the result is that they are physically and emotionally exhausted from the demands of patient care.[69] The norm for clinicians seems to be that the skillful ways they take care of others are not translated into taking good care of themselves. Plagued by fatigue, lack of exercise, stress, poor eating habits, no time for family, and any number of other stressors, their own needs are often the last to be met.[91,94]

To be responsible stewards of our personal resources, we must embody our commitment to promote our flourishing, diminish the harms of self-denial, and uphold our commitment to integrity by engaging in radical self-honesty and choosing compassionate actions that are wholesome and healthy. Without this commitment, our efforts to restore or preserve integrity or to advocate effectively for others or ourselves will be thwarted. Self-stewardship includes all the things we do, consciously and unconsciously, that contribute to our experience of well-being and create a state of equilibrium within the changes that define our life.

To survive and thrive, we need certain practical basics.[95,96] Consistent with Maslow's theory,[73] we need secure housing, adequate food, safety, nurturing relationships, and meaningful work to create a solid foundation for our lives. When our needs are met, we may take these basics for granted; when unmet, however, they can completely dominate our awareness, causing us to become overwhelmed or afraid. Thus, we must meet these needs before we can pursue a holistic approach to self-stewardship.

Self-stewarding begins with making a commitment to all dimensions of integrity—biological, psychological, relational, spiritual, social, and moral/ethical. It leverages the moral imperative to commit to care for our own wholeness with the same level of concern that we direct toward others, including those we are entrusted to care for in our professional roles.[97] This means giving priority to our needs beyond the most basic; it extends to include creative and expressive outlets, pleasurable and meaningful time with others, participating in spiritual and religious practices and rituals, communing with nature, or stimulating our mind in ways that are nourishing. All can contribute to a sense of wholeness and stability. When we are depleted and our systems are imbalanced, our ability to respond to difficulties narrows and we are more likely to react rather than respond, to become unregulated and over-aroused.

As humans, we have a limited supply of energy each day. Yet, unless we find ourselves in unusual circumstances of adversity, we may check off as many items on our "to do" list each day as we can before collapsing into bed at night. This pattern of overextension, particularly among clinicians, is the cultural norm. While caring for patients who have more complex physical, emotional, and spiritual needs than ever before, we are balancing competing interests in our own personal and professional lives. Our commitment to our own well-being can easily drift into neglect and lead to stress, isolation, and habits that undermine our quality of life. Pushed beyond our limits, we are more likely to make poor decisions or experience lapses of integrity.

Commitment to an ongoing plan for self-stewardship is foundational to our well-being and integrity as clinicians. The first step is to acknowledge our limitations; only then can we learn to manage our internal resources.

A simple self-assessment tool invites us to regularly pause to notice whether we are **H**ungry, **A**ngry, **L**onely, or **T**ired.[98] If the answer to any one of these states is yes, **HALT**. Unmet needs require our attention. When we are hungry, our blood sugar level may drop, making us vulnerable to reactive responses. When we are angry, even if we suppress our feelings as unprofessional, we are more likely to respond from our automatic defensive brain systems rather than our higher-functioning selves. When we are lonely, we may isolate ourselves or withdraw from relationships, and our unrecognized needs to connect, to be seen and heard, can contribute to impulsive or reactive decisions. When we are tired, we are likely to have less bandwidth to respond to situations that create confusion and challenge our integrity. Many clinicians consider it "a badge of honor" to have the stamina to keep going without sufficient sleep, yet recent evidence suggests that when we are sleep-deprived we function as if we were legally intoxicated.[99] Any one of these states may create the conditions that imperil integrity, foster reactivity, or lead to poor decisions. As self-stewards and clinicians of integrity, we must honor our commitment to ourselves, our patients, and our profession by acknowledging and addressing them, even in the face of pressures to deny or press on despite them. All clinicians and organizational leaders must devise, commit to, and implement an individualized self-stewardship plan. Without investment in our own well-being, our ability to work skillfully with moral adversity and suffering and to engage in constructive and sustainable systemic solutions is woefully diminished. While self-stewardship begins as an individual responsibility, healthcare organizations also have a corollary responsibility to create enabling conditions to avoid end stage conditions such as burnout or moral decline. It is unlikely that the organizations where clinicians practice will match individual investments in their well-being and integrity, and it is no longer acceptable for them to sidestep their responsibility to address the modifiable factors in the system that degrade clinician health, well-being, and engagement. Investments in both are needed to optimize patient, family, clinician, and organizational outcomes.

Engage in Ongoing, Transformational Learning

Clinicians of integrity are committed to lifelong learning. Any time that we are confronted with moral adversity, it is an opportunity for self-reflection, insight, and learning. Pausing to take stock of the situation, one's own process, the bigger picture, and the consequences of one's behavior and choices requires the courage to be honest with oneself and a willingness to examine patterns that support or disable our integrity and well-being. Doing so in a generous and compassionate way allows us to learn from what we did well and determine whether any adjustments are warranted in the future. Since we tend to focus on our shortcomings, it is important that this process be balanced so that we can notice and honor our strengths and capabilities while also learning from our missteps, misunderstandings, or biases so that we can take corrective action in the future. A commitment to seeing clearly and honestly the internal and external factors that contribute to our moral suffering is essential to a process of moral repair (see Chapter 8). Ongoing transformational learning must leverage both individual and collective insight, wisdom, and principled action. Concurrently, mechanisms for team and organizational surveillance, review, education, and course corrections are vital in creating alignment and synergy.

Reflecting on questions in a constructive manner can help to illuminate what we can do as individuals to foster moral resilience. Acting to do so is a moral imperative for clinicians of integrity—but it is not enough. Individual strategies must be supported and reinforced by collective strategies undertaken by clinical teams and the organizations in which they practice. These collective efforts, up to and including the system level, are the focus of Chapter 10 on healthcare architecture and complete the groundwork for transforming healthcare and creating a culture of ethical practice as envisioned in Chapter 11.

References

1. Browning DM. Fragments of love: explorations in the ethnography of suffering and professional caregiving. In Berzoff J, Silverman P, editors, Living with dying: a handbook for end-of-life healthcare practitioners. New York: Columbia University Press; 2004:21–42.
2. Kleinman A. The illness narratives: suffering, healing and the human condition. New York: Basic Books; 1988.
3. Portions of this chapter are from C. H. Rushton, A. Kaszniak, and J. Halifax (2013). "Addressing moral distress: Application of a framework to palliative care practice." J Pall Med, 16(9), pp. 1080–88. Adapted with permission.
4. Sulmasy DP. Killing and allowing to die: another look. J Law Med Ethics. 1998;26:55–64.
5. Teasdale JD, Chaskalson M. How does mindfulness transform suffering? I: The nature and origins of dukkha. Contemporary Buddhism. 2011;12:89–102.
6. Teasdale JD, Chaskalson M. How does mindfulness transform suffering? II: The transformation of dukkha. Contemporary Buddhism. 2011;12:103–124.
7. Sull DN, Houlder D. Do your commitments match your convictions? Harv Bus Rev. 2005;83(1):82–91, 118.
8. Kabat-Zinn J. Full catastrophe living: using the wisdom of your body and mind to face stress, pain and illness (revised edition). New York: Bantam Books; 2013.
9. Shapiro SL, Carlson LE. The art and science of mindfulness: integrating mindfulness into psychology and the helping professions. Washington, DC: American Psychological Association; 2009.
10. Nielsen L, Kaszniak AW. Awareness of subtle emotional feelings: a comparison of long-term meditators and non-meditators. Emotion. 2006;6:392–405.
11. Ortner CN, Kilner SJ, Zelazo PD. Mindfulness meditation and reduced emotional interference on a cognitive task. Motiv Emot. 2007;31:271–283.
12. Wadlinger HA, Isaacowitz DM. Fixing our focus: training attention to regulate emotion. Pers Soc Psychol Rev. 2010;15:75–102.

13. Lutz A, Brefczynski-Lewis J, Johnstone T, Davidson RJ. Regulation of the neural circuitry of emotion by compassion meditation: effects of meditative expertise. PLoS One. 2008;e1897.
14. Rushton CH, Kaszniak AW, Halifax JS. Addressing moral distress: application of a framework to palliative care practice. J Palliat Med. 2013;16:1080–1088.
15. Farb NA, Segal ZV, Mayberg H, Bean J, McKeon D, Fatima Z, et al. Attending to the present: mindfulness meditation reveals distinct neural modes of self-reference. Soc Cogn Affect Neurosci. 2007;2:313–322.
16. Goleman D, Lippincott M. Without emotional intelligence, mindfulness doesn't work. Harv Bus Rev. Sep 8, 2017. https://hbr.org/2017/09/sgc-what-really-makes-mindfulness-work.
17. Condon P, Desbordes G, Miller WB, DeSteno D. Meditation increases compassionate responses to suffering. Psychol Sci. 2013;24:2125–2127.
18. Weng HY, Fox AS, Shackman AJ, Stodola DE, Caldwell JZ, Olson MC, et al. Compassion training alters altruism and neural responses to suffering. Psychol Sci. 2013;24:1171–1180.
19. Garland EL, Farb NA, Golden P, Fredrickson BL. Mindfulness broadens awareness and builds eudaimonic meaning: a process model of mindful positive emotion regulation. Psychol Inq. 2015;26:293–314.
20. Epstein RM. Mindful practice. JAMA. 1999;282:833–839.
21. Ludwig DS, Kabat-Zinn J. Mindfulness in medicine. JAMA. 2008;300:1350–1352.
22. Smith SA. Mindfulness-based stress reduction: an intervention to enhance the effectiveness of nurses' coping with work-related stress. Int J Nurs Knowl. 2014;25:119–130.
23. Cohen-Katz J, Wiley SD, Capuano T, Baker DM, Shapiro S. The effects of mindfulness-based stress reduction on nurse stress and burnout: a quantitative and qualitative study. Holist Nurs Pract. 2004;18:302–308.
24. Farb N, Daubenmier J, Price CJ, Gard T, Kerr C, Dunn BD, et al. Interoception, contemplative practice, and health. Front Psychol. 2015;6:763.
25. Price CJ, Hooven C. Interoceptive awareness skills for emotion regulation: theory and approach of Mindful Awareness in Body-Oriented Therapy (MABT). Front. Psychol. 2018; 9:798. .
26. Donald JN, Atkins PWB, Parker PD, Christie AM, Ryan RM. Daily stress and the benefits of mindfulness: Examining the daily and longitudinal relations between present-moment awareness and stress responses. J Res Personality. 2016; 65: 30–37
27. Hadash Y, Ruimi L, Bernstein A. (2023). Looking inside the black box of mindfulness meditation: investigating attention and awareness during meditation using the mindful awareness task (MAT). Psychological Assessment, 2023;35:242–256.

28. Taylor SE, Klein LC, Lewis BP, Gruenewald TL, Gurung RA, Updegraff JA. Biobehavioral responses to stress in females: tend-and-befriend, not fight-or-flight. Psychol Rev. 2000;107:411–429.
29. Levy KN, Hlay JK, Johnson BN, Witmer C. An attachment theoretical perspective on tend-and-befriend stress reactions. Evol Psycho Sci. 2019;5:426–439.
30. Bakal D. Minding the body: clinical uses of somatic awareness. New York: Guilford Press; 2001.
31. Rushton CH, Kaszniak AW, Halifax JS. Addressing moral distress: application of a framework to palliative care practice. J Palliat Med. 2013;16:1080–1088.
32. Eisenberg N, Eggum ND, Di Giunta L. Empathy-related responding: associations with prosocial behavior, aggression, and intergroup relations. Soc Issues Policy Rev. 2010;4:143–180.
33. Ogden P, Minton K, Pain C. Hierarchical information processing: cognitive, emotional, and sensorimotor dimensions. In Ogden P, Minton K, Pain C, editors, Trauma and the body: a sensorimotor approach to psychotherapy. New York: WW Norton; 2009: 3–23.
34. van der Kolk B. The body keeps the score: brain, mind, and body in the healing of trauma. New York: Penguin Books; 2015.
35. Gentsch A, Kuehn E. Clinical manifestations of body memories: the impact of past bodily experiences on mental health. Brain Sci. 2022;12:594.
36. Epstein EG, Hamric AB. Moral distress, moral residue, and the crescendo effect. J Clin Ethics. 2009;20:330–342.
37. Webster GC, Baylis FE. Moral residue. In Rubin SB, Zoloth L, editors, Margin of error: the ethics of mistakes in the practice of medicine. Hagerstown, MD: University Publishing Group; 2000:17–230.
38. Siegel DJ. The developing mind: how relationships and the brain interact to shape who we are. 2nd ed. New York: Guilford Press; 2015.
39. Fazio LK. Pausing to consider why a headline is true or false can help reduce the sharing of false news. Harv Ken Sch Misinfo Rev. 2020;1:2.
40. Robinson MD, Wilkowski BM. Personality processes in anger and reactive aggression: an introduction. J Personality. 2010;78:1–8
41. Yanguas J, Pinazo-Henandis S, Tarazona-Santabalbina FJ. The complexity of loneliness. Acta Biomed. 2018;89:302–314.
42. Belle D. Poverty and women's mental health. Am Psychol. 1990;45:385–389.
43. Dimitroff SJ, Kardan O, Necka EA, Decety J, Berman MG, Norman GJ. Physiological dynamics of stress contagion. Sci Rep. 2017;7:6168.
44. Fredrickson BL. The broaden-and-build theory of positive emotions. Philos Trans Royal Soc Lond B Biol Sci. 2004;359:1367–1377.
45. Hanson R. Buddha's brain: the practical neuroscience of happiness, love and wisdom. Oakland, CA: New Harbinger; 2009.

46. Rozin P, Royzman EB. Negativity bias, negativity dominance, and contagion. Pers Soc Psychol Rev. 2001;5:296–320.
47. Frederickson BL. Positivity. Oxford: Oneworld; 2009.
48. Major BC, Le Nguyen KD, Lundberg KB, Fredrickson BL. Well-being correlates of perceived positivity resonance: evidence from trait and episode-level assessments. Pers Soc Psychol Bull. 2018;44:1631–1647
49. Kaszniak AW, Rushton CH, Halifax J. Leadership, morality and ethics: Developing a practical model for moral decision-making. MindRxiv. April 17, 2018. mindrxiv.org/8qby6. doi:10.17605/OSF.IO/8QBY6.
50. Carse A, Rushton CH. Harnessing the promise of moral distress: a call for re-orientation. J Clin Ethics. 2017;28:15–29.
51. Jazaieri H, Lee IA, McGonigal K, Jinpa T, Doty JR, Gross JJ, et al. A wandering mind is a less caring mind: daily experience sampling during compassion meditation training. J Posit Psychol. 2016;11:37–50.
52. Segal ZV, Williams JM, Teasdale JD. Mindfulness-based cognitive therapy for depression. New York: Guilford Press; 2002.
53. Roemer L, Williston SK, Rollins LG. Mindfulness and emotion regulation. Curr Opin in Psych. 2015;3:52–57. ISSN 2352-250X,
54. Decety J. A social cognitive neuroscience model of human empathy. In Harmon-Jones E, Winkielman P, editors, Social neuroscience: integrating biological and psychological explanations of social behavior. New York: Guilford Press; 2007:246–270.
55. Stevens F, Taber K. The neuroscience of empathy and compassion in pro-social behavior. Neuropsychologia. 2021;159:107925.
56. Ruedy NE, Schweitzer ME. In the moment: the effects of mindfulness on ethical decision making. J Bus Ethics. 2010;95:73–87.
57. Kriakous SA, Elliott KA, Lamers C, Owen R. The effectiveness of mindfulness-based stress reduction on the psychological functioning of healthcare professionals: a systematic review. Mindfulness. 2021;12:1–28.
58. Frankl V. Stimulus/response: alleged quote. Vienna: Viktor Frankl Institut; n.d. www.viktorfrankl.org/e/quote_stimulus.html.
59. Parson NC, Wurtz HM, Lowrey M, Santos, CC, "Life will go on with the beauty of the roses": the moral dimensions of coping with distress through autobiographical writing during Covid-19. SSM - Mental Health. 2022;2:100156. ISSN 2666-5603.
60. Teshome BG, Desai MM, Gross C P, Hill KA, Li F, Samuels E A, et al. Marginalized identities, mistreatment, discrimination, and burnout among US medical students: cross sectional survey and retrospective cohort study. BMJ. 2022; 376:e065984 .
61. Newman A, Le H, North-Samardzic A, Cohen M. 2020. Moral disengagement at work: a review and research agenda. J Bus Eth. 2020;167: 535–570.

62. Bandura, A. Moral disengagement: how people do harm and live with themselves. New York: Worth; 2016.
63. Rushton CH. Ethical discernment and action: the art of pause. AACN Adv Crit Care. 2009;20:108–111.
64. Fetters MD, Churchill L, Danis M. Conflict resolution at the end of life. Crit Care Med. 2001;29:921–925.
65. Back AL, Bauer-Wu SM, Rushton CH, Halifax J. Compassionate silence in the patient–clinician encounter: a contemplative approach. J Palliat Med. 2009;12:1113–1117.
66. Singer T, Lamm C. The social neuroscience of empathy. Ann NY Acad Sci. 2009;1156:81–96.
67. Marsh AA. The neuroscience of empathy. CurrOpin Behav Sci. 2018;19:110–115.
68. Lamm C, Batson CD, Decety J. The neural substrate of human empathy: effects of perspective-taking and cognitive appraisal. J Cogn Neurosci. 2007;19:42–58.
69. Teper R, Segal Z V, Inzlicht M. Inside the mindful mind: how mindfulness enhances emotion regulation through improvements in executive control. Curr Direct iPsych Scie, 2013;22: 449–454.
70. Halifax J. The precious necessity of compassion. J Pain Symp Manage. 2001;41:146–153.
71. Holtz H, Heinze K, Rushton C. Inter-professionals' definitions of moral resilience. J Clin Nurs. 2017, 27(3-4):e488–e494
72. Rest JR. Background: theory and research. In Rest JR, Narváez D, editors, Moral development in the professions: psychology and applied ethics. Hillsdale, NJ: Lawrence Erlbaum; 1994:22–26.
73. Rushton CH, Penticuff JH. A framework for analysis of ethical dilemmas in critical care nursing. AACN Adv Crit Care. 2007;18:323–328.
74. Beauchamp TL, Childress JF. Principles of biomedical ethics. 8th ed. New York: Oxford University Press; 2019.
75. Austin W. The ethics of everyday practice: healthcare environments as moral communities. Adv Nurs Sci. 2007;30:81–88.
76. Taylor, CR. Everyday nursing concerns: unique? trivial? or essential to healthcare ethics? HEC Forum. 1997;9:68–84.
77. Walker MU. Moral contexts. Lanham, MD: Rowman & Littlefield; 2003.
78. Gallagher A. The teaching of nursing ethics: content and method. In Davis A, Tschudin V, De Raeve L, editors, Essentials of teaching and learning in nursing ethics: perspectives and methods. London: Churchill Livingstone; 2006:223–229.
79. Walker MU. Moral repair: reconstructing moral relations after wrongdoing. New York: Cambridge University Press; 2006.
80. Lederach JP. The moral imagination: the art and soul of building peace. New York: Oxford University Press; 2005.

81. Morton KR, Worthley, JS, Testerman JK, Mahoney ML, Defining features of moral sensitivity and moral motivation: pathways to moral reasoning in medical students. J Moral Ed 2006;35:387–406.
82. Milliken A. Nurse ethical sensitivity: an integrative review. Nurs Ethics. May 2018;25(3):278–303
83. Kross E, Grossman I. Boosting wisdom: distance from the self enhances wise reasoning, attitudes, and behavior. J Exp Psychol Gen. 2012;141:43–48.
84. Eisenberg N, Eggum ND. Empathic responding: sympathy and personal distress. In Decety J, Ickes W, editors, The social psychology of empathy. Cambridge, MA: MIT Press; 2009:71–83.
85. Klerk J. Nobody is as blind as those who cannot bear to see: psychoanalytic perspectives on the management of emotions and moral blindness. J Bus Ethics. 2017;141:745–761.
86. Nathaniel A. Moral distress among nurses. American Nurses Association: Ethics and Human Rights Issues Updates. 2002;1:3–8.
87. Halfon MS. Integrity: a philosophical inquiry. Philadelphia, PA: Temple University Press; 1989.
88. Tessman L. Moral failure: on the impossible demands of morality. New York: Oxford University Press; 2015.
89. Rodney P, Kadychuk S, Liaschenko J, Brown H, Musto L, Snyder N. Moral agency: relational connections and support. In Storch JL, Rodney P, Starzomski R, editors, Toward a moral horizon: nursing ethics for leadership and practice. Toronto, Canada: Pearson; 2013:160–187.
90. Rushton CH. Moral resilience: a capacity for navigating moral distress in critical care. AACN Adv Crit Care. 2016;27:111–119.
91. Perlo J, Balik B, Swensen S, Kabcenell A, Landsman J, Feeley D. IHI framework for improving joy in work. Cambridge, MA: Institute for Healthcare Improvement; 2017. http://www.ihi.org/resources/Pages/IHIWhitePapers/Framework-Improving-Joy-in-Work.aspx.
92. Thomas TA, McCullough LB. A philosophical taxonomy of ethically significant moral distress. J Med Philos. 2015;40:102–120.
93. Gazelle G, Liebschutz JM, Riess H. Physician burnout: coaching a way out. J Gen Intern Med. 2014;30:508–513.
94. National Academies of Sciences, Engineering, and Medicine. Taking action against clinician burnout: a systems approach to professional well-being. Washington, DC: National Academies Press (US); 2019: chapter 4, Factors contributing to clinician burnout and professional well-being. Available at https://www.ncbi.nlm.nih.gov/books/NBK552615/.
95. Kenrick DT, Griskevicius V, Neuberg SL, Schaller M. Renovating the pyramid of needs: contemporary extensions built upon ancient foundations. Perspect Psychol Sci. 2010;5:292–314.
96. Maslow AH. A theory of human motivation. Psychol Rev. 1943;50:370–396.

97. American Nurses Association. Code of ethics for nurses with interpretive statements. Silver Spring, MD: ANA; 2015.
98. Nowinski J, Baker S, Carroll K. HALT (hungry, angry, lonely, tired). In Mattson ME, editor, Twelve step facilitation therapy manual. Mansfield Center, CT: National Institute on Alcohol Abuse and Alcoholism, National Institutes of Health; 1999:79–86.
99. Williamson AM, Feyer AM. Moderate sleep deprivation produces impairments in cognitive and motor performance equivalent to legally prescribed levels of alcohol intoxication. Occup Environ Med. 2001;57:649–655.

8

Strategies to Restore Integrity

Cynda Hylton Rushton

PRESERVING OUR INTEGRITY is the fundamental goal of responding to violations of our ethical standards and ideals. Being in alignment with our integrity is a process of becoming integrated, deeply connected to our own moral compass and foundational moral commitments so that we have the ground upon which to stand and from which to navigate the complexities of life—to assess, listen, reassess, and act clearly. The process of integrity-preserving action involves body, heart, and mind to inform discernment and action. Mindfulness practices can assist in clearing the mind of distractions and calming the nervous system so that we can perceive ourselves or the situation more clearly. All of us, as human beings, are continually subject to lapses of integrity. Despite our best efforts, we are all vulnerable under certain circumstances. Myriad conditions can contribute to acting in ways contrary to our moral commitments and moral core. This includes circumstances that simultaneously imperil our professional Codes of Ethics. Being aware of these conditions is vital in taking steps to protect against lapses and preserve moral wholeness.

Heed the Call of Conscience

At its core, moral suffering and the signals it sends are the expression "of conscientious moral concern, of fidelity to moral commitments that are seen as imperiled or compromised."[1] It is a troubled call of conscience. Heeding this call under conditions of moral pressure and constraint or uncertainty, conflict, or confusion[2] requires being able to stand for, and

Cynda Hylton Rushton, *Strategies to Restore Integrity* In: *Moral Resilience*. Second Edition.
Edited by: Cynda Hylton Rushton, Oxford University Press. © Oxford University Press 2024.
DOI: 10.1093/oso/9780197667149.003.0009

give voice to, one's commitments and values. Responding to the call of conscience requires discernment to determine whether or when to act and the degree of resistance, acquiescence, or protest to engage in if there is persistent disagreement or if one's own position is not realized.[1] Heeding the call of conscience empowers clinicians to embrace their commitment to be faithful to their personal and professional values and ideals while acknowledging the real challenges of power, voice, and psychological resilience within the organizations where they practice.

The signals of moral stress or the various forms of moral suffering must be understood as a call of conscience, a state of moral apprehension and responsiveness.[1] One must be attuned to that aspect of oneself that evaluates one's own motivations and actions and engenders emotions of dignity or shame or a sense of wholeness or distress—one's sense of conscience. As described earlier, the pathways for recognizing the engagement of conscience involve activation of the autonomic nervous system and the unconscious memory residing in the body. They involve connecting to the physical, emotional, and mental dimensions of conscience and noticing the patterns of responses—muted, angry, numbed, dismissive, cynical, aggressive, "routinized," and so on. Cultivating awareness of the body's signals of alignment or threats to integrity opens an important avenue that alerts one to an occasion for discernment into the meaning and significance of the signals of conscience.

Conformity to ethical values or commitments preserves wholesomeness, engenders feelings such as contentment, honor, and self-respect, and leads to their embodiment reflecting intentions and integrity-preserving ethical action. In contrast, conflicts of conscience occur in response to the perception of conflicting ethical demands without a clear path to resolution, one that does not compromise fundamental values or integrity. The perception of dissonance in one's values and actions often contribute to feelings of powerlessness, a common feature of moral suffering. When one's ethical perception or conscience is activated, emotions become aroused in response to a negative or positive appraisal of the situation as aligned with one's convictions, values, or internalized norms.[3,4] When one acts contrary to one's ethical values or when integrity is compromised, feelings of remorse, guilt, self-disgust, humiliation, shame, regret, or moral outrage may occur, instigating self-focused actions aimed at relieving personal and/or moral distress. Moral outrage may be the appropriate response to unethical or capricious actions; however, if ungrounded and unconscious, it can become a vehicle for detrimental actions that ultimately threaten other core values or relationships, or cause collateral or unintended consequences[5] Some have suggested that moral outrage may, in some circumstances, be self-serving as a means for broadcasting one's position or to elevate one's character or identity as a righteous or trustworthy person.[6]

Mediating conflicts of conscience, when there are two competing moral demands, requires acknowledging that neither one can be met without a partial rejection of the other. The unmet obligation remains present even when the other is prioritized as the path that, all things considered, upholds integrity to the greatest extent or causes the "least worst" consequences. In such instances, consensus regarding the facts, values, or moral analysis is often absent, and constraints or pressures compelling the decision are common. Seldom clear-cut, such situations tend to be punctuated by uncertainty or doubt about whether one has done the right thing or caused harms that one regrets.[7] Choosing one course of action over another in clinically challenging situations creates a moral residue of regret or guilt. While this is inevitable under such conditions, construing it as a signal of compromised integrity can undermine acknowledgment of one's conscientious effort and diligence to bring about the best outcome in a complex ethical context. The moral residue involved in moral distress, for example, has been viewed as the accumulation over time of negative emotions associated with allowing one's integrity to be compromised.[8,9] Moral residue in this sense is predicated on the belief that one has participated in a moral wrong because a morally desirable option was available but not acted upon.[5] While this may be the case in some instances, it can obscure the reality that even when we have done our best, there may be residual negative feelings that we associate with it. Such realities may be unavoidable given the complexity of making ethical decisions in clinical practice. Morley and Ives make the important distinction that "finding an ethical resolution is not the same as personal satisfaction or personal resolution."[7(p388)] They propose that accepting the feelings of guilt and regret associated with moral residue as fundamental to being a moral agent may "ultimately mitigate . . . the accumulation of negative emotions and moral distress."[7(p388)] In these instances, accepting the reality of the situation does not necessarily imply agreement with the choice or the outcome. It can signify a realistic appraisal of the situation and its constraints and limitations.

Failure to acknowledge the consequences of moral trade-offs can ultimately erode integrity. For the person whose decision prevails, self-righteous or arrogant confidence in its defense can become an insidious process, dampening moral sensitivity and character. Integrity can also be eroded for the people who hold an opposing view or prioritize values differently, when they recoil in response to the assertion of a "right" answer to an inherently complex problem. In both instances, acknowledging and appreciating the moral residue is vital to preserving integrity through a process of moral repair. Violations of integrity and conscience invite a range of responses:

> (1) finding a compromise that preserves integrity particularly when there is factual confusion, uncertainty, conceptual ambiguity, and moral complexity;[10] (2) raising a conscientious voice to bring awareness to or criticize a practice or violation of an ethical standard; (3) refusing to participate on the basis of conscience violations; (4) responsible whistle-blowing arising from clarity, non-reaction, and ethical resolve rather than anger and retaliation; and (5) conscientious exiting from institutions or situations where isolated or repeated instances that result in moral distress or outage are unaddressed, unresolved, or continue to compromise integrity.[5(p85)]

Explore Moral Compromise

As discussed in Chapter 4, we live out our values, commitments, and character within a web of relationships to others who are affected by them directly or indirectly. Relational integrity requires balance, accommodation, and compromise to find solutions that serve the interests of others while recognizing that there are legitimate limits to doing so. Moral compromise involves a modification or re-interpretation of a moral principle or ideal in a particular circumstance, which includes the possibility of acting in opposition to a moral consideration that arises from one's values, commitments, or character.[10] When there is factual confusion, uncertainty, conceptual ambiguity, and moral complexity, moral compromise is a legitimate response. In some situations, there is a genuine range of ethically permissible options and a path forward that creates space for all perspectives.[10] Such a path can leave no one diminished and disregard no one's fundamental integrity, although it may require conscious re-configuration. Moral compromise may be considered under conditions of scarcity, when moral complexity involves pragmatic choices, or in situations where reasonable people disagree. Professional duty and self-interest, for example, may be in conflict with broader notions of fairness or equity.

Winslow and Winslow[10] propose that integrity-preserving compromise involves four elements: (1) sharing a common moral language that illuminates areas of conceptual, factual, semantic, or moral understanding and interpretation; (2) mutual respect as demonstrated in intent, process, structure, communication, and so on; (3) humility, "honest acknowledgement of moral perplexity," and complexity, including the limits of moral certainty; and (4) defining legitimate limits of compromise in non-coercive processes, and agreeing that there are limits to certitude of facts, concepts, or legitimacy of moral claims. They propose that it is possible to avoid intractable conflict or inaction when the process is enacted with mutual respect and understanding. Finding an integrity-preserving path amid moral uncertainty, conflict, or ambiguity means that all parties must be willing to make reasonable concessions to preserve the integrity of all.[10(309–317)] Central to this process is determining what each person affected by the decision can live with, respecting what is sincerely vital for their wholeness.

Compromise in this sense does not suggest that people will necessarily be convinced by the justification of another's perspective or that they will fully abandon their own. Rather, the goal is to respect, more fully understand, and accept the differing point of view of others. Acceptance of others' views and reasons does not imply agreement but rather a willingness to concede in certain ways to avoid intractable conflict, paralysis, or inaction. Through this process, with all things considered, the permissible trade-offs can be acknowledged, and the people involved can find a path that is imperfect but acceptable.

Rarely do we achieve sustained moral harmony. Nor should we pursue harmony through creating moral chaos by attempting to avoid or suppress divergent points of view or demand conformity. Moral compromises can also come to constitute forms of self-betrayal. Morally hostile environments increase the likelihood of self-betrayal when we are insufficiently attuned to the contours of our own values and commitments and when such factors as avoiding conflict or pressure to conform distract us from pursuing integrity-preserving compromise. To create an environment where integrity is upheld to the greatest extent possible for everyone, deliberate practices are needed. At an organizational level, moral compromise can be supported through processes and structures that create accountability for decision makers. Daniels and Sabin[11] have proposed four principles:

1. *The process is public and transparent.* The decision-making process and the reasons for decisions are openly shared in a trustworthy manner.
2. *Relevant reasons are mutually agreed upon.* To the extent possible, all stakeholders who will be affected by a decision give input into determining the range of relevant reasons that should be considered. While it is unlikely that everyone's views will be reflected in the final decision, it is still possible to respect the justification or reasons for different courses of action without abandoning one's own values.
3. *Decisions are revisable.* As understanding, knowledge, and evidence evolve, decisions should be reconsidered using a systematic process to consider their implications and potentially revise decisions.
4. *There are enforcement mechanisms.* A systematic institutional due process that reflects the desired norms, includes a forum in which contrary points of view can be heard, considered, or acted upon, and establishes a consistent range of enforcement responses.

Elements of these principles have been proposed as guides for ethics consultation, especially in addressing clinical cases involving medically ineffective treatment.[12] Taken together, a process for understanding the complexity and nuance of clinical and organizational decisions contributes to an infrastructure that fosters integrity-preserving compromise.

Give Voice to Moral Adversity

Clinicians often experience a call of conscience that leads them to give voice to their experience of threatened integrity, sometimes by expressing protests of varying content and intensity.[1] Perceived lapses of integrity or conscience violations can be expressed in a variety of ways. For example:

- *"They (patients, families, surrogates) want us to DO EVERYTHING!"*
- *"They (doctors, legal, ethics committee, policy, or regulators) are making us do what we believe compromises our conscience." Or "They are keeping us from doing what we believe to be correct."*
- *"I can't stand to witness the patient's suffering anymore."*
- "They *don't care." (This could be directed at a particular patient, family member, clinical discipline, leader, or the entire organization.)*
- *"It's no use! Nothing ever changes around here."*
- *"It's FUTILE!"*

Most often such protests are communicated using the familiar refrain "*Why are we doing this?*" Or "*No one listens!*" And rarely do we express such phrases with curiosity; most often we use a tone of indignation, disgust, and anger directed toward individuals (patient, family, clinician, leader) or groups (families, clinical teams, organizations). When clinicians voice this refrain as a form of protest reflecting moral outrage, what is deeply at stake is their integrity, giving rise to searing questions: *"Do I see myself as a person of integrity? Am I fulfilling the ethical mandates of my profession?"* As their distress and discomfort escalate, clinicians express their laments as wanting things to be different, hoping for a different outcome. Feeling frustrated or helpless, they may view their ongoing efforts to preserve their integrity as futile given their participation in actions that threaten or violate their personal or professional values or integrity (outlined in Chapter 2). Along with this, they may also experience guilt or regret that they have betrayed their patients and themselves because they have been ineffective in bringing about results that reflect their character and values.

When voiced, such protests do not, in and of themselves, protect or restore clinicians' integrity. The protests may continue without meaningful shifts in conversation or action at the individual, collective, or systemic levels. When voiced repeatedly, such protests too often reveal that their concerns are not being addressed or adequately resolved.[1] Their language reflects their fears and illuminates the depth of moral compromise or threat they are experiencing. In situations where their ability to respond to constraints is limited, mounting distress or systemic pressures may put clinicians at risk of acting counter to their personal and professional values. In these instances, acting with integrity requires recognizing threats or violations of integrity, raising concerns through protest, and pursuing deliberate and principled action to bring about the result that reflects the most favorable alignment of essential values. But even with such efforts, clinicians may simultaneously confront the very real systemic constraints and obstacles that contribute to pressure, despair, and resistance to doing the right thing and thwart the preservation or restoration of their integrity.

Finding common phrases inadequate to convey their concerns, some clinicians struggle to find expressions of their concerns in ways that are socially and professionally acceptable. They may not be able to articulate their moral concerns or to do so in a way that is congruent with their professional norms. Their perpetual protests are not enough to ensure effectiveness in addressing the concerns and may result in intensified denial or dismissiveness. If the reality of clinician suffering is unacknowledged or the culture criticizes or ostracizes those who speak about their own suffering, the expressions may instead focus on the suffering of the patient or family or the systemic constraints rather than acknowledging one's own suffering.

For example, clinicians caring for a neurologically devastated patient with minimal brain stem function may lament that the treatments being delivered are causing the patient to suffer. Whether the patient can actually be harmed or benefited in such circumstances remains debatable: since suffering requires the ability to perceive it, patients in such states may not actually be able to perceive the suffering that is associated with medical or nursing procedures or treatments.[13] Instead, what may be operating is a sense that the treatment itself is harming the dignity of the person rather than physically causing pain or suffering that the patient is able to perceive. Participating in such actions, especially when they appear senseless, challenges the core values and integrity of the clinicians providing treatment. But instead of speaking directly about their own suffering, which they may feel is professionally unacceptable, clinicians may shift the focus of their lament to concerns about the patient or family or the policies they perceive to constrain their choices. Blame and resentment often follow.

Such patterns of protest and the narratives that accompany them may obscure the very real suffering of those administering treatments. Externalizing the source of their distress may foster an alternative narrative but fail to acknowledge the individual suffering or its consequences. It may also reflect an orientation to "moral residue as a failure to reconcile the irreconcilable rather than a failure of moral character or a sign that one is an incompetent moral agent."[9(p220)] Patterns such as these may also signal deep systemic fractures in the practice environment that contribute to the real or perceived constraints on clinicians' authentic expression of their experience and accompanying suffering. Harnessing the collective lament as a signal of imperiled integrity arising from systemic failures that create moral adversity is one of the potential benefits of perceiving our moral suffering and using it to fuel principled and non-reactive action.

Speak Up with Clarity

Cultivating a clear and compelling voice is vital for clinicians to overcome moral adversity. "Having a voice—being able to assert appraisals, raise concern, protest meaningfully, with background trust that one's perspective counts and can have an impact—is crucial to overcoming the sense of moral powerlessness and isolation so often tied to moral distress."[1(p23)] However, because the risk remains that the ethical concerns clinicians articulate may be discounted and dismissed as personal laments or complaints, it is important to create safe environments where clinicians can "give voice to conscience in meaningful ways . . . as a call or appeal to others with whom they hope to achieve greater shared moral understanding and alignment in practice."[1(p24)] Heard in this context, expressions of moral adversity enter into "the space of reason," where they can be "contested, debated, emended, checked against others' perceptions and perspectives."[1(p24)] This sort of rigorous examination allows for validation, affirmation, and at times correction.

Likewise, discernment in monitoring the tone and content of discussions about the situation—recognizing signs of self-righteous indignation, overstatements, or exaggerations of facts or values—is vital in assessing the willingness of those involved to consider other points of view or to cooperate or collaborate.[5] We should ask ourselves what we must do to stand up and speak with integrity, starting with *"What are my intentions in sharing my perspective? How will my values be visible in my words or actions?"* and moving on to *"What choices are possible? What can be done, all things considered?" "What objections may be raised about my perspective?" Is there a space for integrity-preserving compromise? Am I voicing my concerns with confidence and integrity?"* Pausing to create space to explore such questions before responding invites greater clarity and insight.

Adopt Strategies for Response and Repair

Morally resilient clinicians can cultivate their capacities for recognizing the signals of moral stress, distress, or injury before they become full-blown. With greater mindful awareness, clinicians can be more proactive in noticing the signals of dysregulation, depletion, and distress and in developing the moral/ethical efficacy they need to cultivate moral resilience.

Research suggests that when we focus on the impact of the situation on ourselves, we are more likely to experience empathic over-arousal and distress and expend our energy to relieve our own distress.[14,15,16] In contrast, taking the perspective of the other person tends to modulate empathic arousal and shift the focus to those steps that will serve both ourselves and the other person.[16] The capacities for mindfulness, awareness, self-regulation, and moral efficacy allow us to respond to threatening situations and reduce negative consequences to ourselves and others. Individual strategies can help us remain grounded and whole amid whatever moral adversity arises in our clinical practice. Strategies to support these capacities are outlined in Chapter 7.

Be Resolute with Properly Bounded Courage

Being morally courageous is the ability to translate our intentions, values, and behaviors into integrity-preserving action. It connects us to our heartfelt wisdom of who we essentially are and how we embody our true nature and manifest that sensibility amid conflict and confusion or threats to integrity. Arguably both a virtue and a way of being that can be intentionally cultivated, moral courage is a necessary component of integrity and propels us toward wholeness amid moral adversity.[17] Courage is needed when honest conversation about clinical concerns is met with ridicule, indifference, or dismissiveness. It takes courage to speak up about a medical error when it would be easier to remain silent. Being courageous means overcoming our tendency to rationalize (*"No one else is doing anything about it, so why should I?"*) or justify our actions or lack of action (*"Just let it slide"*). It also involves overcoming our attachment to our own positions so we can remain silent and listen to the perspectives of others. Alternatively, courage is required to remain silent when our words or actions may produce temporary benefit but cause longer-term harms to others or ourselves. Moral courage invites us to transcend the apathy, cynicism, complacency, and fear that accompany complex ethical challenges. It asks us to decide not to participate in gossip, bullying, or taking credit for the accomplishments of others and to be willing to mindfully revise or let go of our position or agenda to serve a higher purpose.

Moral courage is defined as "the voluntary willingness to stand up for and act on one's ethical beliefs despite barriers that may inhibit the ability to proceed toward right action."[18(p1431)] It engages a robust notion of moral agency predicated on the motivation to act with integrity while discerning the relevance of diverse values and commitments that inform principled action. Moral courage engages our confidence to act wisely in accordance with our values and commitments by overcoming our fears, persevering, and withstanding difficulty despite risks; it is a willingness to go beyond "compliance" or maintaining the status quo to wisely enact decisions that serve the highest ethical values or commitments.[19]

Being morally courageous does not imply an expectation of sustained heroic action, particularly when circumstances are refractory to intervention, it make heroic action a form of self-harm.[20] There is, however, a clear expectation of engagement in determining the boundaries of properly nuanced courage in the context of challenging clinical complexity. This appraisal is rarely static. In some instances, one may choose to exercise courageous action in high-risk situations; in others, discernment may temper the contours and expectations of moral courage. Moral efficacy includes a well-honed moral imagination and the ability to discern and act upon what is required—and to determine the threshold of effort to bring about a shift in awareness or action that is necessary to preserve integrity. Without cultivating moral courage or what Joan Didion called "moral nerve" (the non-negotiable virtue when standing above the abyss of harm),[21(p145)] we risk lapsing into moral apathy, disengagement, or cynicism.[22] Denying the moral issue, or being complicit in the recurring circumstances that create it, renders intermittent courageous actions by individuals within a system impotent in redressing its root causes.

Cultivating moral courage requires us to recognize an occasion for moral action and to sustain our effort to restore or preserve personal or relational integrity. It requires us to listen to our call of conscience, that inner knowing that coaxes us toward making integrity-preserving choices by acknowledging our feelings of inadequacy, guilt, or regret and pointing us toward judgments that are in alignment with our highest ideals and moral commitments. When fear is present, naming its source and the nature of ethical conflict can help us to distinguish between a false threat and a real threat that needs to be acted upon. Anne Lamott says, "Courage is fear that has said its prayers."[23(p239)] The call of conscience invites us to befriend our fear and wisely stand up in a principled manner for our core values or principles despite opposition, threats of retaliation, or other negative consequences. It can propel us to take the next step and accept the results even when our effort does not reduce our fear or produce the result we were intending. Being courageous includes taking responsibility for one's choices and actions and their consequences to oneself and others; in egregious circumstances, it also includes the exercise of principled moral outrage or justified exit from recalcitrant and toxic situations or environments.

Like other emergent processes, moral courage can be fostered or undermined by individual and interpersonal factors, culture, and elements of the moral ecosystem where one practices. Creating norms of professional behavior can help clinicians to skillfully discern occasions to exercise their moral courage. Nurses who have had experience speaking up are more likely to address substandard practice by physicians. Dinndorf-Hogenson[24] found that perioperative nurses reported a high degree of moral courage in situational threats to patient safety, while nurses with a higher fear of reprisal were less likely to speak up about safety breaches. As with other elements of moral resilience, individual capability is supported when the work environments are responsive and open and designed to support the exercise of moral courage without negative consequences or retaliation. This includes surveillance mechanisms that detect overt or covert threats or retaliation against those who speak up and accountability structures that address such lapses in ethical behavior.

Acknowledge Our Limitations

Likewise, acknowledging the limitations of our power and influence is vital in preserving our internal resources and leveraging them in realistic and beneficial ways. When we are unable to accept the limits of our role, influence, or authority, our suffering is often intensified. When we use the available resources and pathways for action in ways that reflect our integrity, our conscientiousness is revealed, regardless of whether it brings about the desired result. Frequently, clinicians experience profound suffering when they believe their efforts were for naught because they were unsuccessful in effecting the outcomes they preferred. Noticing when we are "efforting," trying too hard or expending disproportionate effort to bring about our desired result offers an opportunity to pause for inquiry and discernment. Often, we realize that our ethical responsibilities have been at least partially fulfilled by the actions we have taken to articulate the ethical concern, speak up about it, and take various actions aimed at addressing it. Shifting our perspective to acknowledge our contributions in recognizing an occasion for moral action and taking deliberate steps to address it matters from a moral point of view as an act of integrity rather than moral failure. Discounting our efforts by focusing only on situations when our desired outcome prevailed diminishes our moral agency and conscientiousness and ignites patterns of self-judgment and deficiency. Being morally resilient involves being realistic, generous, and forgiving toward our limitations and ourselves, and accepting the inevitability that moral residue is likely to persist when irreconcilable moral trade-offs must be made. While some clinicians may navigate these situations on their own, others will benefit from intensifying personal, professional, and organizational resources to support them when they determine and enact ethical decisions that result in moral residue, uncertainty, ambiguity, or a sense of being persistently unsettled.

Connect to Meaning and Purpose

Meaning involves interpreting an event of moral adversity to discern its significance and inform the narrative that we share about our experiences. As humans, we are oriented to create meaning to explain what is happening or has happened. Meaning provides the background against which we discern the contours and requirements of integrity by connecting us to our intention and purpose. It is a function of the heart that fuels our capacity to connect to our intentions and purposes and to be inspired and motivated by them. By doing so we can create more spaciousness to see things in new ways and to discover possible pathways that have been unseen or undiscovered. When we ground ourselves in our purpose and what we stand for even when fear, resistance, or threats are present, energy and strength are liberated, and we can leverage it toward addressing our moral suffering and finding integrity-preserving solutions. In crisis, it can be the fuel for sustaining engagement and creativity while navigating the treacherous landscape, complete with its ambiguity and uncertainty. As Victor Frankl asserted, having purpose makes adversity bearable and allows us to process and integrate it into our lives rather than be disabled by it.[25]

Each one of us creates our own meaning, individually and socially, in relationship with others. It has relevance to our moral values and commitments, belief systems, experiences, and expectations of ourselves and others. A vehicle for connecting with ourselves, others, and the broader world, it engages past and present experience to forecast the future. Rachel Naomi Remen claims that meaning arises for clinicians through their "service to life, befriending the life in other people and the gratitude for the privilege of 'being with' the full range of human experience."[26]

Consider Alternative Meanings

The significance that moral adversity holds for us is not absolute; we are able to shift the meaning toward narratives that uncover constructive, life-giving alternatives. Exploring these realities within a moral community, can offer safe and brave spaces for clinicians to process their experiences, individually and collectively. In debriefings of ethically challenging and morally distressing situations, clinicians are asked to narrate the meaning of the situation. Consider a case involving prolonged treatment for a patient with a life limiting diagnosis that was punctuated by repeated complications, protracted pain, and despite his requests for continued treatment the medical team concluded that his treatment was medically ineffective. Inevitably, the narrative begins with a detailed story of powerlessness, despair, and often anger. After many moments of bearing witness and acknowledging their experience, they are asked, "*Is there anything about this situation that produced benefit or meaning—for you, the patient, or the family?*" Often in the first moments there is silence; then, with some gentle prodding, another narrative emerges. It often begins with "The patient got what *he* wanted—he wanted to live as long as he could even though we knew he would die." Sometimes clinicians will have insights about themselves or the patient such as, "This patient was a fighter—he never gave up." Then they are asked, "*What did you do that made a difference to this patient?*" Often, nurses describe the meticulous physical care of the patient's body, preventing skin breakdown despite months in the ICU, the moments that they listened to the patient's story late at night, their vigilant attention to the patient's and the family's emotional and spiritual needs, and their unrelenting advocacy to ensure that the patient was kept fully informed. Shifting toward a space of seeing and remembering the difference their care has made offers a pivot point in their interpretation of the experience. Clinicians often carry a heavy burden of responsibility for the outcomes of their efforts. Being realistic about the boundaries of their responsibility and exploring ways to let go of what is not their personal responsibility or to reallocate the responsibility among everyone involved helps to lighten their burden. Discovering an alternative narrative that reveals another perspective that is also true can help clinicians release some of the residue they carry.

Debriefings can also offer alternative meanings and, when skillfully facilitated with a standardized format, provide a safe space for reflection and insight.[27,28] For example, from a physiologic point of view the clinician may be exactly right about the outcome for the patient (the patient was dying), and by not forcing a decision about life-sustaining therapies gave the gift of time to the patient to make sense of their disease and life and for family members to fulfill their promises as spouses, parents, siblings, or children and to create meaning in the midst of grief and sorrow. In some instances, team members can share both positive and negative feedback directly from the patient or family members. Hearing the patient/family experiences, especially the gratitude and appreciation they express even when outcomes they desire do not occur, can help remind clinicians of the benefits of their efforts. Debriefings can also allow clinicians to self-correct, discover underlying contributory factors, reveal gaps in the system, and explore key questions such as *"What can we learn from this case to address the systemic issues that contributed to the distress experienced by the healthcare team? What patterns do we see that offer opportunities for intervention?" "What will we do differently next time?"* Answering these questions allows us to create meaning amid adversity while acknowledging both the positive and negative aspects of the case.

Meaning thus created can connect us as clinicians to why we have chosen our profession and provide us with the grounding and energy we need to continue. This is not unreflective meaning that denies the reality of the situation or of the ethical, clinical, and organizational challenges it entails. Rather, it is insightful, penetrating meaning that supports more realistic expectations of ourselves, our colleagues, the people we serve, and the organizations where we practice—and it provides the energy we need to address gaps in the system that require reforms. While debriefings can offer positive environments for processing difficult emotions and ethically challenging situations, they may not be sufficient to fully heal the distress that clinicians experience.[29,30] Engaging in moral exploration, as in debriefings, can help clinicians navigate cognitive dissonance to find alternative ways to create meaning. They may, for example, encounter new information or viewpoints that contradict what they held to be true or engage self-doubt either because certain truths were withheld or there is a genuine need to reevaluate. To resolve such differences, clinicians of integrity enter a process of discovery, seeking to arrive at a more nuanced understanding of the values, beliefs, or commitments involved. As they consider their colleagues' diverse perspectives, they explore what the situation, with its difficulties, teaches them about themselves and others. Learning through conflict in this way reconnects clinicians with their professional values and basic goodness and restores the integrity essential to their personal and professional well-being.[5]

There are times, however, when our experience of moral adversity creates a sense of meaninglessness—a feeling that it is impossible to construct meaning from the experiences we confront. In the throes of suffering, when it is often difficult to conceive of an alternative narrative or meaning, we must create space to be with our negative feelings without experiencing shame or guilt. Meaning arises when we are ready and able to make the shift.

Engage in Moral Repair

Broadly speaking, "moral repair is restoring or creating trust and hope in a shared sense of value and responsibility."[31(p28)] A variety of methods for moral repair can restore individual integrity, reduce personal distress and moral suffering, and reestablish meaning salience and a sense of wholeness. In the context of clinical practice, the process of moral repair involves interventions aimed at restoring well-being, moral agency, and self-efficacy; cultivating mental and emotional stability; engaging inherent resilience; and enhancing communication, ethical discernment, and discourse. Alignment of various methods requires skillful assessment and design. There is not a "one size fits all" recipe for moral repair, and many times it requires a multi-pronged approach. Rarely are single opportunities sufficient to restore trust and hope when harms have been experienced. Rather, sustained, consistent, and reliable interventions and mechanisms are necessary over time. Walker[31] offers a comprehensive process for designing methods of moral repair that can be applied at the level of individuals and organizations. Discernment is necessary to tailor individual, group, and system interventions to the needs of the clinicians involved and to the root causes of their suffering.

Understand and Engage the Phases of Suffering

As we struggle to repair or mitigate the consequences of moral adversity and suffering, Reich's three phases are useful in organizing the support systems and processes needed to address moral suffering.[32] These three phases are not necessarily linear; individuals may experience different phases of suffering simultaneously or may vacillate or remain in them for varied periods of time. Methods of moral repair must differ for each phase and in response to the unique needs and capabilities of people involved.

Phase 1: Voiceless Suffering

The first phase, voiceless or mute suffering, requires interventions that acknowledge the preconscious, inchoate awareness of distress, anxiety, or negative emotions. While somatic signals may be present, this phase reflects an inability to articulate and communicate one's suffering or even to name it. Miller writes, "Those things about which we cannot speak or will not speak do not simply disappear because we don't discuss them. In fact, they gain some of their power over us because we don't have the language to vent them. They remain crouching in the shadows of our lives, unpredictable, a locus of rage, of despair, of fear, looking for an opportunity to be heard."[33(p21)] Suffering in this way undermines one's autonomy, moral agency, self-esteem, and integrity.

Silence is one response to preconscious suffering. It may reflect denial, avoidance, indifference, or an inability to perceive the signals of our suffering. Reich asserts that this type of suffering is not equated with "suffering in silence" "but of knowing a suffering that reduces one to a silence in which self-disclosure about one's suffering cannot occur."[32(p86)] Unspeakable and unnamed, suffering becomes isolating and lonely. In the absence of language—words, concepts, and practices—to relate what we perceive at a deep and soulful level, responses to suffering vary widely. Biological patterns of disrupted sleep, eating, or physiologic balance may be recognized in response to voiceless suffering. Behavioral patterns reflecting hyperarousal (hypervigilance or irritability) or hypoarousal (depression or exhaustion) may also be present. Addictive patterns may surface or intensify. Affective or emotional expressions of voiceless suffering may manifest in angry outbursts, cynicism, numbness, withdrawal, or sadness. Some clinicians may begin to behave in seemingly unprofessional ways, making jokes about a patient's condition, assigning demeaning nicknames, or depersonalizing and objectifying the patient as no longer a "real" person but rather a "vegetable" or "drug seeker." Other clinicians may engage in overt actions to avoid their suffering by taking aggressive steps to ensure that the patient "doesn't die on my shift" or to distance themselves from situations that are distressing, cause dissonance, or ignite negative emotions. Adopting an attitude of resignation or moral apathy can cause a person to remain immobilized in voiceless suffering. While the nature of one's suffering may not be recognized, becoming preoccupied with its symptoms may prove a distraction from its source. Noticing the subtle cues of voiceless suffering in oneself or others is necessary for moral repair to begin.

While some clinicians withdraw from their patients and colleagues, others behave aggressively. They may construct a wall of defensiveness, demean, or bully others, or become cynical and angry. Their outcries appear to be unrelated to the actual source of their suffering and may be misinterpreted by onlookers, but underneath the behaviors they are an expression of how unspeakable the suffering is. Clinicians may attempt to disguise their suffering by appealing to the comfort of rules and procedures to avoid direct confrontation with their distress. For example, a nurse caring for an elderly woman with dementia at the end of her life refuses to administer opioids to relieve respiratory distress without the addition of a benzodiazepine despite her family's request to allow her to be aware of their presence for as long as possible. While the woman is not agitated, the nurse resists the family's request, perhaps to avoid witnessing the woman's prolonged dying process in favor of a more sanitized death facilitated by the additional medication. Some clinicians may resent others who appear more professionally disengaged or non-reactive, perhaps as a way of distancing themselves from their own uncomfortable feelings. These patterns can result in preoccupation with their suffering as the pain overwhelms other aspects of living and undermines their capacity to exercise their moral agency, develop understanding, or create meaning.[32]

When clinicians cannot express their thoughts and feelings, their suffering becomes voiceless and remains preconscious and inaccessible. In this phase, clinicians cannot articulate their suffering, understand it, discover its meaning, empathize with it, or share their plight with others. This voiceless phase continues until some threshold is achieved and the individual is liberated enough from suffering to discover ways of expressing it.[32] Interventions in this phase focus on identifying more subtle signals of suffering and creating safe, supportive, nonjudgmental spaces for reflection, inquiry, and dialogue. Primarily, a compassionate presence, listening and bearing witness to the experience without consoling or attempting to fix the clinician's suffering, has the potential to invite others into discovering a way forward. To progress out of this phase, the sufferer must believe that change is possible. Creating the conditions for readiness to shift is needed to initiate the process of moral repair. Readiness is a unique process for each person that includes a willingness to step into a new understanding of what has transpired and to experience the reality of it. It has its own timetable and contours that cannot be prescribed or managed but rather invited to emerge.

Phase 2a: Expressive Repair

The second phase of suffering involves the emergence of conscious awareness and the search for language to describe the sources and consequences and communicate about their suffering. The experience of suffering instigates a struggle to discover a voice to express the search for meaning of one's suffering. Initially, the vocabulary to express one's suffering can be quite impoverished, lacking insight or clarity or be animated by strong emotions. For clinicians who elect to share their feelings, suffering that was incomprehensible can come into conscious awareness by talking with others. For clinicians who cannot give voice to their experiences, "creating a container of humble presence and 'invested concern'" may be needed to alleviate their suffering, "despite limits to comprehending its source."[34] Despite efforts to create such spaces, some clinicians still will not be able to articulate their experiences or feel safe enough to share them publicly. Even when language is accessible, the capacities for insight and reflection may be disabled by the degree of suffering clinicians are experiencing and have yet to feel or understand.

Having language to express what has been unspeakable is a potent countermeasure to the fears and anxieties clinicians experience. Language allows us to recount the events, describe what happened, express our thoughts and feelings, and establish a common understanding. Many times, the clinician's first response to suffering is the plaintive lament, "*Why are we doing this?*" or some other phrase repeated more loudly and persistently as the clinician insists on being heard, on being able to understand the rationale for decisions or treatments, or being helped to make sense of a dissonant situation.[1] In voicing their suffering, whether as a lament, protest, or complaint, clinicians frequently offer a narrative of their experience. Relating the story of their suffering can invite them to better understand their experience, to reexamine and reframe it in ways that give it meaning or to provide a new perspective, and perhaps to lessen the anguish it caused. Clinicians sometimes retell exquisitely detailed stories of their moral suffering months or even years after the event. In such instances, telling or retelling the story is a way to deconstruct the experience and to reconstitute it in a way that it makes sense and has meaning.

Phase 2b: The Power of Narrative

In this second phase of expressive suffering, moral repair can take the form of spoken, written, or other expressive techniques that include retelling and at times rehabilitating the well-rehearsed scripts or unexamined narratives we use to describe our ethical conflicts, moral distress, outrage, or injury. These techniques allow us to acknowledge our distress, work with it in a way that allows the painful aspects to be noticed, examined, and released, and reframe the experience more constructively. They represent actual or perceived events with selective detail, involve interpretation, and connect the persons depicted in the story to one another and to the storyteller. Narrative also offers a means of transforming the experience of mute suffering into a form that allows us to more fully embrace it, understand it, and put it into perspective; in some cases, we can create a new story that launches us into a new phase of relationship with our experience.[32] This process is enhanced with a foundation of mindful awareness, patience, and compassion toward the situation and ourselves. These qualities create a foundation that restores moral agency and the person's ability to choose their response and interpretation rather than being held hostage to it.

A narrative can serve a second, equally valuable purpose: it can invite others to affirm our search for meaning of the experience. Having compassionate others share in the exploration of our experience and bear witness to it can fuel our sense of moral agency, diminish isolation, and enable new insights. Although an opportunity for self-reflection and growth exists throughout this process, under some circumstances retelling a story of moral suffering can also lead to re-traumatization. For this reason, skilled facilitators and professionals who can address such circumstances are important to avoid inadvertent, though well-intentioned, harms.[33,34] Using a trauma-informed approach can help mitigate these outcomes with mindful awareness of the diversity of trauma that the people involved may bring to the situation.[35,36]

Expressive writing and journaling can also be useful for processing adverse events and creating meaning and understanding; in some cases we can rewrite the narrative in a way that restores moral agency, releases the residue, and promotes healing.[37] Nurses have been shown to benefit from expressive writing as a means of reducing the effects of job-related stress and traumatic events.[38] Journaling about an adverse event helps to begin a healing process in three ways: (1) exposure to difficult feelings over time eventually renders them less intense and more manageable; (2) cognitive restructuring reduces the angst associated with moral adversity by cultivating new ways to relate to it; and (3) writing down the details can strengthen the ability to self-regulate troubling emotions and reduce their painful residue.[38,39]

Phase 2c: Narrative Repair

Another promising intervention to restore personal and relational integrity involves what has been called "narrative repair."[40] Designed to constructively engage with pervasive narratives that hold individuals or groups captive to often unconscious and oppressive stories about themselves and their identities, narrative repair aims to shift and replace these stories with new narratives or "counter-stories" that demand respect and consideration.

Nelson[40] gives the example of how an oppressive narrative of nurses as being "touchy-feely, emotional, subservient, and nonscientific" can constrain their moral agency and self-worth unless a counter-story that more accurately reflects their role is created to resist that characterization and ultimately repair their imperiled integrity. The first step in the process is to identify the moral, social, and normative fragments that have been woven together to create the oppressive identity and to discern how these fragments have misrepresented individuals or groups. Nelson's example of nurses identified assumptions about the value of gender-related work that discount caring practices and privilege and define medical practice as more scientific and therefore more valuable, and so on. These long-standing patterns were exacerbated during the COVID-19 pandemic as nurses were subject to policies and practices that further undermined their identity and societal contribution despite the significant risks they undertook.[41]

The second step involves retelling the story about an individual or group in such a way that morally relevant details that were suppressed in the original narrative emerge. For Nelson, this takes the form of recasting the role of nurses to include more robust descriptions of their educational preparation, contribution, and value. The goal is to make moral sense of the situation by rewriting the narrative that surrounds it in a way that restores moral agency, self-esteem, and wholeness. Rewriting the nursing narrative following the pandemic, for example, includes re-imagining the fractured social contract to create a social covenant with more realistic and balanced commitments by the public and healthcare organizations.[41] Resisting the dominant narrative, according to Nelson, involves three levels: (1) refusing to adopt it, denying its relevance to one's identity without expectation that others will adopt the counternarrative; (2) repudiation, leveraging self-understanding to oppose others who inappropriately apply the dominant narrative to oneself; and (3) publicly and systematically contesting its validity.

Engaging in a narrative repair process can be particularly useful in restoring relational integrity when the source of the moral distress, outrage, or injury involves interpersonal relationships and a cultural context that has solidified destructive norms, patterns, or policies. It can also be useful in recognizing and understanding the broader societal and cultural patterns that have contributed to moral suffering. In the context of nursing, the assumption that nurses will always do "whatever it takes" to meet the needs of their patients, including sacrificing their health and wellbeing, may offer a path to begin to shift it[42]. (see chapter 9 for further evidence).

In the second phase of suffering, as in the first, it is vital to create opportunities for clinicians to explore their experiences with compassion and respect. Depending on the intensity and context surrounding their moral suffering, clinicians may find individual methods that support their own well-being, or they may opt for group settings facilitated by persons skilled in moral repair. Using mindful awareness to notice and recalibrate in response to the somatic signals of their moral suffering offers clinicians' new skills to support self-regulation when they are confronted with moral adversity. For some, group dialogue may provide the needed insights or motivation to pursue strategies aimed at fostering well-being and moral resilience. For others, group work may involve a variety of techniques to deepen their engagement with their suffering in a way that serves their own unique process. If the moral distress or injury is chronic and intense, clinicians may benefit from guidance from mental health professionals, counselors, or clergy who are skilled in working with clients with varying degrees of distress and diverse manifestations.

Phase 3a: Transformation

In the third phase, transformation of suffering is possible when the act of creating a new meaning brings forth a new identity. This occurs when individual clinicians incorporate the essence of their suffering into their own personal narrative, identity, and character by engaging in a reciprocal and supportive process with compassionate others and with themselves. Transformation does not imply denial or complacency but rather an honest acknowledgement of the moral suffering without hiding the sources and consequences of it. The process can be a vehicle for expanded personal awareness and generosity and compassion toward oneself and others. Building on and deepening the strategies identified for the previous phases of suffering, this third phase may require additional internal and external resources. Continuing to discover meaning in moral suffering by exploring some of the larger existential questions clinicians face adds depth to the process. Reich[32] offers insight into the questions healthcare professionals may need to reflect upon to make sense of both their own suffering and the suffering they witness or inflict upon those they hope to benefit. Making sense of questions such as *"How can I see myself as a healer in the face of profound suffering and death?"* [32] or "How do I forgive those who have hurt or harmed me or whom I have harmed?" offers an opportunity to shift one's narrative and choose a counter-story that more accurately reflects one's intentions, character, and integrity. This is not an easy or rapid process. It may involve cyclical stops and starts or uneven progress that evolves over time. Throughout the process, sustained compassion, understanding, and support are essential. It may also be necessary to explore methods for responding to the situations that have compromised or violated one's integrity, including a range of ways to address the residue and harm associated with moral suffering and injury. Table 8.1 offers common responses to imperiled integrity that may arise in the moral repair process. Each response offers an opportunity to examine its source and to explore its relevance and potential for releasing the residue of single or accumulated harms or betrayals. Chapters 7, 10 and 11 offer additional guidance.

Phase 3b: Experiential, Council Process

The type of transformation Reich suggests occurs as part of the Upaya Institute's *Being With Dying* professional training program, an eight-day program that examines suffering from a variety of vantage points using

Table 8.1. Potential Responses to Threats or Violations of Integrity

- Accept responsibility for one's part in the situation
- Let go of the offense or violation and release its grip.
- Blame, shame, or reproach the offender(s).
- Turn away: Push those we no longer trust to the margins.
- Demand acknowledgment of responsibility or wrongdoing by others.
- Request apology, repentance, or amends.
- Pardon or excuse.
- Establish the truth and have it recorded.
- Create ways to commemorate the event that precipitated the violation.
- Devise ways to prevent future wrongdoing or lapses of integrity.
- Forgive.

Source: Walker MU. Moral repair: reconstructing moral relations after wrongdoing. New York: Cambridge University Press; 2006 (Adapted)

contemplative practice, inquiry, small group councils, and experiential dialogue.[43] It is offered and evaluated on an ongoing basis. The facilitators of the program have borne witness as many clinicians have discovered new meaning in their own suffering. Often they arrive depleted, despairing, and distressed; by the end of the program, their perspectives on their patients, and their colleagues and their own lives have shifted.[39] With a foundation of mindfulness, participants explore the contours of suffering within the safety and discipline of the council process, where everyone listens wholeheartedly, speaks authentically and from the heart, resists offering commentary or advice, and invites whatever is true to be witnessed and honored.[44] Many participants are able to create new meaning in their work, renew their commitment to their professions, and gain insights and skills to support them in their roles. Some reorient their identity as clinicians by acknowledging their limitations, anger, or numbness. Others recommit to their original intentions for becoming a nurse or a physician or let go of resentments or regrets that no longer serve a useful purpose for them.

Not everyone can transform their suffering into something meaningful, but the possibility is open to clinicians who desire to work with their situations with compassion and dedication. Whether one can do so depend on many factors, such as one's readiness and internal and external resources. Importantly, inviting clinicians into a space of vulnerability requires organizational investment in the resources that support their engagement in such explorations with solidarity in purpose and psychological safety. Mediating factors such as the boundaries of professional roles, organizational culture, the impact of hierarchy, and experience must also be acknowledged and engaged in the healing process.

Throughout the phases of suffering, multi-faceted modalities and processes are vital in creating a container for healing and growth. Innovative public health projects such as Theater of War: Frontline and The Nurse *Antigone* present dramatic readings of ancient Greek plays for diverse audiences—in person and on Zoom—featuring professional actors and choruses of frontline nurses and clinicians to help frame powerful, guided discussions about the unique challenges faced by nurses and other clinicians before, during, and after the COVID-19 pandemic.[45,46] By presenting emotionally charged, ethically complex scenes from ancient plays, the projects create a brave space for open, candid dialogue and reflection, fostering compassion, a renewed sense of community, and positive action.[47] They utilize the power of performance and live storytelling to dissolve hierarchies and generate a shared vocabulary for professional audiences to discuss stigmatized subjects such as the impact of the pandemic on clinicians.[46,48] The Theater of War Productions model does not feel like medicine; yet it is an effective intervention for medical professionals, who are often reluctant to express vulnerability, acknowledge error, or seek resources or support.[46,48] The methodology offers a healthy alternative to standard medical debriefings and creates a dynamic way for clinicians to step back from their professional roles, bear witness to their own experiences, and come together as a community—without having to narrate their trauma—by discussing and interpreting performances of ancient plays.[47] Innovative methods to engage clinicians' moral suffering and open new doorways for healing are an essential component for ethical practice environments.

A Shared Responsibility

Walker[31] proposes that there is a communal responsibility for repairing the relationships, processes, and decisions that imperil integrity and create moral adversity and suffering. These shared responsibilities include creating and upholding ethical standards and having respectful and fair processes in place for addressing violations of them. Embedded in this are processes for ensuring that those who violate them take responsibility and, in some instances, reparative action and for ensuring that the person(s) whose integrity has been imperiled is supported and the violation is validated and if possible repaired. Rebuilding trust and relational integrity will require courageous leadership, patience, and sustained organizational commitment. The mechanisms for organizational intervention are discussed further in Chapters 10 and 11. Further innovation in this area is warranted to align such practices within a culture of ethical practice.

References

1. Carse A, Rushton CH. Harnessing the promise of moral distress: a call for re-orientation. J Clin Ethics. 2017;28:15–29.
2. Morley G, Bradbury-Jones C, Ives J. What is 'moral distress' in nursing? A feminist empirical bioethics study. Nurs Ethics. 2020;27(5):1297–1314.
3. Gross JJ. Antecedent- and response-focused emotion regulation: divergent consequences for experience, expression, and physiology. J Pers Soc Psychol. 1998;74:224–237.

4. Rushton CH, Kaszniak AW, Halifax JS. A framework for understanding moral distress among the inter-professional team. J Palliat Med. 2013;16:1074–1079.
5. Rushton CH. Principled moral outrage: an antidote to moral distress? AACN Adv Crit Care. 2013;24:82–89.
6. Jordan J, Hoffman M, Bloom P, et al. Third-party punishment as a costly signal of trustworthiness. Nature 2016;530: 473–476.
7. Morley G, Ives J. Reflections on how we teach ethics: moral failure in critical care. AACN Adv Crit Care. 2017;28:384–390.
8. Epstein EG, Hamric AB. Moral distress, moral residue, and the crescendo effect. J Clin Ethics. 2009;20:330–342.
9. Webster GC, Baylis FE. Moral residue. In Rubin SB, Zoloth L, editors, Margin of error: the ethics of mistakes in the practice of medicine. Hagerstown, MD: University Publishing Group; 2000: 217–230.
10. Winslow BJ, Winslow GR. Integrity and compromise in nursing ethics. J Med Philos. 1991;16(3):307–323.
11. Daniels N, Sabin JE. Accountability for reasonableness: an update. BMJ (Clinical research ed.). 2008;337:a1850.
12. Bosslet GT, Pope TM, Rubenfeld G, Lo B, Truog R, Rushton C, Curtis JR, Fords DW, Osborne M, Misak C, Au DH, Azoulay E, Brody B, Fahy B, Hall J, Kesecioglu J, Kon AA, Lindell K, White DB. An official ATS/AACN/ACCP/ESICM/SCCM policy statement: responding to requests for potentially inappropriate treatments in intensive care units. Am J Resp and Cri Care Med. 2015;191(11): 1318–1330.
13. Fins JJ, Master MG, Gerber LM, Giacino JT. The minimally conscious state: a diagnosis in search of an epidemiology. Arch Neurol. 2007;64;1400–1405.
14. Eisenberg N, Fabes RA, Murphy B, Karbon M, Maszk P, Smith M, et al. The relations of emotionality and regulation to dispositional and situational empathy-related responding. J Pers Soc Psychol. 1994;66:776–797.
15. Eisenberg N. Distinctions among various modes of empathy related reactions: a matter of importance in humans. Behav Brain Sci. 2002;25:33–34.
16. Lamm C, Batson CD, Decety J. The neural substrate of human empathy: effects of perspective-taking and cognitive appraisal. J Cogn Neurosci. 2007;19:42–58.
17. Lachman VD. Moral courage: a virtue in need of development? MedSurg Nurs. 2007;16:131–133.
18. Martinez W, Bell SK, Etchegaray JM, Lehmann LS. Measuring moral courage for interns and residents: scale development and initial psychometrics. Acad Med. 2016;91:1431–1438.
19. Sekerka LE, Bagozzi RP, Charnigo R. Facing ethical challenges in the workplace: conceptualizing and measuring professional moral courage. J Bus Ethics. 2009;89:565–579.
20. Hamric AB, Arras JD, Mohrmann ME. Must we be courageous? Hastings Cent Rep. 2015;45(3):40–42.

21. Didion J. Slouching towards Bethlehem. New York: Farrar, Straus and Giroux; 1968.
22. Halifax J. Standing at the edge: finding freedom where fear and courage meet. New York: Flatiron Books; 2018.
23. Lamott A. Traveling mercies: some thoughts on faith. New York: Anchor Books; 1999.
24. Dinndorf-Hogenson GA. Moral courage in practice: implications for patient safety. J Nurs Regul. 2015;6:10–16.
25. Frankl VE. Man's search for meaning: an introduction to logotherapy. New York: Simon & Schuster, 1984.
26. Remen RN. The healer's art. n.d. Cited February 10, 2018. www.rachelremen.com/learn/medical-education-work/the-healers-art/.
27. Keene EA, Hutton N, Hall B, Rushton C. Bereavement debriefing sessions: an intervention to support health care professionals in managing their grief after the death of a patient. Pediatr Nurs. 2010;36:185–189.
28. Morley G, Grady C, McCarthy J, Ulrich CM. Covid-19: ethical challenges for nurses. Hastings Center Report. 2020;50(3): 35–39.
29. Rose SC, Bisson J, Churchill R, Wessely S. Psychological debriefing for preventing post-traumatic stress disorder (PTSD). Cochrane Database Syst Rev. 2002;2:CD000560.
30. Sijbrandij M, Olff M, Reitsma JB, Carlier IV, Gersons BP. Emotional or educational debriefing after psychological trauma. Br J Psychol. 2006;189:150–155.
31. Walker MU. Moral repair: reconstructing moral relations after wrongdoing. New York: Cambridge University Press; 2006.
32. Reich WT. Speaking of suffering: a moral account of compassion. Soundings. 1989;72:83–108.
33. Miller S. Finding hope when a child dies: what other cultures can teach us. New York: Fireside; 2002.
34. Carse A. Vulnerability, agency and human flourishing. In Taylor CR, Dell'Oro R, editors, Health and human flourishing: religion, medicine, and moral anthropology. Washington, DC: Georgetown University Press; 2006:33–52.
35. Lanphier E, Uchenna E. Anani Trauma Informed Ethics Consultation. Am J Bioethics. 2022;22(5): 45–57.
36. Lanphier E, Uchenna E. Anani enriching the theory and practice of Trauma Informed Ethics Consultation, Am J Bioethics. 2022;22(9):W7–W9,
37. Smyth JM, Pennebaker JW. Exploring the boundary conditions of expressive writing: in search of the right recipe. Br J Health Psychol. 2008;1:1–7.
38. Sexton JD, Pennebaker JW, Holzmueller CG, Wu AW, Berenholtz SM, Swoboda S, et al. Care for the caregiver: benefits of expressive writing for nurses in the United States. Prog Palliat Care. 2009;17:307–312.
39. Cochran KL, Mealer M. An evaluation of a narrative expressive writing program for nurses during the COVID-19 pandemic. J Nur Admin. 2023;53(4):228–233.

40. Nelson HL. Damaged identities, narrative repair. Ithaca, NY: Cornell University Press; 2001.
41. Fry-Bowers E, Rushton C. Who will be there to care if there are no more nurses? Hastings Center Bioethics Forum. 2021. https://www.thehastingscenter.org/who-will-be-there-to-care-if-there-are-no-more-nurses/.
42. Fry-Bowers E, Rushton C. Reimagining nursing's social contract with the public. Am Nurs J. 18(9), 3-8
43. Rushton CH, Sellers DE, Heller KS, Spring B, Dossey BM, Halifax J. Impact of a contemplative end-of-life training program: Being With Dying. Palliat Support Care. 2009;7:405–414.
44. Zimmerman J, Coyle V. The way of council. 2nd ed. Seattle, WA: Bramble Books; 2009.
45. Theater of War Productions' website: theaterofwar.com.
46. Rushton C, Doerries B, Greene J, Geller G. In the tragedy of this pandemic, dramatic interventions can heal moral suffering. Lancet. 2020;396(10247):305–306.
47. Doerries, B. The theater of war: what ancient Greek tragedies can teach us today. New York: Knopf; 2015.
48. Batman E. Can ancient Greek tragedy get us through the pandemic? The New Yorker, September 2020.

9

Building the Evidence Base for Moral Resilience

Katie Nelson, Katherine (Katie) Brewer, Heidi Holtz, and Katherine Heinze

AS THE CONCEPT of moral resilience has taken hold, an empirical measure is needed to validate the conceptual relationships and outcomes. Conceptual definitions of moral resilience are generally congruent with Rushton's.[1] However, the operational definition and the empirical referent vary (e.g., workplace engagement, moral distress, burnout, etc.), and this tends to situate moral resilience in response to negative phenomena, hence limiting the expanse of what it means to have and exercise moral resilience. It has also been conflated with general resilience, which lacks specificity to examine the pillars of moral resilience directly. Researchers, including Rushton, have defaulted to using the Connor-Davidson Resilience Scale (CD-RISC), which measures general resilience within an individual's physical and mental realms, in the absence of a validated measure to examine moral resilience.[2,3] The concept of resilience as described by Connor and Davidson more closely relates to the "bounce-back" factor than to a processing of emotions and experiences through a moral lens; that is, resilience measured by the CD-RISC is likely measuring more of the person's general physical and emotional stamina. Resilience, as measured by the CD-RISC, acts as a shield against harmful experiences and emotions; this instrument does not assess the metaphorical healing or transformation of moral stress or suffering that distinguishes moral resilience. (see Chapter 5).

Katie Nelson, Katherine (Katie) Brewer, Heidi Holtz, and Katherine Heinze, *Building the Evidence Base for Moral Resilience* In: *Moral Resilience.* Second Edition. Edited by: Cynda Hylton Rushton, Oxford University Press.
 DOI: 10.1093/oso/9780197667149.003.0010

Though a useful tool for measuring general resilience, the CD-RISC does not wholly account for the recognition of moral adversity and the ethical processing of emotions and experiences, nor does it account for the connectedness and awareness nurses often use to process morally distressing experiences.[4] It is more a tool for measuring resilience as the concept of *withstanding* as opposed to measuring moral resilience as a concept of integrity and *wholeness* with the potential for positive transformation. As discussed in Chapter 6, moral resilience as defined in our work is more complex and nuanced within the moral domain of resilience.

Moral resilience as a concept focuses on responses to moral adversity and ethical challenges and emphasizes preserving or maintaining one's integrity while facing morally challenging situations.[1] No human is spared from grappling with moral complexity, crises of conscience, or moral suffering. However, healthcare professionals often encounter further moral complexity related to their professional obligations—above and beyond typical life challenges. These are outlined in previous chapters.

In healthcare settings, moral stressors may occur at the individual, team, or systems level.[5] At the individual level, healthcare professionals have reported moral complexity related to situations such as ignoring patient concerns.[6,7,8] futile (that is, medically ineffective or risky) treatments;[5,8] unethical behavior toward patients;[7,8,9] and the role of surrogates in patients' healthcare decision-making.[10] At the team level, situations such as witnessing unethical behavior, unsafe conditions,[6] and lack of respect for autonomy[11] have been linked to distress in healthcare professionals. From a systems perspective, burnout, diminished ability to show compassion toward patients and families, and absenteeism are associated with having personal values that a healthcare professional does not perceive as aligned with organizational values[7,12,13] and government and institutional policies[6] that are perceived to be at odds with patients' and healthcare professionals' well-being. More detail is included in Chapters 2 and 3.

When healthcare professionals encounter these morally complex situations, their integrity may be threatened or violated, and serious consequences such as moral injury, burnout, and job turnover may ensue.[12,13,14] Despite experiencing moral complexity in their respective professions, many healthcare professionals exhibit features of moral resilience and can maintain integrity in the face of ethical challenges.[15,16] Each person has a unique set of capacities, strengths, and resources that may be enhanced and nurtured, providing that person with a wider range of response options and increased efficacy to face challenging situations.[15,16,17,18,19]

The concept of moral resilience has been included in various studies, with most examining moral resilience among a health-oriented caregiving population.[20] Moral resilience was understood as a contributing factor to workplace well-being through variables such as burnout or turnover intention and/or included as an independent variable alongside measures of moral suffering (such as moral distress); therefore, the true impact of moral resilience was unclear.[20,21,22,23,24,25] Without a valid and reliable measure of moral resilience, it would not be possible to gauge the existing level of moral resilience among healthcare professionals or to measure the effectiveness of interventions designed to enhance moral resilience in this population. The clear need to measure moral resilience in an empirically sound manner led to the development of the Rushton Moral Resilience Scale (RMRS).[25]

The Rushton Moral Resilience Scale©™

The initial development of the RMRS©™ was done with input from a variety of interprofessional healthcare researchers and clinicians, including chaplains, nurses, philosophers, physicians, and social workers. It was important to examine the conceptual basis of moral resilience and develop a measurement tool among practitioners in differing disciplines with a focus on care and human response to health and wellness. Every profession or specialty has a unique perspective and responsibility, but all healthcare professionals need to be equipped to maintain integrity in the face of moral adversity and complexity. As such, it would have been shortsighted to focus exclusively on nurses or physicians, for example, and still expect an interdisciplinary team's collective moral resilience to flourish.

RMRS Development Process

The first step in developing the RMRS was to establish conceptual domains of moral resilience to ensure that scale items represented the totality of moral resilience concepts, which could be generally applied to interprofessional healthcare workers. Toward that end, over 180 practicing physicians, nurses, clergy, and moral resilience experts were asked to write down how they would define moral resilience; responses were analyzed and sorted into domains (Table 9.1).

Table 9.1. Definitions by conceptual domain

Moral Resilience Construct	Definition
Personal Integrity	• Moral wholeness • A state of balance, harmony, and solidarity. • Clarity about who one essentially is and what one stands for in life and work. • Staying true to one's values and commitments amid moral adversity
Relational Integrity	• Distinguishing one's own values, views, and interests from others'. • Maintaining one's own beliefs and values while remaining open and flexible to the beliefs and values of others. • Reflects the interplay between upholding one's personal values and one's professional commitments as outlined in professional Codes of Ethics
Buoyancy	• Ability to recover from threats to one's integrity. • Gaining new perspectives while facing ethical challenges. • Being courageous while facing ethical challenges. • The possibility to grow in response to moral adversity
Self-Regulation	• Noticing one's own mental, emotional, and somatic state. • Observing what is happening without being overwhelmed or distracted. • Shifting from upset and anxiety to balance and insight.
Moral Efficacy	• Confidence in one's capacity to respond to ethical challenges effectively. • Communicating what one believes is morally/ethically justified despite facing resistance. • Navigating moral conflict in a way that reflects one's values • Taking principled and reasoned action
Self-Stewardship	• Giving sufficient attention to one's own well-being. • Acknowledging one's needs and limitations • Serving others while keeping others' needs in proportion. • Responding with compassion to one's limitations

Source: Heinze KE, Hanson G, Holtz H, et al. Measuring healthcare interprofessionals' moral resilience: validation of the Rushton Moral Resilience Scale. J Palliat Med.

After establishing the conceptual domains of moral resilience, the RMRS was established and tested in three stages: (1) item development, (2) item refinement after focus group discussions, and (3) item testing for validity and reliability.[26] Rushton and colleagues initially wrote 100 items for the scale, which were subsequently reviewed for content validity by 6 individuals with content expertise in resilience, philosophy, and ethics. In the second stage of development, the remaining 95 items were further refined with the aid of 22 practicing healthcare interprofessionals representing the target population in a focus group setting. After item refinement, the remaining 34 items were administered to 702 healthcare interprofessionals along with related scales to establish convergent validity. After testing, the final version of the scale contained 17 items.

Common factor analysis revealed four distinct factors: Responses to Moral Adversity, Personal Integrity, Moral Efficacy, and Relational Integrity. Initial psychometric testing of the RMRS yielded the following reliability indices: Responses to Moral Adversity ($\alpha = .78$), Personal Integrity ($\alpha = .50$), Relational Integrity ($\alpha = 0.78$), and Moral Efficacy ($\alpha = 0.69$), with a total scale alpha of .84.[26] Items that represented all six of the original domains were included. Correlations were calculated between the RMRS and the Connor-Davidson Resilience Scale-10 (CD-RISC-10)[2] and the RMRS and the Maslach Burnout Inventory-Human Services Survey (MBI-HSS).[27] As theorized, the RMRS had a positive correlation to general resilience and a negative correlation to burnout, establishing convergent validity of the RMRS beyond constructs measured by the CD-RISC-10 and MBI-HSS.

Current Research Using RMRS©™

Since publication of the RMRS, research teams have begun initiating projects utilizing the scale to varying degrees. Most have undertaken survey-based empirical studies, feasibility trials,[28] and translation of the scale—all evidence of moving toward intervention development.

Antonsdottir et al. conducted a cross-sectional, online survey of interdisciplinary healthcare professionals (N = 702) to examine predictive factors of burnout and their relation to moral resilience factors.[14] They found that religious preference, number of years in the profession, practice location, race, patient age, profession, and education level had varied significant relationships with burnout factors, including depersonalization, emotional exhaustion, and personal accomplishment. The RMRS subscales demonstrated a protective relationship with burnout and turnover intention after controlling for all work and demographic characteristics. These findings corroborated moral resilience as an important avenue for reducing the impact of burnout.

Rushton et al. conducted a cross-sectional, online survey of interprofessional healthcare workers (N = 595) to elicit experiences of moral resilience, moral injury, and other stressors amid the COVID-19 pandemic.[29] In the overall sample, prevalence of clinically significant moral injury was 32.4% and highest among nurses (38.1%). They also found moral resilience, religion, and having more than twenty years in the profession were protective from moral injury. Not only did moral resilience significantly predict moral injury ($p = .0001$), it also was shown to moderate the effect of years of experience on moral injury ($b = 0.87$, 95% CI = 0.20, 1.55). These findings elucidated the negative correlation between moral resilience and moral injury, suggesting that cultivating moral resilience through intervention may be useful for healthcare workers in mitigating the impact of ethical challenges faced at work.

Building on the previous study, Nelson et al. conducted a mixed-methods analysis, focusing specifically on healthcare workers who provided qualitative comments in the survey about their lived experiences.[30] In total, 55% (N = 328/595) added comments, of which 41% had clinically significant moral injury scores. Three themes and 10 themes were synthesized using the Reina Trust and Betrayal Model©™,[31] which focuses on how trust is built and broken with organizations. Responses underscored the betrayal many felt from their organizations, which contributed to reduced capacity and moral resilience. To this end, the study team offered five remedies: (1) counseling/emotional support, (2) peer support, (3) education and ethical support, 4) wellness offerings, and 5) spiritual/faith support as possible avenues for circumventing organizational challenges and bolstering moral resilience and trust between leaders and frontline healthcare workers.

Rushton et al. performed a secondary analysis of nurses from their overall study (N = 344/595), whereby the objective was to understand nurses' perceptions of their organizations' effectiveness and its impact on their moral resilience and moral injury scores.[32] In total, 4 of 10 nurses had clinically significant moral injury symptoms, and the average RMRS score was 28.93 (SD = 5.02). RMRS scores were lower in this sample of nurses compared to all other studies using the measure. As theorized, moral injury was negatively correlated with moral resilience scores ($p < .05$)—consistent with the pattern seen in the full sample of interdisciplinary healthcare workers. After controlling for all variables in the analytic model, the results showed (1) for every unit increase in organizational effectiveness, moral injury decreased by .40 points ($b = -.40$, 95% CI = $-.52$, $-.28$), and (2) for every one unit increase in moral resilience, moral injury decreased by 1.14 points ($b = -1.14$, 95% CI = -1.22, -.80). Both organizational effectiveness and moral resilience uniquely contributed to moral injury scores. Study findings contributed to an important discussion regarding the need to pair individual strategies for enhancing moral resilience with system-level actions and behaviors to bolster organizational effectiveness.

Thomas et al. conducted a cross-sectional analysis of pediatric critical care healthcare professionals ($N = 337$) to examine factors contributing to their moral distress.[33] Overall, 85.8% of respondents reported experiencing moral distress; nurses and respiratory therapists reported higher levels than physicians and advanced practice providers. They also found the primary cause of moral distress was the experience of specific challenges to professional integrity and lack of organizational support. Overall, moral distress was significantly inversely associated with moral resilience. In total, 76% of participants reported being confident in their ability to reason through ethical dilemmas in their role and 78.9% in their ability to think clearly when confronting an ethical challenge in the workplace. This contributed to a call for organizations to proactively recognize and respond to potentially morally distressing events by establishing psychologically safe forums for interdisciplinary colleagues and leaders to foster greater moral resilience and relational integrity.

Spilg et al. conducted a cross-sectional, online survey of healthcare workers during the first wave of the COVID-19 pandemic in Canada.[34] Their goal was to (1) examine whether moral resilience moderates the association between exposure to morally distressing situations and ensuing moral distress, and (2) identify factors associated with stronger moral resilience. They found that those who worked directly with patients experiencing COVID-19 had higher levels of moral distress ($p < .02$). Moral resilience moderated the relationship between exposure to distressing events and moral distress ($p < .001$). It was also correlated with lower stress, anxiety, and depressive symptoms ($p < .001$). Other factors associated with increased moral resilience included being male, older, no mental health diagnosis, greater sleep, and higher social support. Their recommendation was that future interventions may benefit from focusing on reducing both frequency and intensity of exposure to moral adversity rather than focusing on one or the other, to cultivate the capacities of moral resilience to holistically function as a protective factor.

Holtz et al. conducted a qualitative analysis using semi-structured interview data collected from fourteen emergency department nurses.[35] The aim of the study was to understand their perceptions of psychological trauma experienced during COVID-19 and potential protective mechanisms used to build moral resilience. The mean RMRS score was 45.9 (SD = 4.6) in the sample. Despite high levels of moral resilience, participants anecdotally stated they could not prevent psychological trauma from occurring. Two key themes identified were (1) losing identity as a nurse and (2) hopelessness and self-preservation. Stressors ebbed as the COVID-19 pandemic evolved, but the culmination of continued stress and moral injury exceeded their ability to fully adapt, which ultimately impacted their moral resilience outcomes.

Swavely et al. conducted a similar study[36]—a mixed-methods analysis among a sample of twenty-two registered nurses working in medical-surgical units and critical care units during COVID-19. Mean RMRS scores were 48 (SD = 5.8) for critical care nurses, and 53 (SD = 10) for medical-surgical nurses, respectively. Quantitative results were used to support the four qualitative themes identified: (1) phases of traumatic stress response to perceived risks; (2) honoring their sacrifice; (3) professional self-identity; and (4) sustaining resilience in a stressful work environment. Findings contributed to the literature on the need for organizational-level support for nurses to mitigate traumatic stress and threats to their core values.

Albaqawi and Alrashidi conducted a cross-sectional study among a sample of 393 nurses in the Hail Region, Saudi Arabia, to determine the relationship between perceived stress and moral resilience.[37] Mean RMRS©™ scores were 2.74 (SD = 0.30) indicating high moral resilience. They found a significant difference between gender and moral resilience, with females being more morally resilient than males. There was not a significant relationship between perceived stress and moral resilience, which led the researchers to conclude that being morally robust enables nurses to respond to ethical issues and other challenges regardless of any underlying stress occurring in the workplace.

Dr. Laura Quigg utilized the RMRS in her dissertation study, which comprised a mindfulness self-care program for critical care nurses' resilience and well-being during COVID-19.[38] She used a pre-/post-test design with thirty participants and found significant changes in RMRS scores after four weeks. There were significant changes in three of the RMRS sub-scales: Response to Moral Adversity ($p < .001$), Relational Integrity ($p = .003$), and Moral Efficacy ($p = .012$). Changes in Response to Moral Adversity were the most significant, which may have been due to the self-regulatory skills fostered through the mindfulness intervention and should be explored further in future studies.

Kovanci et al. tested the reliability and validity of a Turkish version of the RMRS among a sample of 255 clinical nurses.[39] Following the translation-back technique, their confirmatory factor analysis yielded the following reliability indices: Responses to Moral Adversity ($\alpha = .75$); Personal Integrity ($\alpha = .55$); Relational Integrity ($\alpha = 0.77$); and Moral Efficacy ($\alpha = 0.62$), with a total scale alpha of . 83. These results were consistent with original study findings, suggesting that the translated scale is a valid measure for the Turkish language and culture. Researchers have translated the RMRS into several other languages as well, including Dutch, Chinese, and Portuguese, with others in process.

Revised Rushton Moral Resilience Scale©™

In establishing reliability and validity of the RMRS it became apparent that further work was needed to (1) improve reliability of the Personal Integrity sub-scale; (2) ensure relevant content was holistically captured in each of the four sub-scales; and (3) shorten the overall scale. Rushton et al[40]. utilized a cross-sectional survey design to accomplish these aims in a cohort of interprofessional healthcare workers, which was derived from a larger study.[34] They began by conducting an item analysis to determine poorly functioning items, which resulted in one item from the Personal Integrity sub-scale being dropped, leaving sixteen items in total. The team then created two sub-samples of 646 and 651 participants, respectively, to perform a series of three confirmatory factor analyses: (1) in sub-sample 1, using all items that performed well in the item analysis; (2) in sub-sample 1, using the four sub-scales reduced to four items each; and (3) in sub-sample 2, to validate the shortened scale. Reliability of the revised RMRS-16©™ is as follows: Response to Moral Adversity ($\alpha = .73 - .74$), Personal Integrity ($\alpha = .76 - .78$), Relational Integrity ($\alpha = .78$), and Moral Efficacy ($\alpha = .72 - .76$); overall reliability is .86.[40] The final higher-order factor analysis determined that calculating an overall moral resilience score may also be justifiable depending on the needs of future RMRS-16 users. Finally, in establishing criterion validity, they found expected correlations between the RMRS-16 and other measures. It was significantly negatively associated with the Measure of Moral Distress for Health Care Professionals (MMD-HP),[41] Perceived Stress Scale (PSS),[42] Generalized Anxiety Disorder (GAD-7),[43] and the Quick Inventory of Depressive Symptomatology-Self-Report (QIDS-SR);[44] the RMRS-16 was significantly positively associated with the Brief Resilience Coping Scale (BRCS)—a measure of general adaptive tendencies.[45]

Future Directions

Moral resilience is a promising protective resource to mitigate the detrimental effects of moral adversity in healthcare. Cultivating the capacities that comprise the conceptual underpinnings of our definition of moral resilience has the potential to restore moral agency and reduce the consequences of unacknowledged and unrelieved moral suffering. Programs such as the Mindful Ethical Practice & Resilience Academy (MEPRA) were derived from this idea and have yielded significant changes among nurses. MEPRA has demonstrated significant improvements in ethical confidence and competence, mindfulness, resilience, and work engagement while it showed decreases in depression, anger, emotional exhaustion, and turnover intention.[3,46] While the RMRS©™ had not yet been validated for the program's evaluation, core elements of moral resilience are woven throughout the curriculum. Future studies using the newly validated RMRS-16 offer opportunities to examine the impact of interventions on overall moral resilience and/or specific sub-scales based upon research questions being investigated. Defining relevant cutoff scores will also advance comparisons of responses of different roles, disciplines, and other demographics, and inform the development of targeted interventions.

A theme that has emerged from several recent conceptual and empirical studies of moral resilience is the need to understand the dynamic interplay among individuals, teams, and the broader healthcare ecosystem. Relational integrity is integral to team cohesion, respect, and collaboration. When present, the integrity of everyone is supported. During times of diminished connection and communication, efforts to enhance the dimensions of moral resilience that impact relational engagement are needed.[47] Further conceptual work should help to deepen our understanding of this dimension of moral resilience and create strategies for enhancing it within team-based settings. The Relational Integrity sub-scale of the RMRS-16 may be useful for assessing the impact of team-based interventions on key outcomes of interest.[47]

Moral resilience is situated at the individual level to amplify individual capacities to transform moral suffering and potentially learn and grow, yet much of this growth happens outside the workplace—a limitation within the current measure of moral resilience. Healthcare workers often process experiences after leaving work, and this processing may be impacted by sociocultural contexts and the communities where they reside. Over the last twenty years there has been a growing societal disconnection, a sharp decrease in actual person-to-person interaction in communities, as social media have developed and replaced real interaction, becoming a major disruptor in community-level coping and resilience.[48] The abrupt onslaught of the COVID-19 pandemic further exacerbated the divisions and disconnect that have been growing over time. Reactions across society and direct or indirect experiences nurses had within their communities likely influenced how they were able to process the moral adversity and moral suffering that ensued. Moral suffering and trauma escalated among healthcare workers due to the compounding factors of not only caring for critically ill patients but also navigating scarce resources, fear of personal safety, and feelings of betrayed trust by their organizations.[49] As outlined in this book, moral resilience is conceptualized within a culture of ethical practice. Research on the impact of organizational actions—by measuring ethical culture,[50] ethical climate,[51] or organizational effectiveness[32]—may offer important insights. More fully accounting for the impact of one's external environment on developing and/or strengthening moral resilience is a next horizon. The concept of collective moral resilience, or "the response to moral distress which emerges from the shared capacity within a group,"[52] offers a promising avenue for further inquiry. Collective moral resilience encompasses the overarching societal values, norms, and practices that shape and influence clinicians' responses to their experiences in providing care and the subsequent moral adversity they face as a result. However, we must currently rely on measures that include elements of personal and relational integrity as proxy measures to capture this concept.

Conclusion

The concept of moral resilience has evolved over time, and the growing evidence base supports it as a promising strengths-based approach to preserving and restoring healthcare workers' integrity. As the healthcare and socio-political environments become seemingly more complex, researchers and clinicians have found that moral resilience may have the greatest potential for benefit as part of a multi-faceted approach to dismantling systems and processes rendering moral adversity and suffering[53]. Individuals and healthcare organizations should align in their efforts to maximize collective moral resilience and overall capacity across communities. This must involve enhancing conditions that foster integrity, and when threatened, ensuring that systems, processes, and resources are in place to properly restore it and prevent suffering.

References

1. Rushton CH. Moral resilience: transforming moral suffering in healthcare. New York: Oxford University Press; 2018.
2. Connor KM, Davidson JRT. Development of a new resilience scale: The Connor-Davidson Resilience Scale (CD-RISC). Depress Anxiety. 2003;18:76–82.
3. Rushton CH, Swoboda SM, Reller N, et al. Mindful ethical practice and resilience academy: equipping nurses to address ethical challenges. Am J Crit Care. 2021;30(1):e1–e11.
4. Defilippis T, Curtis K, Gallagher A. Moral resilience through harmonized connectedness in intensive care nursing: a grounded theory study. Inten Crit Care Nurse. 2020;57:102785.
5. Riedel P-L, Kreh A, Kulcar V, et al. A scoping review of moral stressors, moral distress and moral injury in healthcare workers during COVID-19. Int J Environ Res Public Health. 2022;19(3):1666.
6. Nia HS, Shafipour V, Allen K-A, et al. A second-order confirmatory factor analysis of the Moral Distress Scale-Revised for nurses. Nurs Ethics. 2019;26(4):1199–1210.
7. Lamiani G, Dordoni P, Argentero P. Value congruence and depressive symptoms among critical care clinicians: The mediating role of moral distress. Stress Health 2018;34(1):135–142.
8. Bartholdson C, Molewijk B, Lützén K, et al. Ethics case reflection sessions: enablers and barriers. Nurs Ethics 2018;25(2):199–211.
9. Ramos AM, Barlem ELD, Barlem JGT, et al. Cross-cultural adaptation and validation of the Moral Distress Scale-Revised for nurses. Rev Bras Enferm. 2017;70(5):1011–1017.
10. Liu X, Xu Y, Chen Y, et al. Ethical dilemmas faced by frontline support nurses fighting COVID-19. Nurs Ethics. 2022;29(1):7–18.
11. Abdolmaleki M, Lakdizaji S, Ghahramanian A, et al. Relationship between autonomy and moral distress in emergency nurses. Indian J Med Ethics. 2019;4(1):20–25.
12. West CP. The value of values alignment in healthcare. J Intern Med. 2023;293(6):666–667.

13. Pavlova A, Paine S, Sinclair S, et al. Working in value-discrepant environments inhibits clinicians' ability to provide compassion and reduces well-being: A cross-sectional study. J Intern Med. 2023; 0: 1–20.
14. Antonsdottir I, Rushton CH, Nelson KE, et al. Burnout and moral resilience in interprofessional healthcare professionals. J Clin Nurs. 2021;31(1–2):196–208.
15. Rushton C. Moral resilience: a capacity for navigating ethical challenges in critical care. AACN Adv Crit Care. 2016;27(1):111–119.
16. Prentice TM, Gillam L, Davis PG, Janvier A. Always a burden? Healthcare providers' perspectives on moral distress. Arch Dis Child Fetal Neonatal Ed. 2018;103(5):F441–F445.
17. Lützén K, Ewalds-Kvist B. Moral distress and its interconnection with moral sensitivity and moral resilience: viewed from the philosophy of Viktor E. Frankl. J Bioeth Inq. 2013;10:317–324.
18. Traudt T, Liaschenko J, Peden-McAlpine C. Moral agency, moral imagination, and moral community: antidotes to moral distress. J Clin Ethics. 2016;27(3):201–213.
19. Morley G, Field R, Horsburgh CC, Burchill C. Interventions to mitigate moral distress: a systematic review of the literature. Int J Nurs Stud. 2021;121:103984.
20. DeGrazia M, Porter C, Sheehan A, et al. Building moral resiliency through the nurse education and support team initiative. Am J Crit Care. 2021;30(2):95–102.
21. Clark P, Crawford TN, Hulse B, et al. Resilience, moral distress, and workplace engagement in emergency department nurses. West J Nurs Res. 2021;43:442–451.
22. Faraco MM, Gelbcke FL, Brehmer LCD, et al. Moral distress and moral resilience of nurse managers. Nurs Ethics. 2022;29(5):1253–1265.
23. Tolksdorf KH, Tischler U, Heinrichs K. Correlates of turnover intention among nursing staff in the COVID-19 pandemic: a systematic review. BMC Nurs. 2022;21:174.
24. Woods M. Moral distress revisited: the viewpoints and responses of nurses. Int Nurs Rev. 2020;67:68–75.
25. Rushton CH. Transforming moral suffering by cultivating moral resilience and ethical practice. Am J Crit Care. 2023;32(4):238–248.
26. Heinze KE, Hanson G, Holtz H, et al. Measuring healthcare interprofessionals' moral resilience: validation of the Rushton Moral Resilience Scale. J Palliat Med. 2020;24(6):865–872.
27. Maslach C, Jackson SE, Leiter MP. Maslach Burnout Inventory manual, 3rd ed. Palo Alto, CA: Consulting Psychologists Press; 1996: iv, 52.
28. Van Schaik MV, Pasman HR, Widdershoven G, et al. CURA-An ethics support instrument for nurses in palliative care. Feasibility and perceived outcomes. HEC Forum. 2023;35(2):139–159.

29. Rushton CH, Thomas TA, Antonsdottir IM, et al. Moral injury and moral resilience in health care workers during the COVID-19 pandemic. J Palliat Med. 2022;25(5):712–719.
30. Nelson KE, Hanson GC, Boyce D, et al. Organizational impact on health care workers' moral injury during COVID-19: A mixed-methods analysis. J Nurs Adm. 2022;52(1):57–66.
31. Reina D, Reina M. Trust and betrayal in the workplace: Building effective relationships in your organization. Oakland, CA: Berrett-Koehler; 2015.
32. Rushton CH, Nelson KE, Antonsdottir I, et al. Perceived organizational effectiveness, moral injury, and moral resilience among nurses during the COVID-19 pandemic: secondary analysis. Nurs Manage. 2022;53(7):12–22.
33. Thomas TA, Davis FD, Kumar S, et al. COVID-19 and moral distress: a pediatric critical care survey. Am J Crit Care. 2021;30(6):e80–e98.
34. Spilg E, Rushton CH, Phillips J, et al. The new frontline: exploring the links between moral distress, moral resilience, and mental health in healthcare workers during the COVID-19 pandemic, BMC Psychiatry. 2022;22(19):1–12.
35. Holtz HK, Weissinger GM, Swavely D, et al. The long tail of COVID-19: implications for the future of emergency nursing. J Emerg Nurs. 2023;49(2):198–209.
36. Swavely D, Romig B, Weissinger G, et al. The impact of traumatic stress, resilience, and threats to core values on nurses during a pandemic. J Nurs Adm. 2022;52(10):525–535.
37. Albaqawi H, Alrashidi MS. Perceived stress and its relationship to moral resilience among nurses in the Hail Region, Saudi Arabia. Makara J Health Res. 2022;26(3):159–164.
38. Quigg L. Evaluating a brief mindfulness-based self-care intervention on critical care nurses' resilience and well-being during the COVID-19 pandemic. [Doctoral dissertation]. Los Angeles: University of California–Los Angeles; 2022.
39. Kovanci MS, Ozbas AA. Examining the effect of moral resilience on moral distress. Nurs Ethics. 2023; 30(7-8):1156-1170.
40. Rushton, CH, Hanson, GC, Boyce, D, Holtz, H, Nelson, KE., Spilg, EG, Robillard, R. Reliability and validity of the revised Rushton Moral Resilience Scale-16 for healthcare workers. J Adv Nurs, 2023, *80*(3), 1177–1187.
41. Epstein EG, Whitehead PB, Prompahakul C, et al. Enhancing understanding of moral distress: the measure of moral distress for health care professionals. AJOB Empir Bioeth. 2019;10(2):113–124.
42. Perera MJ, Brintz CE, Birnbaum-Weitzman O, et al. Factor structure of the Perceived Stress Scale-10 (PSS) across English and Spanish language responders in the HCHS/SOL Sociocultural Ancillary Study. Psychol Assess. 2017;29(3):320–328.
43. Spitzer RL, Kroenke K, Williams JBW, Löwe B. A brief measure for assessing generalized anxiety disorder. Arch Intern Med. 2006;166(10):1092–1097.

44. Brown ES, Murray M, Carmody TJ, et al. E.S., The quick inventory of depressive symptomatology-self-report: a psychometric evaluation in patients with asthma and major depressive disorder. Ann Allergy Asthma Immunol. 2008;100(5):433–438.
45. Sinclair VG, Wallston KA. The development and psychometric evaluation of the Brief Resilient Coping Scale. Assessment. 2004;11(1):94–101.
46. Rushton C, Swoboda S, Reimer T, Boyce D, Hansen G. The Mindful Ethical Practice & Resilience Academy (MEPRA): sustainability of impact. Am J of Crit Care. 2023;32(3):184–194.
47. Rushton, C., Manbaumann, C. A web of mutuality: relational integrity in critical care nursing. AACN Adv Crit Care. 2023, 34(4), 381-390.
48. Valkenburg PM, Beyens I, Meier A, et al. Advancing our understanding of the associations between social media use and well-being. Curr Opin Psychol. 2022;47:101357.
49. Brewer KC. Institutional betrayal in nursing: A concept analysis. Nurs Ethics. 2021;28:1081–1089.
50. Rushton CH, Brooks-Brunn JA. Environments that support ethical practice. New Horiz. 1997;5(1):20–29.
51. Ozdoba P, Dziurka M, Pilewska-Kozak A, et al. Hospital ethical climate and job satisfaction among nurses: A scoping review. Int J Environ Res Public Health. 2022;19(8):4554.
52. Delgado J, Siow S, de Groot J, et al. Towards collective moral resilience: the potential of communities of practice during the COVID-19 pandemic and beyond. J Med Ethics. 2021;47:374–382.
53. Rushton, C, Transforming moral suffering by cultivating moral resilience and ethical practice. Am J Crit Care.2023, 32 (4): 238–248.

10

Designing Sustainable Systems for Ethical Practice

Cynda Hylton Rushton and Monica Sharma

Moral Adversity in Healthcare

Rapid change in healthcare has imperiled its moral compass.* Healthcare institutions and systems declare their commitment to core ethical values, yet many clinicians struggle to understand institutional policies and decisions that appear inconsistent with their normative values as professionals. This disconnect threatens the integrity of the organization, especially when unclear expectations and decision-making processes, ineffective communication, and lack of transparency lead to the breaking of trust.[1] Leaders in healthcare organizations struggle to balance commitments to patients, families, staff, and governing boards and at the same time are compelled to pursue externally reported measures of effectiveness, seemingly abandoning their mission and values. Complex financial, regulatory, policy, and societal pressures contribute to unrecognized drifts in norms of ethical behavior. Clinicians and healthcare leaders may be unaware of the gradual accumulation of pressures that slant their conclusions, make them morally insensitive to ethical issues, allow them to normalize ethically suspect behavior, or cause them to justify their decisions to maintain the status quo.[2]

* Acknowledgment: Portions of this chapter were adapted from Sharma M. Radical Transformational Leadership: Strategic Action For Change Agents. San Francisco, CA: North Atlantic Books; 2017. Used with permission.

Cynda Hylton Rushton and Monica Sharma, *Designing Sustainable Systems for Ethical Practice* In: *Moral Resilience*. Second Edition. Edited by: Cynda Hylton Rushton, Oxford University Press. © Oxford University Press 2024.
DOI: 10.1093/oso/9780197667149.003.0011

A countermeasure to the current reality is to create a new paradigm grounded in respect, compassion, and wisdom that is sustained by a culture of ethical practice. Focusing attention on the behaviors and ethical practices of individuals will enable shifts in structures and systems to create a culture that deliberately supports ethical action with sound ethical discernment and deliberation. Such a culture can support the cultivation of moral resilience and restore integrity for clinicians and organizations alike, ensuring that patients and families receive safe, high-quality, person-centered care. Concurrently, virtuous healthcare organizations can foster ethical standards and best practices that inspire everyone to uphold them.[3]

Building a culture that fosters moral resilience and ethical practice requires individuals, leaders, and organizations to design solutions together. No single element can produce meaningful and lasting change. Norms within an organization reflect the implicit or explicit patterns, rules, or standards that are typical or expected. Within the organization, ethical values and commitments are codified in its policies, code of ethics or conduct, budget processes, and other mechanisms adopted by the governing board and senior leadership. These in turn are reflected in the priorities the organization sets and the decisions and actions it takes; arguably, the budget of an organization may be the most important ethical documentation of its values and its conscience.[3] Embedded in these are the sanctions and rewards the organization imposes on its leaders and members when they align with or violate values and norms. Myriad normative patterns develop governing social interactions, communication (who talks to whom), how conflicts are managed, who has formal and informal authority, and so on. It is the interplay between formal and informal normative patterns that creates the moral ecosystem where clinicians practice.

Creating the culture we desire for ethical practice requires a multipronged approach that takes into account "the role of leadership, the relationship between individual and team resilience, the balance between personal and professional obligations on resilience, and understanding the role of culture."[4(p60)] This approach must also consider the interplay between clinical ethics and organizational ethics, including business and corporate ethical frameworks, policies, and processes;[2,5] it must also examine how adaptive systems break down in response to adversity, and what steps can be taken to anticipate and respond to it.[6]

This chapter provides a conceptual basis for designing individual, team, and system interventions to cultivate individual moral resilience and a culture that enables ethical practice.[7] It broadens the lens of inquiry to focus on culture, inviting a more robust view of the elements that support ethical practice as well as individual, team, and organizational integrity. Consistent with a social ecological view of resilience (discussed in Chapter 5), there is a dynamic interplay and synergy among individuals, organizations, communities, society, and the broader ecosystem. As Haidt notes, "Moral systems are interlocking sets of values, virtues, norms, practices, identities, institutions, technologies, and evolved psychological mechanisms that work together to suppress or regulate self-interest and make cooperative societies possible."[8(p314)]

The examples offered in this chapter and the next are intended to stimulate reflection, creativity, and innovation, not to prescribe a particular course of action or to exclude innovative efforts that have been developed using different frameworks. The approach described here does not suggest a single method or solution; rather, it offers a process that is dynamic by intent and thus suitable for use in complex, demanding environments.[7] Attention to inclusion of all elements of the model is necessary to achieve the desired results.

A Culture of Ethical Practice

An ethical culture stimulates ethical conduct[9] and creates the conditions that prevent lapses in ethical behavior.[10] In essence, a culture of ethical practice is composed of the values, norms, systems, and structures that support moral agency, dignity, integrity, and moral resilience. As a multidimensional concept, ethical culture also includes transparency; normative expectations that are clear and consistently upheld by leaders and employees; conditions that enable and support ethical conduct; safety to raise and discuss ethical concerns; and clear and fairly and consistently applied sanctions for unethical behavior and rewards for ethical conduct.[10] It aligns individual and organizational norms, decision-making practices, budgetary allocations, and priorities to create an environment where ethical values and commitments are lived and used as robust benchmarks rather than just talked about or relegated to meaningless plaques hung on the wall. In such a culture, financial incentives and expenditures are driven by ethical values and commitments, not by compliance or data alone. The synergy between individuals, teams, and the organization results in a shared commitment to high-quality, safe, compassionate care and respectful, fair, and equitable practices and processes.

Ethical culture is fundamentally socially constructed and mediated. In healthcare, such a culture embraces individuals who receive care as well as those who deliver it. Leaders and clinicians contribute to the formal and informal socialization processes within an organization, beginning with orientation and later through training, mentorship, social networks, career development, and other mechanisms.[11] In turn, these processes communicate and reinforce vital messages about what is valued, sanctioned, and expected. When there is coherence and alignment, trust is fostered; when there is dissonance, trust is broken.[12] Work cultures that discourage or prevent moral solidarity leave people to fend for themselves; as people grow weary of the struggle to maintain their integrity, they can succumb to habitual moral isolation, fatigue, alienation, and indifference. Demotivated or disgruntled staff are more likely to demonstrate lapses in ethical conduct, including intentionally discrediting or undermining the organization.[13,14]

An ethical culture prioritizes ethical practice as central to the organization's mission, governance, leadership, and operations.[2,15] The organization's mission is the touchstone whereby institutional processes, structures, decisions, and procedures are evaluated and aligned.[2,3] Moral and ethical values, commitments, and principles are the criteria for evaluating behaviors that foster or undermine integrity at all levels;[16] these and other criteria are used to determine what constitutes ethical conduct within an organization.[17] In healthcare organizations, ethics reflects a broader normative system established by society, the organization, or the institution and is often expressed within a code of conduct, policies, and internal control and monitoring systems. The integrity of the people who create, administer, and monitor the organizational internal control system that alerts leaders and the governing board to lapses in ethical values and norms is essential to creating an environment where individuals and the organization can thrive.

When there are clear, normative expectations of ethical conduct and guidelines rather than rigid, proscriptive rules, everyone is inspired to uphold them.[2] Empowering individuals to behave ethically requires mechanisms that allow them to recognize and speak up about ethical concerns and to take principled action to address them. Building such a culture also requires that an organization establish norms and responsibility for ethical dialogue, invest in resources to support decision-making and conflict management, and design systems to detect and address ethical issues through processes such as performance improvement, ongoing monitoring, reporting systems, and incentive, risk management, and human resource processes. Critically important but often missing is an approach that leverages universal values (dignity, compassion, equity) by intentionally designing systems and processes to systematically shift underlying structures, norms, and policies to align with them and produce the desired results.[7]

Responses to Moral Adversity and Suffering

While there are numerous studies documenting the incidence, sources, and impact of moral distress in clinicians, over three decades of scholarship and practice have yielded a limited number of interventions that have been proven effective in mitigating the detrimental effects of this distress.[18,19,20,21,22,23,24,25] Each of these interventions, taken individually, has had local impact, much to the credit of its creators; yet, despite concerted efforts, sustainable and scalable results have been largely absent. We have the technology and the resources, so what is missing? People are asking thoughtful questions and seeking answers to them: *What does it take for clinicians to have integrity despite unwarranted labels and criticism? What is it in the healthcare culture that prevents clinicians from speaking up about ethical concerns? How do we restore the integrity and joy in the delivery of healthcare?*[26,27,28,29,30] *How do clinicians deal with unrealistic expectations of patients, families, payers, and organizations?* These are just a few of the questions that must be addressed if we are to shift our current reality toward an alternative grounded in integrity, compassion, and fairness.

The limitations of our current responses render them inadequate given the enormity and complexity of the issues we face in healthcare and society. Complex issues require skillfully designed solutions. In finding reasons for and explaining the deeper causes of moral suffering and moral distress, we generally focus our energy on reducing the anxiety and dissonance that accompany them. We can lapse into finger-pointing and blame. We may view the moral disagreements and conflicts that arise in clinical practice as a series of individual challenges and failures without paying attention to the underlying factors and forces within society and healthcare that have created the conditions for moral adversity in the first place. Thus, the approaches we take may be necessary but only partial. However, when we see the concerns of clinicians as symptoms of a more fundamental, deeper-rooted crisis, we can mount a more holistic and profound response that is likely to move us forward in a more sustainable way. We ponder why, when there are so many "good" people with "good" intentions, we cannot make a significant dent in solving these recalcitrant problems. The answer is clear and simple—but not simplistic: we have been neglecting the deeper dimensions of the problem, focusing on surface-level interventions to solve complex challenges, and arriving at partial, unsustainable solutions.

Figure 10.1 a, b, c shows three partial ways we embark on strategic action related to addressing moral adversity in healthcare. These include: a: tactics implemented only, b: policy and process only, and c: personal development only. Figure 10.2 depicts a holistic approach that can generate sustainable outcomes and impacts; this approach is at the heart of this chapter and is described in detail in the pages that follow.

Partial Response #1: Tactics Implemented Only

In fast-paced clinical environments, we are impatient for instant solutions to address what appears to be the presenting problem and immediately develop tactics or superficial fixes, including programs and processes, without fully understanding the scope or depth of the problem. Partial Response #1 (Figure 10.1a) identifies some of the factors that produce moral adversity and offers specific solutions with available technologies (the inner sphere).

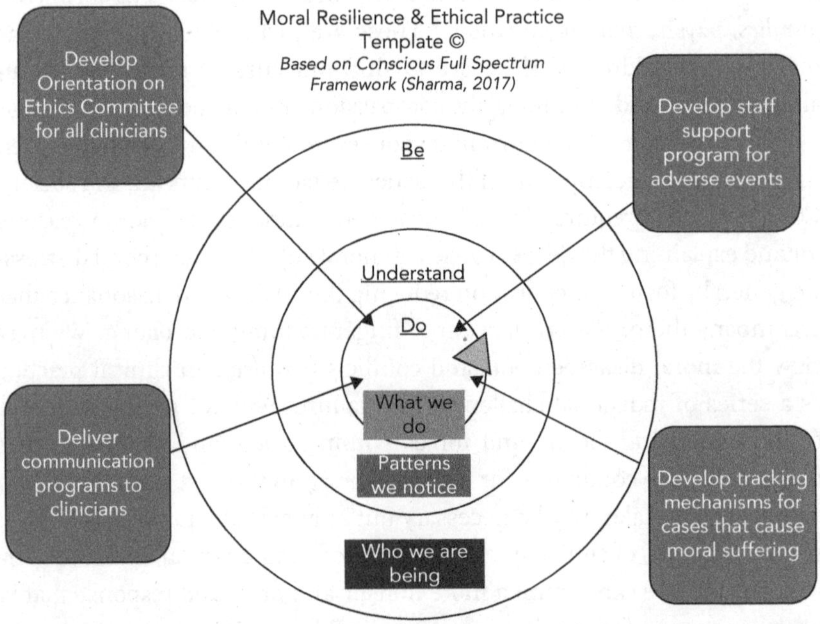

FIGURE 10.1A. Three partial ways we embark on strategic action related to addressing moral adversity in healthcare. a: Tactics Implemented Only. b: Policy and Process Only. c: Personal Development Only. a: shown here: Tactics Implemented Only.

Assumptions about what will fix the problem include identification of knowledge deficits and lack of skills or sufficient systems. Partial responses may include orientation to the role of the ethics committee for all employees, developing staff training programs to address adverse events, delivering programs to build communication skills to address ethical conflicts, or devising tracking mechanisms for cases that cause moral suffering or distress.

Each one of these tactics is a step toward enhancing the culture of ethical practice within the organization. However, when tactics are focused on one aspect of a specific problem, that aspect may be influenced but the underlying problem itself remains unresolved.

Partial Response #2: Policy and Patterns Only

Another common way we approach solutions is reflected in Partial Response #2 (Figure 10.1b).

We identify the factors and structures that empower or disempower clinicians and their integrity and define ways to address cultural or systemic factors that contribute to them (middle sphere). Results in the middle

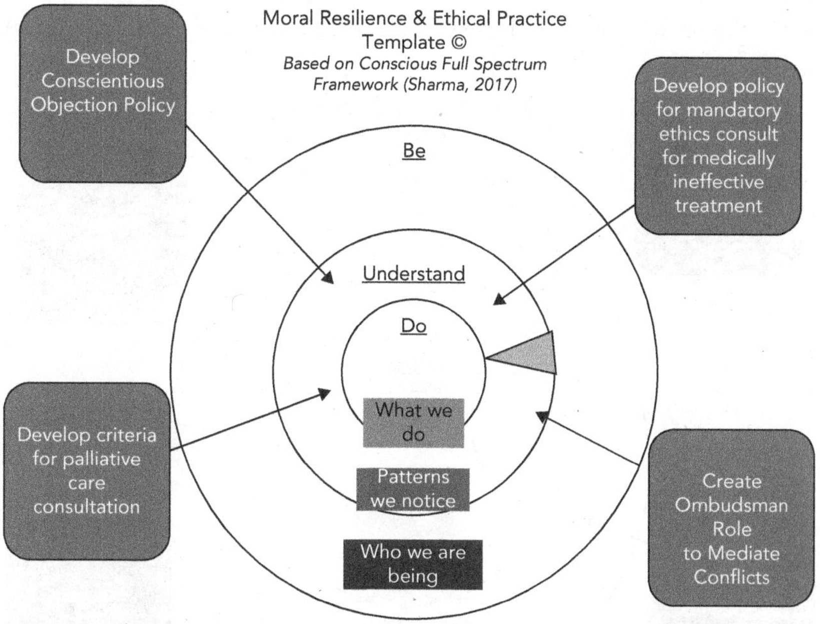

FIGURE 10.1B. Three partial ways we embark on strategic action related to addressing moral adversity in healthcare. b: Policy and Process Only.

sphere require that there are shifts in key dimensions of the clinical culture, including ethical norms, policies, procedures, and so on. Policies that acknowledge the integrity of clinicians, such as those addressing conscientious objection or refusal, are an important vehicle that contributes to ethical practice.[31] Additionally, developing mechanisms to address a source of moral distress, such as mandatory ethics consultation for cases involving medically ineffective treatment[32] or consultation by a palliative care service when treatment goals are unclear,[33] are steps in the process of change. Similarly, creating an ombudsman role to mediate ethical conflicts can help to deepen an ethics infrastructure.[11,34]

However, focusing on policies and patterns only is also a partial response. While none of these responses is wrong, they are likely to produce some results but alone may not be sufficient to shift the culture or produce sustainable change. At the same time, we may not notice whether these norms, policies, or procedures are aligned with our essential values or commitments. Inadvertently we may be fostering processes that exacerbate rather than remediate the patterns and ultimately derail the results we desire.

Partial Response #3: Personal Development Only

Examining the issue from the point of view of personal discovery as the solution to the broader problem is reflected in Partial Response #3 (Figure 10.1c).

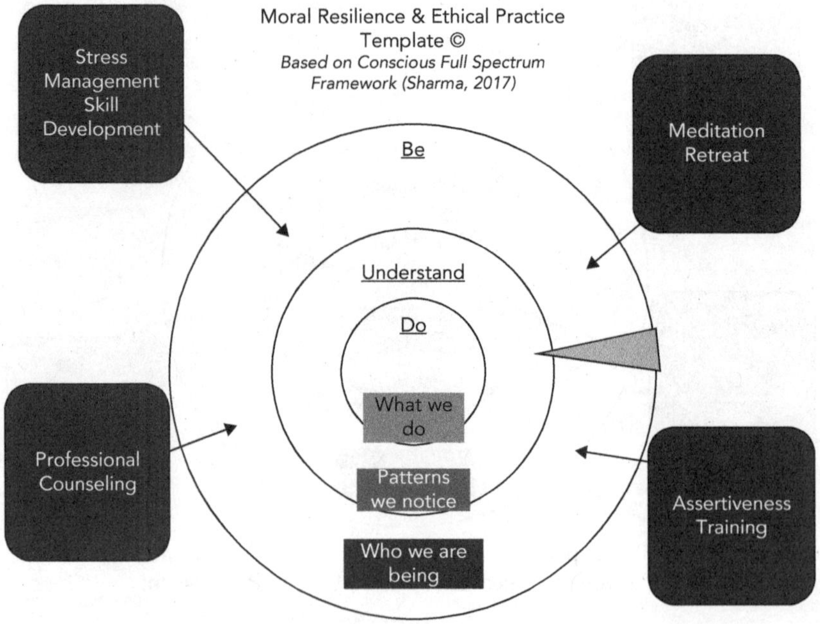

FIGURE 10.1C. Three partial ways we embark on strategic action related to addressing moral adversity in healthcare. c: Personal Development Only.

Focusing on cultivating personal capacities to address moral adversity is a necessary foundation for a culture of ethical practice. This may include developing stress management or assertiveness skills, attending a meditation retreat, or pursuing professional counseling to address one's responses to moral suffering (outer sphere of the figure).

While each of these may provide additional personal support, in the context of sustainable organizational and systemic change, they too are partial solutions. Over the last two decades, numerous consciousness-based training programs have been initiated, and books on personal self-awareness have proliferated. They have paved the way for different perspectives and actions and have contributed to greater self-awareness. These individual skills are necessary to build capacity within individuals to participate in large-scale design. However, self-discovery alone cannot transform the workplace or society unless we also respond to systemic challenges. We must leverage our essential values and wisdom with self-awareness and self-regulation to design solutions and system shifts in a more comprehensive, sustainable manner.

Limitations of Partial Responses

Partial responses produce some results that may be useful in solving specific problems caused by one variable without interrelated factors. As such, they are not wrong and should not be criticized or abandoned. However, their limitations must be acknowledged, and the necessary steps taken to identify gaps and create more robust solutions. Partial responses are relatively ineffective in solving complex problems with multifactorial etiologies. The sources of moral adversity, for example, are diverse and far-reaching. Likewise, the sources of moral distress are not limited to a single factor or systemic problem. Many of the factors that impact clinician and organizational integrity are interdependent and not easily dissected from individual, team, and organizational factors and the cultural norms and systems that maintain the conditions that manifest them. Cultivating a virtuous healthcare organization requires integrating both individual and organizational conscience to enable clinicians and leaders to live out their moral and ethical values and commitments.[3]

An Approach for Sustainable Results

Our responses to diverse conditions must be designed to help people innovate, generate breakthroughs, and sustain the specific change that is needed to establish the desired result[7]—in this case, shifting the culture to enable and sustain integrity amid moral adversity. When we focus our energy on solutions to the presenting problem or symptom, we can inadvertently overlook the bigger context of the situation, its root factors, and the possibilities for change. In clinical practice, this would be like treating the patient's symptom rather than the underlying disease or applying our knowledge of how the body works without understanding the unique characteristics of the person; neither necessarily leads to health or healing. What we need is a broader topography that reveals relational patterns, organizational structures and systems, and societal/global context and forces. Concurrently, we must source our design from our universal values of dignity, compassion, and equity and our inner capacities throughout design and implementation. We must return to these anchors over and over throughout the process.

Figure 10.2 represents a framework for a response involving the alignment of the three overlapping spheres to foster moral resilience and create a culture of ethical practice.

The triangle, with the broadest base in the space of our inner capacities, provides the fuel for design and action and transcends each individual sphere to align purpose, values, and action into a coherent whole. Such alignment represents a Conscious Full Spectrum Response (CFSR).[7]

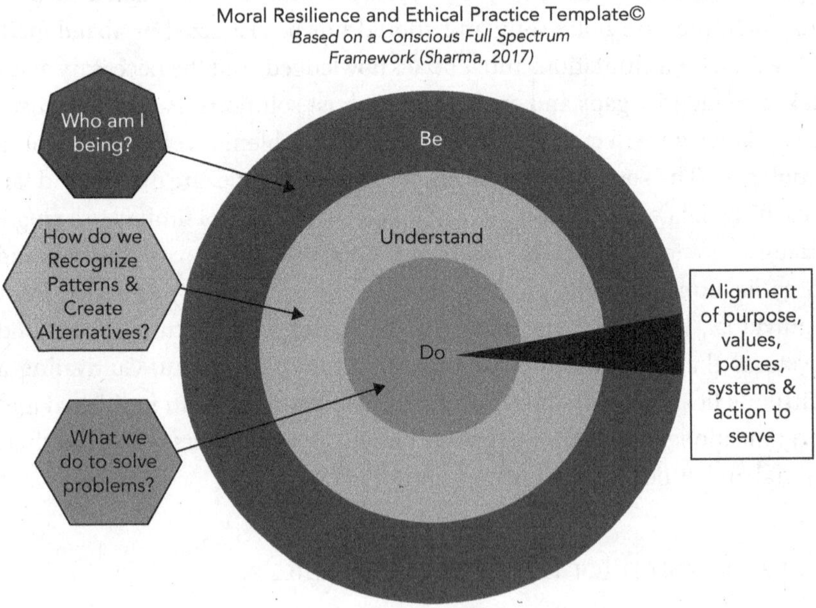

FIGURE 10.2. Moral resilience and ethical practice template.

The outer sphere, *be*, invites individuals to identify and embody the values and commitments that make up their moral compass and the essence of who they are. Embodying what one stands for grounds one's moral compass and informs choices and behavior. Mindfully exploring the somatic, emotional, and cognitive signals vital to the preservation or restoration of one's integrity is fundamental to self-awareness and self-regulation. Likewise, insight and discernment emanate from the space of being. This outer sphere is closely aligned with the elements necessary to cultivate moral resilience described in Chapters 7 and 8. *Being* encompasses the other two spheres to infuse understanding and action with essential values and wisdom rather than exclusively relying on knowledge or expertise. The middle sphere, *understand*, leverages the values, commitments, insights, and discernment that arise from the space of being, resulting in ethical policies and programs. It consists of recognizing patterns of behaviors and creating alternatives that can produce a culture of moral resilience and ethical practice when enacted in the inner sphere, *act*. The inner sphere is where specific tactics, programs, or initiatives are implemented. Unlike other methods of design, the CFSR approach is an "inside-out" approach sourced in universal values.

The success of this framework depends upon new ways of noticing, listening, engaging, and interpreting; expanding our conceptual and relational repertoire; and addressing our assumptions and biases, both positive and negative. In the context of moral adversity, it also involves examining deeper patterns of relationships within the context where moral and ethical conflicts find expression in day-to-day clinical practice and either support or disable relational integrity. In this space, attention to norms for relational integrity is essential (see Chapter 4). Pattern recognition depends upon new methods of recognizing the symptoms and root factors that result in moral adversity and moral suffering and tracking their impact, as well as the often invisible, interrelated patterns of power, financing, or political agendas that shape the situations and actions that impact the delivery of healthcare. Examining these deeper patterns requires new skills and practices and the support and solidarity of like-minded others.

Some of the non-linear shifts needed to transform clinical care to support integrity and create a culture that fosters ethical practice are proposed in Table 10.1. This is not an exhaustive list but rather illustrative of the sorts of shifts needed to begin the process of transformational change. These shifts must occur within and be responsive to the unique culture

Table 10.1. Potential Shifts to Create a Culture of Ethical Practice

From	To
Resigned	Engaged
Inattentive	Mindful
Victimized	Capable
Alienated	Collaborative
Silenced	Being heard
Excluded	Included
Lack of worth, disrespect	self-esteem, dignity
Sensing disparity	Experiencing fairness

and circumstances where changes are desired. In healthcare organizations, for example, many employees are disengaged and feel victimized and constantly distracted. Their stress and distress create separation, exclusion, and widening disparities rather than cultivating mindfulness, collaboration, inclusion, and fairness. These patterns contribute to a culture of silence, unworthiness, and disrespect rather than enabling employees to constructively use their voice to foster self-esteem and dignity. Shifts in the individual's way of *being* simultaneously impact systems in a dynamic synergy that is inseparable from the results ultimately produced. As discussed in Chapter 5, via our mirror neurons we are acutely attuned to one another, often mimicking each other's energy, intention, and tone. A shift in one person has the power to activate a shift in others. Sourcing our *understanding* of the patterns that are present from the *being* sphere informs insight, decisions, and action. Creating space to recognize patterns and their connection to who we are and the values of the organization where we serve is itself is a powerful change in how we typically do business. This begins to shift the patterns of defining the problem, its solutions, and desired results.

The inner sphere, *act*, engages the *being* and *understanding* spheres to inform the way we execute decisions, interact, and design solutions. It involves the skillful application of a variety of frameworks, tools, and techniques to solve problems and support individual moral resilience and ethical practice. Clinicians and organizational leaders are often well versed in developing and taking problem-focused action; we are constantly finding solutions to the myriad challenges we face each day. However, these well-established patterns can be both an asset and a liability. They can lead us to prematurely conclude that we know the solution before we have fully examined the whole situation. One of the challenges is to resist adopting a solution without carefully assessing whether it aligns with our essential values and contributes to the intended outcome. We commonly rush to act before we fully explore the values driving the solution and understand the patterns of behavior, decisions, or actions that are creating the conflict or concern. Choosing expedience over intentional and disciplined alignment with values and pattern recognition can easily derail meaningful and long-lasting results.

The tools and techniques to design solutions must be aligned with the outer sphere and the shifts identified in the middle sphere. When the outer, middle, and inner spheres align as one seamless whole, rather than a set of partial, fragmented interventions, sustainable results are possible. This new paradigm is about the ability to design and generate responses that integrate our individual and collective capacities to address complex situations by understanding the factors and patterns that create them. Each sphere focuses our attention on different dimensions of reality, but each must be used in relationship with the others as part of an integrated whole-systems framework. The outer sphere that engages our values, ethics, and creativity merges with the middle sphere—the capability to synthesize information, detect patterns, and create alternatives—and these in turn inform the inner sphere skills that foster personal mastery, ethical competence, and design innovation.

The capacities, methods, and skills of the past are insufficient to meet today's challenges. We must cultivate an expanded repertoire or "five minds" as a foundation for action:[35] the disciplinary mind to solve problems; the synthesizing mind to make sense of the invisible patterns affecting reality as well as endless incomprehensible bits of information; the creative mind to forge innovative alternatives; and the ethical and respectful minds to leverage our inner values and wisdom for action that honors our diversity and shared humanity. This expanded repertoire is synergistic with the framework shown in Figure 10.2 and the CFSR approach it depicts.

The Conscious Full Spectrum Response

Used worldwide for large-scale change, the CFSR is designed to align universal, non-negotiable values, purpose, commitments, and actions.[7] Sharma defines universal values as "dignity, equity and compassion, all emanating from our inherent oneness"[7(p3)] that apply to everyone and transcend cultural and religious norms. Instead of reacting to a single incident or series of incidents, CFSR invites diverse stakeholders to employ a rigorous and disciplined process for change. This involves new frames of reference—questions, concepts, and frameworks; new knowledge and skills; and new ways of behaving and relating. Cultivating individual moral resilience and a culture that enables ethical practice requires interventions at the individual, team, and organizational levels to address and transform the intensity and consequences of moral adversity experienced by interprofessional clinicians. Orienting toward transformation implies moving toward a horizon, a vision. Transformation does not imply denying the challenges but rather using them as fuel to create an alternative future. It requires the intention and commitment to design and nurture a vision that provides purpose and direction and is sourced from universal values and wisdom. It leverages our capacity to envision moral adversity as an opportunity for insight, change, and growth—as an opportunity to respond in ways that maximize the potential for principled and lasting change.

What we have learned is that we need to cultivate our ability to source action from the deepest place within ourselves and generate appropriate actions to meet challenges.[7] Sourcing our actions from values such as dignity, compassion, and equity that apply to everyone and exclude no one establishes the foundation for ethical practice. Importantly, we begin our work by looking within at our attitudes, opinions, and spirit that inform our decisions in the face of opposition, ridicule, or rejection. For example, we may ask, "*How do I summon the courage to speak up in situations where power imbalances are prominent? How can we ensure access to life-enhancing preventive and promotive health services without discriminating based on race, religion, or class? How can we allocate resources for those in need who do not have spaces and platforms to express themselves? How do I cultivate my inner capacities and resilience to be mindfully engaged in my clinical practice?*" Answering these questions requires us to draw upon the individual capacities for moral resilience described in Chapter 7. They provide the foundation to design solutions that weave together the wisdom of our bodies, hearts, and minds to produce meaningful and sustainable results.

The practices of mindfulness, self-regulation, self-awareness, and discernment engage our imagination and creativity to co-create new paradigms and solutions. If we are not connected to our purpose and values as individuals, we are likely to repeat the patterns and solutions of the past that only partially address the complexity inherent in ethical practice. We may inadvertently reinforce and solidify patterns, norms, and structures that keep the status quo firmly in place.

In clinical environments, there is a powerful bias toward seeing cognitive capacities as the primary source of knowledge and influence. We are smart enough, we tell ourselves, to think our way through these complex situations without engaging and leveraging other ways of knowing such as insight, imagination, and relationships. But profoundly important values and aspects of our lives and work are likely to be discounted or overwhelmed if we push for solutions to relieve the anxiety and distress of pressing issues. A focus on cognitive capacities can also lead to patterns of confirmation bias that leverage new evidence to confirm existing beliefs or maintain the status quo.[36] Without an ongoing, intentional, and disciplined connection to who we are and what our essential values are, the solutions we design can inadvertently compromise the commitments that matter most.

Leading from the inside out, leveraging our inner capacities and wisdom, is vital to producing the desired results. Instead of beginning with partial solutions to narrowly defined problems with ideas and tactics that are devoid of the deeper aspects of our work, a CFSR sources all actions and solutions from the space of wisdom that includes our intellect but is not limited to it. This process mirrors the individual capacities for moral resilience that invite us to hold lightly to our ideas, agendas, and solutions to allow new possibilities to emerge.

There is often an urgency to create an "action plan" when pressure is exerted somewhere in the system—either by individuals or collectively—in response to moral adversity. Frustrated with the increasing numbers of chronically, critically ill patients in their intensive care units, clinicians may resort to solutions aimed at managing bed allocation to relieve the dissonance in their values about the lives they are sustaining with their interventions.[19] The moral suffering that ensues may be a symptom of a broader, more complex issue. As Thomas and McCullough warn,[37] our impatience may limit our focus to symptoms of the problem while overlooking patterns that reveal its root causes. It is important to understand that myriad factors are involved in the care of chronically, critically ill patients, for example, such as diverse values and preferences regarding quality and quantity of life, cultural norms for treatment and decision-making, budgetary priorities, and funding for healthcare services, and so on. We cannot act on what we do not see or understand. Resource allocation is a dimension of the underlying problem that must be unpacked, and its patterns at the individual, team, organization, and societal levels must be understood in the context of our shared values and commitments. If we see the issue only as a resource allocation problem that produces moral suffering, we may miss other important dimensions that must also be addressed to make lasting change. Developing a protocol without heeding the other interdependent dimensions can produce some relief in the short term but may produce unintended consequences that impede progress toward a more systemic solution.

Complex systems produce tangible consequences that must be addressed when designing solutions that generate results at the individual and systemic level. In clinical settings, most of our responses are aimed at solving specific problems rather than addressing whole systems.[38,39] Within the complex, interdependent world of healthcare, we cannot yet distinguish, design, and generate responses that integrate the different domains related to the entangled hierarchies of any given situation. The pressures in healthcare today are intensified in ways that everyone is feeling the urgent pressure to survive much less thrive. Instead of accepting this reality as an immutable truth, it must be engaged through a new lens. The urgency of crises is inescapable: we have no option but to learn to do things differently, move beyond our separate silos, and create synergy through design and action. The CFSR offers us a way forward.

Applying the CFSR

Instead of designing partial solutions, the CFSR helps us to address moral adversity within the context of systems. It uses technologies, tools, and techniques within that context to help us align purpose, values, and actions. It brings together who we are, how we function, and what we do into a synergistic whole. In effect, this alignment produces individual, relational, and organizational integrity or wholeness. With such a transformational approach, users can seek to understand the systemic patterns within the issue or episode causing moral suffering as embedded in a larger context that is complex and dynamic. It invites us to view the issue or concern within the moral ecosystem that produces the results it is designed to produce rather than limiting the scope to the types of partial solutions described above.

In what follows, we describe methods and strategies illustrating the results-oriented CSFR process. For each sphere (individual, team, and organization), we set forth a process to explore the underlying values and inner capacities; explicate the shifts necessary to create new patterns and desired results; and identify tools, techniques, and practices to achieve the desired results, engage stakeholders, and build capacity. Each sphere must participate in the CFS process. Lasting change requires us to design and invest differently; sustainable transformation is not possible without realistic expectations and synergistic strategies.

Below we apply the model to the individual, leveraging many of the individual capacities outlined in Chapter 7. How we embody who we are as individuals impacts how we embody our values and commitments collectively within our teams, organizations, and broader systems. Likewise, the patterns we see in ourselves have implications for the actions we will take both individually and in the context of relationships with others. Then we move on to its application for the team and the organization to illustrate how the CFSR process aligns the outer, middle, and inner spheres to create concentric rings of interconnected synergy. Mirroring the process that is occurring at the individual level, the CFSR process in this realm illuminates how the CFSR can be applied in various contexts. The examples provided are illustrative rather than comprehensive in scope.

Interventions for the Individual

Outer Sphere: Be

The outer sphere, *being*, focuses on our inner space of who we really are. This goes beyond our roles and identities to the essence of our being.[7] It illuminates who we are as persons and as professionals, and how we engage with the world and the sources of moral adversity we encounter. This is the space where our essential moral/ethical values and intentions are embodied—where they are lived in every moment. We learn to recognize and trust our inherent power for resilience, creativity, and integrity-preserving action. As described in Chapter 7, methods for accessing this space include the cultivation of self-awareness, self-regulation, and mindfulness; accurate and honest self-assessment; and inquiry into our essential values, intentions, and commitments. In its purest form this is where values such as wisdom, compassion, and fairness reside. Moral agency, courage, and personal integrity are grounded in this space. It is the space from which our worldviews and conscience emanate. Cultivating awareness of our inner landscape, moral sensitivity, sources of discernment, and attunement to conscience provides a robust foundation for understanding and making meaningful contributions. It also demands that we distinguish worldviews that emanate from social, education, or ideology sources rather than our essential values and commitments. Knowing our purpose, what we stand for, and how our essential moral/ethical values and commitments are embodied and reflected in our choices and behaviors are key issues to explore. Examining issues that produce moral adversity from the point of view of personal discovery as the solution to the broader problem might include developing mindfulness, self-awareness, moral sensitivity, and recognition of activators of emotional and moral responses. Part of this discernment involves becoming aware of our fears, vulnerabilities, and default responses; recognizing when we act out of courage even when we are afraid; and noticing when we can draw on our inner strength to act when nonnegotiable values are imperiled.

Middle Sphere: Understand

In the middle sphere, the orientation is toward understanding for the purpose of basing decisions and actions on our very essence—our essential values and commitments. This sphere focuses on cultivating the capacities to see things as they are, to understand carefully and critically the morally and ethically salient aspects of an issue, and to see new possibilities with fresh eyes. This space of humble and wise inquiry extends beyond the mind to include imagination and conscience, and it engages all senses and modes of awareness to understand the truth of the situation. Insight based on moral sensitivity, conscience, and discernment is central. It encompasses the ability to see patterns in oneself and others that inform ethical decisions and behavior. Self-regulatory skills and the capacity for openness and vulnerability amid disagreement, conflict, or confusion are cultivated in the outer sphere and engaged here and throughout the process. Insight enhances transparency with oneself and with others. See Chapter 7 for more details.

Discerning and distinguishing patterns of responding, thinking, speaking, and behaving and the role of memory provide a foundation for the individual (and for the team and organization). For example, noticing one's personal narrative about situations that involve moral adversity and gives rise to moral suffering can reveal patterns of communication among clinicians. Noticing the tone, language, content, and themes in our narratives offers insight into choosing whether we need to revise or shift them in some way. Similarly, we must notice our thought patterns and how memory (personal and professional) is manifested in our work. Without focused attention to distinguish the nuances of clinical cases, we are more likely to project past experiences onto the current reality. We must disrupt the patterns that undermine our individual moral agency and collective cohesion. Understanding involves a more robust inquiry process; we need to shift the questions we ask to facilitate insight and understanding of our personal and professional responsibilities. Understanding in this way invites inquiry based on our essential values where we hold lightly to our assumptions, point of view, or position so that alternatives can arise. It also involves disciplined reflection on ambiguity, confusion, and conflicting points of view. An outgrowth of our understanding is the ability to give voice to our views, discernment, and insights in ways that can be appreciated and acted upon. Self-expression and finding one's voice are important countermeasures to the powerlessness and victimization that many clinicians experience. The result of the middle sphere process is the identification of the shifts that are needed to achieve individual results.

Inner Sphere: Act

The inner sphere focuses on the skills, techniques, and methods we can use to embody the essential ethical values that we espouse and that we are committed to. This sphere is where our problem-solving abilities and tools for ethical analysis reside. The process culminates in ethical action.

Rather than beginning here, the CFSR is a disciplined process that engages other abilities and awareness *first*. Without the ability to skillfully enact our ethical commitments, however, it is not possible to fully live our ethical values. Principled action requires us to use decision-making frameworks, decision aids, and practices to support personal integrity. Specific ethical decision-making methods can be useful in addressing ethical challenges that involve value conflicts among individuals, and ethical frameworks that address broader societal issues such as public health are also necessary.[40,41,42,43,44] Adopting methods such as Mindfulness-Based Stress Reduction (MBSR),[45,46] appreciative inquiry,[47,48] the G.R.A.C.E. process for cultivating compassion,[49] and other tools and techniques[50] must be aligned with the results that we aspire to achieve.

Using one of these frameworks or tools is a necessary component but alone is insufficient to produce sustainable and meaningful change. By intentionally addressing the internal and external root factors of the situations that produce moral adversity and the patterns that keep them intact, we can go beyond just thinking to acting differently and embodying our essential values by making conscious choices. No longer are our actions rote, unreflective, or reactive; there is conscious alignment so that every action reflects the essence of who we are and what matters most.

The alignment of these three spheres—*Be, Understand, Act*—is central to personal integrity (the concept of integrity is discussed at length in Chapter 4). The process of integrating being, understanding, and acting serves as the foundation for collaborative and team discernment, design, and action. While individuals alone cannot change an organizational culture, when there is resonance in our values, commitments, decisions, and actions, there is a release of energy that can be aligned and leveraged. As Margaret Mead said, "Never doubt that a small group of thoughtful, committed citizens can change the world; indeed, it's the only thing that ever has."[51(p261)] Individuals within organizations can include all levels of staff, faculty, leadership, and administration as well as the broader community. When committed people come together around their shared values and commitments, change is possible.

Imagine what could be unleashed if frontline clinicians, managers, and senior leaders participated in a simultaneous CFSR process. This was the case when we worked with leaders at the University of Virginia to launch their Compassionate Care Initiative. Nearly 100 people attended an initial workshop to explore their individual and collective values and to begin to create a shared vision and to leverage it for strategic change.[52] Instead of reluctant compliance, the energy released fuels actions that engages everyone involved as empowered partners in a culture of ethical practice.

Interventions for the Team and Organization

Given the interconnection of individual clinicians and others within the healthcare environment, concurrent attention must be given to relational patterns and structures that influence the integrity of the individual, the team, and the organization. As described in Chapter 4, the dynamics involved shape both the context of relationships and the dimensions of relational integrity that extend locally to the healthcare team and more broadly to the organization. In this context, relational integrity reflects the collective integrity of the entire team or organization as manifested in their alignment of values, intentions, behaviors, and support for their ethical commitments. As such, it leverages each individual's *being* sphere to inform and enhance the team's and the organization's collective ways of being, understanding, and acting. Coming together to focus on team or organizational integrity requires a concurrent exploration of related issues and questions, which are explored more fully in Chapter 11 Although the questions team members ask differ to varying extents from those the organization must consider, they both build upon the questions for the individual.

Outer Sphere: Be

For interprofessional teams and the complex organizations where they practice, the outer sphere engages the collective ways of *being* of the people who make up their membership. This sphere leverages the individual constellation of capacities described in Chapter 7 to create a space where those intentions, values, and commitments can be aligned to create a collective way of being. Without exploration and embodiment of one's own purpose, values, and commitments, alignment with others is likely to be ineffective or inauthentic. This space requires a rigorous process to articulate the ways individuals bring their uniqueness, personal moral compass, and professional values and commitments into relationship with others to create a shared purpose, aligned values, and synergistic actions to foster the results they desire.

Congruent with the outer sphere, *be*, focused on the individual, we begin with reflecting how our modes of *being* within the team and the organization impact the relational integrity of the whole—for example, *"In what ways do my purpose, values, and commitments show up in my interprofessional role? To what extent are these aligned with those of my team members and the organization where I practice? To what extent do the opinions and assumptions of various team members impact moral sensitivity, ethical norms, discernment, and action? To what extent is relational integrity upheld?"* A coherent alignment of our individual ways of *being* into a shared way of being is vital if we are to generate the necessary energy, motivation, and focus for culture change. By recognizing implicit and explicit communication patterns, the ways team members ask for and receive advice and support, and instances of integrity and effective moral agency, we can illuminate the space of being within the healthcare team.

Organizationally, this space requires attention to know how values, norms, and strategic priorities are embodied, from the bedside to the boardroom. It goes beyond talking about values to exploring how to express and embody them in terms of communication, making decisions, and setting priorities. This requires asking questions: *"Are decisions explicitly made in alignment with the organization's stated ethical values? To what extent do leaders articulate and embody the stated values? How do the purpose, values, and commitments of clinicians, managers, and leaders connect to the organization's mission, strategic priorities, and the people it serves?"* Exploring these questions requires insight and discernment to engage and weave together a shared set of essential ethical values, commitments, and vision of the team or organization to create a collective culture with standards and norms everyone agrees to be accountable for.

These in turn create an ethical climate that fosters ethical practice that is sourced from the individual and collective wisdom of the group rather than just the agendas and perspectives of a few. In such a climate of mindful awareness, the assumptions, biases, and conscious and preconscious patterns of engaging or not engaging come into view. Disciplined reflection, discernment, and space for insight and wisdom can arise and provide fertile ground for *being* within teams and organizations/systems.

Each element described above is nested within the broader societal context. The collective ways of *being* of the community where we practice and the society where we live exert influence on the micro-community of the healthcare institution and its members. The degree of alignment or misalignment in terms of purpose, values, and commitments influences the tenor and tone of the relationships, decisions, and behaviors of clinicians. At a time of deep divisions within society, processes must be in place to nonjudgmentally invite people with different opinions and perspectives to bring their essential values and essence as the source for dialogue with others. Doing so invites individuals to show up with their most evolved, conscious selves and to earnestly seek connection rather than alienation or opposition. This is where the discipline of individual practice begins to align with collective intentions, commitment, and shared values to the benefit of the broader community and society. Questions are needed to guide the exploration of *being* within these broader contexts: *"What are the essential moral/ethical values endorsed by the community and embodied by community members to guide access to and allocation of healthcare resources?*

Are the expectations that patients, families, and clinicians hold about treatment of people with chronic or advanced illness transparent? Are the cultural norms of the community and broader society regarding healthcare aligned with the organization's stated values?" Reflecting on these questions leads us toward a "collective moral resilience."[53]

Middle Sphere: Understand

Consonant with the middle sphere of individual exploration, this middle sphere focuses on *understanding* how we relate to each other in response to moral adversity as members of a team, organization, and society. Noticing the interplay among individuals within the healthcare team and organizational leaders, systems, and structures creates opportunities for insight. Bringing that insight into patterns, together with the discernment and wisdom that flow from the *being* sphere, makes it possible to determine the shifts needed to bring about the results we desire. For example, we may ask, *"In what ways are common organizational values such as respect and compassion reflected in how leaders make trade-offs of line items in the budget process? How do treatment patterns that are driven by individual values and perspective impact the integrity of those who must implement them? How do our individual values show up in how we appraise clinical situations?"*

Data gathered at a 2016 symposium on moral resilience suggest that the collective sense of powerlessness among critical care nurses may account for an increase in the intensity of moral distress.[54] This pattern offers insight into what shifts may be necessary to restore the moral agency and confidence of critical care nurses. Such patterns may also provide insight into the patterns that affect other members of the clinical team. These other patterns may reflect the ways interprofessional communication and collaboration affect the identification and resolution of situations of moral adversity; the characteristics of ethically challenging cases that lead to moral suffering or distress; the sources or root factors of the patterns that result in moral suffering; and the ways moral disagreements or conflicts are addressed.

Identifying patterns that undermine integrity and ethical practice at all levels of the organization offers fruitful insights about where there are promising points for change. Understanding organizational patterns that arise when complex systems fail to respond to adversity or change can begin to illuminate areas for intervention. These include patterns of "decompensation, working at cross purposes, or getting stuck in outdated behaviors."[4(p66)] Decompensation occurs when the demands of the system exceed its capacity to adapt. Working at cross-purposes occurs when local teams develop "workarounds" that inadvertently have negative global consequences. Getting stuck in outdated adaptive responses that are uninformed by learning from prior experience or failures can indicate system maladaptation. When organizations become "brittle"[55] and lack resilience, factors such as overemphasis on productivity and efficiency contribute to a culture that requires individuals to compensate for the gaps within the system to keep it functional. Similar factors are common within healthcare systems, and it is often frontline clinicians and staff who are exerting heroic efforts to keep a broken system functioning and who bear the burden of these efforts. Recognizing these patterns and their consequences opens the door for innovation and intentional redesign.

Critically examining the written and unwritten norms, rules, policies, and regulations that deter ethical practice can reveal opportunities for change. In an initiative to identify unhelpful rules in healthcare, the Institute for Healthcare Improvement found that while one-third included habits that result from misinterpretation of external regulations or laws or actual legal or regulatory requirements, nearly two-thirds involved organizational policies that were not mandated by external bodies or laws and were within their control to change.[56] This suggests that identifying the patterns reflected in the norms, behaviors, decisions or policies is a fruitful area of exploration in determining the functions that are barriers to ethical practice. Such an approach may reveal common myths, unexamined habits, or unjustified practices and can contribute to creating a new narrative about ethical practice within an organization.

Designing interventions informed both by our essential ethical values and commitments and by our conscious awareness of the patterns that contribute to moral adversity leads to action that is based in wisdom rather than assumption or reaction. Team and organizational patterns of communication, decision-making, protocols, governance, polices, and regulations all contribute to the culture of clinical practice. Recognizing the implicit and explicit values in each lead to greater awareness of systemic contributions to situations of moral adversity. For example, policies that provide all members of the healthcare team, patients, and families with access to ethics consultations reflect values of inclusion, respect for diverse perspectives, and equity in using resources aimed at leveling the playing field when differences or conflicts arise. We must differentiate the patterns that demonstrate alignment with our values from those that undermine them so that we can make the necessary shifts in our culture. Noticing expressions in the workplace that demonstrate respect, conflict mediation, and moral resilience can help us understand what is needed to preserve or restore integrity. This might include having a regular process for team conferences that focus on acknowledging what is working rather than what is not, and on pausing to notice and express gratitude when teamwork has led to desirable outcomes. For instance, in one institution each time an organ is successfully donated and transplanted, the coordinator for the program sends an email to all those involved, sharing the results, and acknowledging the contribution of each person in the process and ultimate outcome. Designing routine patterns of gratitude and acknowledgment engage positive emotions and contribute to a culture of respect that honors the value of teamwork and collaboration.

Similarly, detecting patterns of violations of implicit and explicit team or organizational values or norms and inquiring into the root factors that create them fosters the understanding that can lead to designing solutions for remediation. Teams and organizations may profess a commitment to respectful communication, yet day-to-day examples of disrespectful, dismissive communication patterns observed between leaders and employees, among interprofessional team members, and with patients and families may suggest otherwise. Policies governing informed consent may be skewed toward a risk-management, efficiency framework rather than a robust notion of shared decision-making that more fully invites patients or their surrogates to understand all the treatment options that are available and feasible, thereby fostering a therapeutic rather than a transactional relationship. When team members interpret current practices as disrespecting patient autonomy, their sense of integrity and team cohesion erode.

Consider the informed consent process, for example. If nurses are limited to witnessing the authorization of treatment and are not included in the consent process itself, unresolved ethical questions about the adequacy of the process often follow. Nurses may communicate their concerns by expressing doubts about the adequacy of the patient's understanding of the available choices and resultant consequences. Being able to name these lapses in alignment with team or organizational values provides a platform for intentional change and forms the basis for identifying the shifts that must be enacted to change the patterns and the results accompanying them. Conversely, highlighting and celebrating instances where integrity is visible is a powerful way to shift patterns. Doing so is a valuable antidote to despair, disengagement, and degraded moral agency.

At the organizational level, it is vital to understand the intended and unintended consequences of how resources are allocated, what values drive budget decisions, and what consequences ineffective ethical decision-making has on individuals, professions, patients, families, community, and the organization. Within this process, it is critically important to understand the assumptions we are making about each other's worldviews based on essential values or roles and the ways that our individual and collective narratives impact the way we engage with one another, the decisions we make, and the actions we take. For example, creating a space where teams and organizational leaders can safety and authentically come together to unpack and understand the assumptions made about each other's roles, decisions, and actions creates a new possibility for understanding and design. While it may be necessary for clinicians to be armored against the assaults on their integrity, they must also have safe spaces where they can take off their armor and engage without fear of reprisal, reprimand, or shame.

Concurrently, it is critically important to detect and understand how power and hierarchy inform the patterns of team and organizational engagement and decision-making. Delving into patterns of decision-making (who is at the table and who is not) can reveal unrecognized patterns that need to be shifted to proactively circumvent common factors contributing to moral adversity. Transparency by the leaders of the organization in responding to the systemic factors and cultural norms that produce moral suffering is a vital dimension of inquiry. Noticing how the system adapts during periods of stress and change can add important insights. If there is a loss of a collective purpose or vision, or communication and decision-making patterns become more rigid, or instances of collaborative efforts wane, or decisions become more centralized reducing input from others or there is reluctance to challenge the leader's behavior, can each produce patterns that impede ethical practice.[4] Recognizing these patterns offers insight into the design of interventions aimed at shifting them.

Within this sphere, critical patterns include how clinical and organizational ethical issues are identified; how the sources of disagreement or conflict are recognized; and how the morally salient features of cases involving moral adversity are brought up and prioritized within the context of interprofessional teams, person-centered care, and organizational norms and processes. For example, noticing the pattern of cases that cause moral distress allows teams and the organization to inquire into the contribution of certain patient, team, or system characteristics to determine the root factors.[57] Similarly, understanding patterns of treatment of patient populations (e.g., people needing critical care or oncology treatment or neonatal/pediatric patients) can reveal opportunities for intervention. Opportunities for intervention (e.g., documenting the changing demographics of pediatric critical care from a primarily intensive care environment to an increasing population of children who are chronically, critically ill) may reveal patterns that contribute to ongoing moral suffering of, in this case, pediatric critical care clinicians.[58] In organizations where the treating team focuses on preserving life at all costs, there are generally patterns of aggressive treatment that can be tracked and documented.[19]

In all instances, noticing and tracking the patterns of organizational support or constraints that either enable or disable ethical practice is equally important. For example, throughput pressures can lead clinicians to normalize practice patterns that result in providing ineffective informed consent for tracheostomy or gastrostomy tube procedures to get patients out of the hospital instead of informing patients and surrogates of the implications of their decisions in the short and longer term.[59,60,61]

Noticing patterns of speaking or not speaking within the interprofessional team or organization and exploring how they are informed by our individual narratives (and vice versa) begins to reveal our default patterns and illuminate opportunities for amplification or change. Such patterns often reflect both informal and formal norms. Discerning how we communicate about our ethical conflicts and what words we use—such as "Why are we doing this?"—can make explicit unrecognized patterns of behavior and decisions. Pausing to name and acknowledge these patterns provides clinicians and others the opportunity to reflect on their meaning and to choose to shift them if they are not constructive or beneficial. Making these patterns and others explicit leads to radical transparency among members of the interprofessional team. These seemingly small shifts can be instrumental in creating an opening for greater collaboration, understanding, and innovation.

More broadly, in today's complex healthcare environment, it is also vital to examine the impact of external factors such as financing, regulation, laws, public policies, and societal norms on the individual and collective practices of clinicians. Some may have enormous impact, both positive and negative, on how ethical issues are identified, addressed, and resolved. These patterns must also be examined and considered to determine the shifts that are needed for sustainable change and to clarify the scope of responsibility and influence of individuals, teams, and organizations. The uncertainty of healthcare financing, for instance, creates an organizational culture of fear and negativity that affects how clinicians, patients, families, and administrators engage with each other. There are implications for how these external pressures create alignment or constraints at the point of care.

Likewise, societal norms related to access to and payment for services can create patterns that impact how healthcare decisions are understood and enacted. In the United States, differences in values and worldview regarding access to medical treatment, what is considered the basic minimum healthcare benefit, methods of curbing costs, and expectations regarding access to expensive therapies with marginal benefit affect the way healthcare decision-making is legislated and enacted. Examining these patterns through the lens of individual and collective values and commitments illuminates how we can align actions with the desired shifts.

Inner Sphere: Act

In this sphere, teams and organizations act to formulate strategies to shift the ethical norms so they foster a culture that supports ethical practice. When practitioners base their interventions on their individual and collective wisdom rather than reaction or ego, they create a new foundation for designing solutions. Instead of responding with partial solutions, it becomes possible to create strategies that align individual, team, and organizational purpose, values, and actions in strategies that serve people rather than control, coerce, or rescue them. This requires awareness of how the problems or concerns arise in day-to-day practice and being explicit about what will visibly change because of the individual, team, or organizational action. Above all, it requires commitment and accountability to implement deliberate steps to bring about the desired result. When clinicians share the value of respect as core to their professional roles, their team, and the organizational mission, they are more likely to identify patterns that undermine this value and those that reinforce it, such as moving from autopilot to intentional patient care planning and decision-making.

End-of-life decisions, for example, are a key contributor to moral distress among interprofessional clinicians.[62,63,64,65,66] Using a standardized assessment tool to proactively identify the patient, family, or team characteristics that may contribute to these situations offers a fruitful method for recognizing and understanding what is needed to proactively avoid conflict or disagreement.[28,67,68] When such efforts are explicitly aligned with the teams or organization's ethical values, norms, and commitments and the underlying patterns that contribute to them, it is possible to design interventions that will systematically and intentionally produce different results. Often what is needed is asking, *"How can we approach what we are currently doing differently?"*

When a team member acts with integrity, we need to call it out and celebrate it just as we celebrate every life saved in clinical care. We must begin to recalibrate the belief that acting with integrity is the norm rather than the exception. We must recognize breaches of ethical practice as deviations from our norms rather than accept them as "just the way things are." We can begin by identifying incidents of integrity supported by system shifts in the patterns and narratives surrounding ethically challenging situations. For example, when clinicians request advice and support from ethics consultants, we can acknowledge that they are not ridiculed or overruled by superiors and their concerns are listened to and responded to in respectful and inclusive ways. Reinforcing the behaviors that we wish to collectively cultivate can become the glue that holds teams together under conditions of adversity. Such efforts can be enhanced by intentionally developing policies and practices that align essential ethical values, arise from understanding the patterns that produce the challenges, and create concordance with the methods used to address them. This may be a fruitful area for ethics committees or other organizational bodies to engage in exploring these issues.

At the team level, convening an interprofessional group to engage their collective commitment to "do no harm," to document the behaviors and decisions that produce beneficial results, and to identify patient, team, and system characteristics that contribute to cases of moral distress can lead to the development of specific criteria that can be systematically and proactively implemented to identify ethically complex situations[48,69] or respond to instances of moral distress.[70] Utilizing peer coaches and mentors at the point of care to help identify the ethical problem and possible solutions contributes to an environment where ethical concerns are normalized and discussed regularly.[71] For such processes to reflect a CFSR, they would need to do the following:

1. Align the elements of outer (*be*) and middle (*understand*) spheres.
2. Define the essential ethical values that will guide the intervention.
3. Determine how one's moral/ethical values and purpose will be manifested (individually and collectively), including each team member's accountability for integrity and ethical practice.
4. Identify and articulate the specific shifts that the intervention is designed to address, along with the details of the program or process.

The process for supporting clinicians who experience moral adversity and suffering may include staff debriefings, action reviews to uncover the patterns that contribute to the moral adversity or moral distress consults,[69] and customized individual and team support systems such as the Resilience in Stressful Events (RISE) team,[72] employee assistance, and a repertoire of strategies to regain balance and foster resilience. So too does using a systematic process for moral repair when situations of moral adversity arise. The key to aligning these strategies using a CFSR is the implicit grounding in the essence and ethical values individually and collectively so that the design and action are infused with wisdom rather than self-interest, reaction, or position. It concurrently leverages understanding the patterns that contribute to the conditions where integrity thrives and those that undermine it. While each strategy has some impact, engaging all spheres of the model simultaneously unleashes the full potential of the CFSR. Leveraging organizational norms of providing safe, quality care engages key administrative and clinical leaders in strategies to uncover the system's contributions to the resolution of moral adversity and to invest resources in a robust ethics infrastructure that includes interventions such as routine ethics consultation for cases that meet clinically determined criteria;[52] facilitated ethics conversations and rounds;[69] and policies that impact end-of-life decision-making or conscientious objection.[31]

Beyond this, organizational leaders must commit to strengthening and aligning performance appraisal, incentives, education, and other organizational levers to support and amplify the behaviors, patterns, and actions they wish to cultivate. This involves identifying and aligning regulatory and legal policies with values, norms, and structures for ethical practice, and then structuring the norms of organizational investment in processes to ensure ethics integration across the spectrum. Examining the extent to which internal staffing policies and external safety regulations impede or promote organizational values of fairness, distributive justice, and respect for all levels of staff, for example, can create an intentional mapping of their relationship and impact on ethical practice. Other important dimensions are establishing mechanisms to address regulatory, legal, and policy alignment with values, norms, and the structure for ethics integration within the organization/system and surveillance mechanisms to identify patterns of practice that are likely to create ethical concerns.

Creating a Culture of Ethical Practice

Creating a culture of ethical practice requires focused interventions and engaged leadership. It demands attunement and alignment of individual and organizational values and the methods used to enact them. A culture of ethical practice is vital to the sustainability, safety, and integrity of the healthcare enterprise. A robust, multi-pronged policy mandate is needed to restore and strengthen individual and collective moral compasses. Creating a culture where patients are respected and not harmed, clinicians experience meaning and nourishment in their work, and leaders are rewarded for acts of integrity and courage will require transformational change. The challenge is to involve all stakeholders and all disciplines in processes that acknowledge divergent views and provide new mechanisms to bring values and actions into alignment.

Clinicians have the expertise and moral obligation to advocate for change. Their involvement is vital to avoid recreating the patterns of the past and to enact a new vision for the future. They contribute an invaluable moral anchor to a beleaguered healthcare system. Individually, clinicians must leverage their fundamental moral/ethical commitments to produce meaningful and sustainable change in their daily practice in areas within their control and authority to address those factors that are modifiable. They can begin by examining their own roles and discerning their own contribution to a culture of ethical practice.

Confining the responsibility for solutions to clinicians alone, however, is misplaced and will only exacerbate the problem, intensify resistance, and undermine long-term solutions. Clinicians have responsibility for their own clinical practice, decisions, and behaviors, and meaningful and sustainable change is only possible when individuals, groups, and organizations work together to transform individual and team distress and the organizational culture in ways that create the conditions in which moral and ethical practice can thrive. Leaders in organizations have an equally important obligation to be full partners in design and implementation and demonstrate their commitment by investing in system design and results that fundamentally shift the patterns that are impediments to ethical practice. Without leadership, the efforts of clinicians at the front line will likely have limited impact. Collectively, clinicians must stand together to fulfill their ethical mandate to participate in creating a culture of ethical practice and work with interprofessional colleagues and health system leaders to create system and policy solutions.

Teams and healthcare organizations must also become aware of the collective contributions that support ethically grounded practice in their institutions. Together, individuals and organizations must align interventions to avoid fragmentation and partial solutions. This will require establishing "learning in action" communities where various groups practice, refine, and embody the elements of the CFSR at each step of the process. This is not a one-off program that will miraculously produce results; it requires a commitment to invest in our learning because we care deeply about cultural change, and it requires that we systematically integrate this learning in everyday actions at work to generate immediate and longer-term results. When resistance, frustration, or disappointment arises, we need to be able to begin again with renewed focus and practice to realign ethical values, clarify purpose, and refine strategies that are not working. Questions that can guide individuals and leaders in these efforts appear in Table 10.2.

The CFSR offers individual clinicians, teams, and organizations a framework for designing change that is ethical, meaningful, and sustainable. Without making intentional and fundamental shifts in our mindsets, patterns, and actions, we are likely to replicate the solutions of the past and thereby intensify the moral suffering that currently exists. Such changes will require a disciplined and sustained commitment to actualizing all the dimensions of the process. This will require adopting synergistic strategies to produce the desired results and create a culture of ethical practice, such as that envisioned in Chapter 11.

Table 10.2. Cultivating a Culture of Ethical Practice: Questions for Individuals and Leaders © 2018

- Do I live the values I espouse as vital to my role?
- What specific behaviors demonstrate this alignment?
- When did I notice myself demonstrating my moral resilience?
- What inner and external resources did I draw upon?
- When ethical conflicts arise, am I able to detect physical, emotional, and cognitive signals of alignment or lack of alignment with my essential values?
- What values or personal resources do I draw upon to address ethical concerns or moral adversity?
- What systems/resources do I use in ethically challenging cases?
- Do I participate in forums to address ethical concerns?
- Do I use ethics consultation?
- What tools or techniques do I use to recognize and define ethical issues?
- Do I notice practice or organizational patterns, expectations, or dynamics that are likely to create ethical concerns?
- Do I make my ethical concerns heard and understood?
- Am I able to recognize my symptoms of moral suffering and distress?
- Do I use resources to address the root factors that contribute to ethical conflict or moral suffering?
- When confronted with ethical issues, do I compromise my integrity by my actions or inactions?
- Do I exercise conscientious objection (voice) or refusal when justified?
- Am I aware of how ineffective ethical decision-making affects me, patients and families, other professionals, and the community?
- Do regulatory, legal, financial, and organizational policies influence the way I respond to ethical issues?

References

1. Meth N, Lawless B, Hawryluck L. Conflicts in the ICU: perspectives of administrators and clinicians. Intensive Care Med. 2009;35(12):2068–2077.
2. Magill G, Prybil L. Stewardship and integrity in health care: a role for organizational ethics. J Bus Ethics. 2004;50(3):225–238.
3. Wildes KW. Institutional identity, integrity, and conscience. Kennedy Inst Ethics J. 1997;7(4):413–419.
4. Institute of Medicine. The future of nursing: leading change, advancing health. Washington, DC: National Academies Press; 2010.
5. American Society for Bioethics and Humanities. Core competencies for healthcare ethics consultation. 2nd ed. Glenview, IL: ASBH; 2011.

6. Hollnagel E, Paries J, Woods DD, Wreathall J, editors. Resilience engineering in practice: a guidebook. Aldershot, UK: Ashgate; 2011.
7. Sharma M. Radical transformational leadership: strategic action for change agents. San Francisco, CA: North Atlantic Books; 2017.
8. Haidt J. The righteous mind: why good people are divided by politics and religion. New York: Vintage Books; 2012.
9. Trevino LK, Weaver GR. Managing ethics in business organizations: social scientific perspective. Stanford, CA: Stanford Business Books; 2003.
10. Kaptein M. Developing and testing a measure for the ethical culture of organizations: the corporate ethical virtues model. J Organ Behav. 2008;29(7):923–947.
11. Cohen DV. Creating and maintaining ethical work climates: anomie in the workplace and implications for managing change. Bus Ethics Q. 1993;3(4):343–358.
12. Reina ML, Reina DS, Rushton CH. Trust: the foundation for team collaboration and healthy work environments. AACN Adv Crit Care. 2007;18(2):103–108.
13. Skarlicki DP, Folger R, Tesluk P. Personality as a moderator in the relationship between fairness and retaliation. Acad Manag J. 1999;42(1):100–108.
14. Kaptein SP. Ethics management: auditing and developing the ethical content of organizations. Netherlands: Springer Netherlands; 1998.
15. Fox E, Crigger B, Bottrell M, Bauck P. Integrated ethics: improving ethics quality in health care. Washington, DC: Veterans Health Administration. Accessed February 11, 2018. http://www.ethics.va.gov/elprimer.pdf.
16. Robichaux C, Parsons ML. An ethical framework for developing and sustaining a healthy workplace. Crit Care Nurs Q. 2009;32(3):199–207.
17. Victor B, Cullen JB. The organizational bases of ethical work climates. Adm Sci Q. 1988;33(1):101–125.
18. American Nurses Association Professional Issues Panel on Moral Resilience. Exploring moral resilience toward a culture of ethical practice. Silver Spring, MD: American Nurses Association; 2017. Accessed February 11, 2018. http://nursingworld.org/ExploringMoralResilience
19. Dzeng E, Dohan D, Curtis JR, Smith TJ, Colaianni A, Ritchie CS. Homing in on the social: system-level influences on overly aggressive treatments at the end of life. J Pain Symptom Manage. 2017;55(2):282–289.
20. Pavlish C, Brown-Saltzman K, Hersh M, Shirk M, Rounkle AM. Nursing priorities, actions, and regrets for ethical situations in clinical practice. J Nurs Scholarsh. 2011;43(4):385–395.
21. Rushton CH, Caldwell M, Kurtz M. CE: moral distress: a catalyst in building moral resilience. Am J Nurs. 2016;116:40–49.
22. Rushton CH, Schoonover-Shoffner K, Kennedy MS. A collaborative state of the science initiative: transforming moral distress into moral resilience in nursing. Am J Nurs. 2017;117(2):S2–S6.
23. Musto LC, Rodney PA, Vanderheide R. Toward interventions to address moral distress: navigating structure and agency. Nurs Ethics. 2015;22(1):91–102.

24. Lamiani G, Borghi L, Argentero P. When healthcare professionals cannot do the right thing: a systematic review of moral distress and its correlates. J Health Psychol. 2017;22(1):51–67.
25. Riedel PL, Kreh A, Kulcar V, et al. A scoping review of moral stressors, moral distress and moral injury in healthcare workers during COVID-19. Int J Environ Res Public Health. 2022;19(3):1666.
26. Johnson Foundation. A gold bond to restore joy to nursing: a collaborative exchange of ideas to address burnout. Racine, WI: Johnson Foundation; 2017. Accessed February 11, 2018. http://www.qpatientinsight.com/uploads/2/0/7/1/20710150/nurses_at_wingspread__final.022217.pdf.
27. Perlo J, Balik B, Swensen S, Kabcenell A, Landsman J, Feeley D. IHI framework for improving joy in work. Cambridge, MA: Institute for Healthcare Improvement; 2017. Accessed February 11, 2018. http://www.ihi.org/resources/Pages/IHIWhitePapers/Framework-Improving-Joy-in-Work.aspx.
28. Rushton C, Swoboda S, Reller N, Skrupski K, Prizzi M, Young P, Hanson G. Mindful Ethical Practice and Resilience Academy: equipping nurses to address ethical challenges. American Journal of Critical Care. 2021;30(1):e1–e11.
29. Johnson Foundation. Physician burnout in America: a roadmap for restoring joy and purpose in medicine. Racine, WI: Johnson Foundation; 2016. Accessed February 11, 2018. http://www.qpatientinsight.com/uploads/2/0/7/1/20710150/healingbringsmejoy_final_print.pdf.
30. Rushton C, Swoboda S, Reimer T, Boyce, D, Hansen, G. The Mindful Ethical Practice & Resilience Academy (MEPRA): sustainability of impact. 2023, American Journal of Critical Care. 32(3):184–194.
31. Lewis-Newby M, Wicclair M, Pope T, Rushton C, Curlin F, et al. Managing conscientious objections in intensive care medicine: an official policy of the statement of the American Thoracic Society. Am J Respir Crit Care Med. 2015;191(2):219–227.
32. Schneiderman LJ, Gilmer T, Teetzel HD, Dugan DO, Blustein J, et al. Effect of ethics consultations on nonbeneficial life-sustaining treatments in the intensive care setting: a randomized controlled trial. JAMA. 2003;290(9):1166–1172.
33. Aulisio MP, Chaitin E, Arnold RM. Ethics and palliative care consultation in the intensive care unit. Crit Care Clin. 2004;20(3):505–523.
34. Bramstedt KA, Molnar M, Carlson K, Bilyeu SM. When families complicate patient care: a case study with guidelines for approaching ethical dilemmas. Medsurg Nurs. 2005;14(2):122–125.
35. Gardner H. Five minds for the future. Boston, MA: Harvard Business School Press; 2006.
36. Nickerson RS. Confirmation bias: a ubiquitous phenomenon in many guises. Rev Gen Psychol. 1998;2(2):175–220.
37. Thomas TA, McCullough LB. A philosophical taxonomy of ethically significant moral distress. J Med Philos. 2015;40(1):102–120.

38. Sabin JE. Using moral distress for organizational improvement. J Clin Ethics. 2017;28(1):33–36.
39. Epstein E, Hurst A. Looking at the positive side of moral distress: why it's a problem. J Clin Ethics. 2017;28(1):37–41.
40. Beauchamp TL, Childress JF. Principles of biomedical ethics. 7th ed. New York: Oxford University Press; 2013.
41. Kass NE. An ethics framework for public health. Am J Public Health. 2001;91(11):1776–1782.
42. Jonsen AR, Siegler M, Winslade WJ. Clinical ethics: a practical approach to ethical decisions in clinical medicine. 7th ed. New York: McGraw-Hill; 2010.
43. Rest J. The major components of morality. In Kurtines W, Gewortz J, editors, Morality, moral development, and moral behavior. New York: Wiley; 1984: 24–38.
44. Robichaux C. Developing ethical skills: from sensitivity to action. Crit Care Nurse. 2012;32(2):65–72.
45. Brown KW, Ryan RM. The benefits of being present: mindfulness and its role in psychological well-being. J Pers Soc Psychol. 2003;84(4):822–848.
46. Guillaumie L, Boiral O, Champagne J. A mixed-methods systematic review of the effects of mindfulness on nurses. J Adv Nurs. 2017;73(5):1017–1034.
47. Haizlip J, Plews-Ogan M. Successful adaptation of appreciative inquiry for academic medicine. AI Practitioner. 2010;12(3):44–49.
48. Harmon RB, Fontaine D, Plews-Ogan M, Williams A. Achieving transformational change: using appreciative inquiry for strategic planning in a school of nursing. J Prof Nurs. 2012;28(2):119–124.
49. Halifax J. G.R.A.C.E. for nurses: cultivating compassion in nurse/patient interactions. J Nurs Educ Pract. 2014;4(1):121–128.
50. Rushton C, Reller N, Swoboda S. Applying E-PAUSE to Ethical Challenges in a Pandemic. AACN Adv Crit Care. 2020;31(3):334–339.
51. Lutkehaus NC. Margaret Mead: the making of an American icon. Princeton, NJ: Princeton University Press; 2008.
52. Fontaine DK, Rushton CH, Sharma M. Cultivating compassion and empathy. In Plews-Ogan M, Beyt G, editors, Wisdom leadership in academic health science centers: leading positive change. London: Radcliffe Publishing; 2014:92–110.
53. Delgado J, Siow S, de Groot J, et al. Towards collective moral resilience: The potential of communities of practice during the COVID-19 pandemic and beyond. J Med Ethics. 2021;0; 1–20.
54. Sofer D. Panel discussion 2: promising system and environmental strategies for addressing moral distress and building moral resilience. Am J Nurs. 2017;117(2):S18–S20.
55. Woods DD. Creating foresight: lessons for enhancing resilience from Columbia. In Starbuck WH, Farjoun M, editors, Organization at the limit: lessons from the Columbia disaster. Malden, MA: Blackwell; 2005:289–308.

56. Berwick DM, Loehrer S, Gunther-Murphy C. Breaking the rules for better care. JAMA. 2017;317(21), 2161–2162.
57. Rushton CH. Defining and addressing moral distress tools for critical care nursing leaders. AACN Adv Crit Care. 2006;17(2):161–168.
58. Shapiro MC, Henderson CM, Hutton N, Boss RD. Defining pediatric chronic critical illness for clinical care, research, and policy. Hosp Pediatr. 2017;7(4):236–244.
59. Brett AS, Rosenberg JC. The adequacy of informed consent for placement of gastrostomy tubes. JAMA Intern Med. 2001;161(5):745–748.
60. Fairfax LM, Christmas AB, Norton HJ, Jacobs DG. Breakdown of the consent process at a quaternary medical center: our full disclosure. Am Surg. 2012;78(8):855–863.
61. Vargas M, Servillo G, Antonelli M, Brunetti I, De Stefano F, et al. Informed consent for tracheostomy procedures in intensive care unit: an Italian national survey. Minerva Anestesiol. 2013;79(7):741–749.
62. Prentice T, Janvier A, Gillam L, Davis PG. Moral distress within neonatal and paediatric intensive care units: A systematic review. *Arch Dis Child.* 2016;101:701–708
63. Dzeng E, Colaianni A, Roland M, Levine D, Kelly MP, et al. Moral distress amongst American physician trainees regarding futile treatments at the end of life: a qualitative study. J Gen Intern Med. 2016;31(1):93–99.
64. O'Neill BJ, Kazer MW. Destination to nowhere: a new look at aggressive treatment for heart failure—a case study. Crit Care Nurse. 2014;34:47–55.
65. Rushton CH, Kaszniak AW, Halifax JS. Addressing moral distress: application of a framework to palliative care practice. J Palliat Med. 2013;16(9): 1080–1088.
66. Rushton CH, Kaszniak AW, Halifax JS. A framework for understanding moral distress among palliative care clinicians. J Palliat Med. 2013;16(9): 1074–1079.
67. Lautrette A, Darmon M, Megarbane B, Joly LM, Chevret S, Adrie C, et al. A communication strategy and brochure for relatives of patients dying in the ICU. N Engl J Med. 2007;356(5):469–78.
68. Pochard F, Azoulay E, Chevret S, Lemaire F, Hubert P, Canoui P, et al. Symptoms of anxiety and depression in family members of intensive care unit patients: ethical hypothesis regarding decision-making capacity. Crit Care Med. 2001;29(10):1893–1897.
69. Helft PR, Bledsoe PD, Hancock M, Wocial LD. An evaluation of unit-based ethics conversations. JONAS Healthc Law Ethics Regul. 2010;12(2):48–54.
70. Hamric AB, Epstein EG. A health system-wide moral distress consultation service: development and evaluation. HEC Forum. 2017;29(2):127–143.

71. Trotochaud K, Fitzgerald H, Knackstedt A. Ethics champion programs: a promising practice to promote moral agency in healthcare settings. Am J Nurs. In press.
72. Edrees H, Connors C, Paine L, Norvell M, Taylor H, Wu AW. Implementing the RISE second victim support programme at the Johns Hopkins Hospital: a case study. BMJ Open Internet. 2016;6(9):e011708.

11

Creating a Culture of Moral Resilience and Ethical Practice

Cynda Hylton Rushton, Monica Sharma, Katherine (Katie) Brewer, and Heather Fitzgerald

CREATING A CULTURE for moral resilience and ethical practice will require a sustained and multi-faceted approach.* To begin the process, we must believe that change is possible and work together to launch a vision of possibility and hope. We must take the long view of culture change so that we can intentionally and incrementally start to shift the patterns that undermine personal and professional integrity and ethical practice by grounding our efforts in our essential values. Intentionally strengthening capacities for moral resilience, building new skills and abilities, and designing organizational interventions to do so will offer hope and support for those at the front lines who are confronted daily by ethical challenges and complexity. To succeed, solutions must align the dynamic interplay among individuals, teams, organizations, and the broader society. In this chapter, we bring together the concepts presented through this book in two sections—strategies for system design and transformational design for sustainable results—and describe key elements of each.

* Acknowledgment: Portions of this chapter were adapted from Sharma M. Radical transformational leadership: strategic action for change agents. San Francisco, CA: North Atlantic Books; 2017.

Cynda Hylton Rushton, Monica Sharma, Katherine (Katie) Brewer, and Heather Fitzgerald, *Creating a Culture of Moral Resilience and Ethical Practice* In: *Moral Resilience*. Second Edition. Edited by: Cynda Hylton Rushton, Oxford University Press.
 DOI: 10.1093/oso/9780197667149.003.0012

Strategies for System Design

Large-scale change is not possible without aligning individual and collective values, wisdom, and commitment to the architecture needed to support ethical practice. In Chapters 7 and 8 we explored the individual capacities for fostering moral resilience and in Chapter 10 the interpersonal, team, and organizational dimensions of those capacities. Here we describe using the Conscious Full Spectrum Response (CFSR) to integrate the three spheres of *Be, Understand,* and *Act* in the context of moral resilience and ethical practice to fuel the dynamic synergies needed to achieve individual, relational, and organizational integrity. The examples reflected in this chapter illustrate the application of the CFSR model—many from our own work. As others adopt the model, more examples will emerge, and we look forward to learning about their experiences and results. We include examples that are not specifically designed using the CFSR to illustrate elements that are aligned with certain aspects of the model but may not reflect all elements. It is vital that the entire CFSR method is used to produce the desired results.[1] The model has been tested worldwide to address complex problems in diverse contexts.[1,2] Figure 11.1 depicts the process required to design a system that supports ethical practice on a moment-to-moment basis; these strategies for organizational change are discussed below.

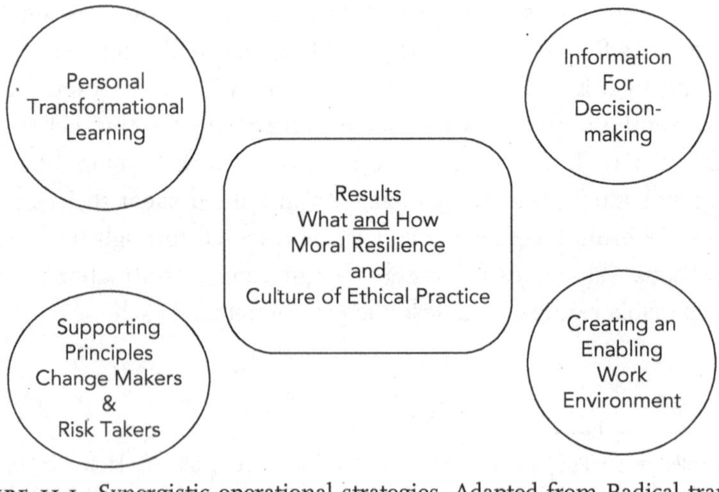

FIGURE 11.1. Synergistic operational strategies. Adapted from Radical transformational leadership: strategic action for change agents (p. 120), by M. Sharma, 2017, San Francisco, CA: North Atlantic Books. Copyright 2017 by North Atlantic Books. Reprinted with permission.

Personal Transformational Learning

A growing body of evidence shows that humans are slow to change, even when change is clearly needed. Transformational learning unleashes the human potential to commit, care, and effect change. By teaching us what we otherwise could not learn without having experienced it, it can fundamentally change who we are and how we view the world. When we take for granted that moral adversity and unhealthy work environments are "part of the job," we reinforce our feelings of powerlessness, victimization, and resignation. When we overlook daily examples of integrity-preserving decisions and compassionate action, we begin to erode respect for the effort, wisdom, and skill routinely manifest in clinical practice. At the same time, our sense of moral agency, confidence, and self-efficacy is tarnished. When our moral sensitivity, conscience, and engagement in our work is eroded, it is more likely that we will adopt an "us-versus-them" attitude that fosters blaming each other and the system for the conditions in which we practice. Aligning our shared values requires that all stakeholders take responsibility for both the process and the results ultimately produced.[3,4]

At faith-based Providence/St. Joseph Health, leaders embarked on a journey to make compassion the basis of strategic action throughout their organization.[5] The organization and people within it embraced compassion as a core value, but some individuals were unable to embody it in day-to-day practice or were unaware of how their suffering might impact others. An interprofessional program enrolling all levels of the organization was deployed to engage leaders, clinicians, and frontline staff in understanding their own suffering to expand their skills cultivating compassion. This led to the engagement of clinicians at the point of care with formal leaders to address the barriers to embodying compassion and expressing it in everyday practice. This in turn led members of the neonatal intensive care unit to leverage their commitment to compassion (*be*) into designing (*understand*) and implementing (*act*) an intervention to address burnout in their unit.

If senior leadership is not engaged, staff may feel that they do not have "permission" to take action to shift the culture in the workplace. No matter how courageous clinicians are as individuals, if the leadership does not cultivate its full potential, there cannot be a change in culture. For senior leaders, engaging in such initiatives requires them to reconnect to their purpose and intentions for service in healthcare—instead of creating committees to study the problem or collect more data. The leaders at Providence/St. Joseph's participated in the same program as other members of the workforce. They were invited, like everyone else, to connect to "who they are" as people as well as leaders. Sometimes people at the point of care overlook or deny the ways their leaders experience suffering and how it impacts their decisions, communication, and behavior.[6,7,8,9] The COVID-19 pandemic was rife with issues for leaders at any level of the organization, those in clinical positions as well as those in administrative roles. Healthcare leaders might experience a tension unlike that of clinicians or other healthcare workers, in that they may have dual identities as clinicians and as administrators. Evidence indicates that this duality presents challenges when they are faced with difficult administrative decisions that might defy their ethical inclinations as clinicians or vice versa.[10] Evidence indicates that nurse leaders also experienced stress during the pandemic, with some evidence hinting that operational and policy decisions related to the pandemic created even more stress among nurse leaders than in nurses at the point of care.[8]

In any event, leaders and those at the point of care are all accountable for their actions. Being able to attune to and understand the suffering of oneself and others creates possibilities for understanding and collaborative solution-finding. Resilience programs in the military have established a clear relationship between leadership and resilience in the people in the organization.[11] When leaders embody compassion, it is a powerful motivator for others to do the same and drives change in visible and sustained ways.[12] Leaders who have chosen to move from control to get things done to empowering others to fully leverage their purpose and contribution are able to establish transformational learning programs.[13]

Unfortunately, we tend to invest in programs that develop technical skills for professional practice rather than in initiatives that focus on transformational learning. Consider how many organizations have adopted one-off programs, requiring mandatory participation, only to find that the impact is unsustainable. Intensified cynicism, resistance, and disengagement often follow. Skills alone will not produce the desired outcomes for clinicians, patients, or organizations. As a founder of quality assessment emphasized, "Systems awareness and systems design are important for health professionals but are not enough. They are enabling mechanisms. It is the ethical dimension of individuals that is essential to a system's success."[14(p137)] Clinicians must invest in their own learning to cultivate moral, emotional, and social intelligence and to expand, enhance, and value their potential contribution to patient care, their team, and the organization. This requires expanding their repertoire of practices, tools, techniques, and skills. It will also necessitate organizational commitment, giving staff time, resources, and safe spaces to integrate well-being practices into their workday as a means of self-stewardship and to develop and practice the skills to address ethical challenges.[15,16] Not unlike an infertile garden, staff who cultivate well-being practices on their own time may amplify their integrity and moral resilience, but then be faced with harsh headwinds in the workplace that severely test it. The seed is strong, but when planted in rocky, inhospitable soil, it does not thrive.[1]

Organizations must commit to giving staff the time and space to cultivate self-stewardship and well-being while at work, but they must also create a climate and culture where integrity and moral resilience are not constantly tested or undermined. Inhospitable work environments and challenging workplace culture with low staffing, reduced resources, angry patients, and pay cuts challenge the stamina and professional commitment of nurses and other clinicians.[17,18,19] Organizations must embrace their role in building strong, nourishing workplaces that preserve integrity, through acts that are seemingly simple but might be financially challenging, such as providing ample staffing, increasing compensation, setting reasonable expectations for patients and families, and elevating the value and prowess of nurses and other clinicians to patient and organizational outcomes.[17,20] Alongside these complex issues, organizational investment is needed in a robust ethical infrastructure that is proactive and responsive to ethical challenges faced by everyone in the organization,

Examples of sustained and conscious organizational efforts to promote moral resilience include those with sustainable funding and programs such as the Mindful Ethical Practice and Resilience Academy (MEPRA).[15,16] It is a twenty-four-hour experiential, discovery learning program for nurses at the point of care. The program, launched in 2016, has demonstrated significant improvements in ethical confidence, competence, mindfulness, resilience, and work engagement while showing decreases in depression, anger, and intent to leave. Most of these improvements were sustained at three and six months after the program.[16] Graduates of MEPRA are using the skills they learned in the program to initiate change in their local practice settings. Through their engagement in the MEPRA Community of Practice, they apply these skills as they use the CFSR framework described in Chapter 10 to design solutions for an issue they wish to change at the unit level. Drawing on their essential values and commitments, they identify the patterns that are producing the conditions that imperil their integrity and the shifts that are needed to achieve the desired results; then they design specific strategies to address these gaps. A critical care nurse, committed to respect for self and others, sought to shift the attitudes of her clinical team from resentment to engagement. She recognized that efficiency pressures were undermining team cohesion. Based on what she learned in MEPRA, she was aware of the power of engaging positive emotions such as gratitude to shift the way she and her colleagues related to each other, especially under situations of stress and moral conflict. She instituted a "gratitude circle" during the daily interprofessional team huddle. After three weeks, she noticed a change in engagement: team members were pausing to express gratitude even when she was not present, positive regard for the contributions of team members increased, and people commented on the positive feelings unleashed by connecting to something they were grateful for. When mired in distress and negativity, clinicians are more likely to resort to autopilot patterns that lead to disconnection and constricted possibilities. These patterns are predictable especially in the aftermath of a global pandemic. Strategies such as these offer an alternative that ignites the basic goodness of members of the team and propels them toward a new pattern of relating with themselves and others. Building on this, she engaged unit charge nurses to institute a "What I Noticed" board to capture and highlight acts of integrity, courage, clinical excellence, and teamwork among their colleagues. At the end of each shift, these moments are written on the board to publicly acknowledge and express gratitude for their contributions. When their contributions are acknowledged, team members feel honored and respected, a key element of a healthy workplace.[21] Leveraging these new patterns is an important tool for engaging others in the process of change.

Building on the MEPRA program, R^3: Renewal, Resilience & Retention of Maryland nurses, a statewide initiative focusing on resilience and ethical practice in nursing students, faculty and practicing nurses was launched in Maryland.[22] Using the CSFR model, eight schools of nursing, five hospitals and the thirty-six-member Nurse Residency Collaborative joined to build capacity, skills, and tools to support individual and system change. Faculty began the journey by exploring their values, moral compass, mindfulness, emotional intelligence, self-stewardship, and other concepts to shift their mindsets and capacities to embody who they are and what they stand for in life and work. From this foundation they built skills to integrate newly developed content and modules into their existing courses and to engage in addressing some modifiable pattern within their organization.[22] Content related to resilience and ethical practice will be integrated into practice from the first day of nursing school through collaboration with the educators from the Maryland Nurse Residency Collaborative of Maryland.[23] Models of academic/practice partnerships have the potential to overcome historical barriers to alignment of initiatives and programs and to synergize and amplify mutually beneficial results.

Providing a framework to guide design helps to empower and enable clinicians and others to unleash their potential despite the challenges they face. In this case, it is a meaningful step toward building a culture where the integrity of the members and the relational integrity of the team are fostered in day-to-day interactions. Starting small and dreaming big creates a new way of responding to the inevitable challenges of clinical practice. Some may say such efforts will do little to move the needle of change, but in reality, sustainable change will require the aligned and concerted efforts of many to create "a new fractal" to shift what may be viewed as deeply embedded patterns and systems.[1] When we begin to resonate with and create new patterns within teams, our organizations, and ourselves, new solutions emerge with the potential to fundamentally change the culture in ways that support ethical practice.

Information for Decision-Making

Personal transformation that manifests in workplace, organizational, and social transformation requires identification of appropriate indicators and an evolving system of measurement. If we only focus on documenting the problem of moral adversity and distress, we will likely miss other salient aspects of the problem and, importantly, the potential solutions. We can overlook the daily examples of integrity-preserving action and the practices that support it. What we choose to measure is what will be amplified: the choice is to balance the focus on the problem and the solutions in a way that propels us toward progress and culture change. Both will be needed to gain a complete view of progress, gaps, and opportunities for innovation and meaningful results. Using methods such as polarity management offers a useful tool to assess and account for this dynamic interplay.[24]

The current set of indicators used for most human and ecological development efforts tells an incomplete story; it often omits stories of innovation, courage, transformation, and profound change. Measures such as the Hospital Consumer Assessment of Healthcare Providers and Systems survey,[25] employee engagement, or safety assessments fail to capture the ways that clinicians are innovating, transforming their workplaces through their efforts. The external pressure to rely exclusively on these scores as benchmarks of organizational effectiveness can distract innovation teams from their essential values and cause them to overlook invisible patterns that must be understood to design solutions. While responses to these measures are routinely collected, the context that influences them is often complex, making it difficult to discern the specific impact of various interventions on them. Programs such as those created by the Institute for Healthcare Improvement (IHI) offer robust models for capturing the often-overlooked elements of change along with traditional measures.[26] They can begin by asking questions of diverse stakeholders such as "*What matters to you?*" to connect to people's moral compass or adapting the *"What is the pebble in your shoe?"* question to understand what is in the way of providing care with integrity.[27] Gathering these data begins to build a more comprehensive view of the issues and their impacts and to measure the success of innovations.[28,29]

One of the challenges is to develop ways to measure the immeasurable—or, perhaps more accurately, the unmeasured. This starts with viewing individuals and their contributions as assets rather than considering them "beneficiaries" or a means to an end. This is where our creativity is needed to distill indicators of well-being, integrity, and system design that are sourced from inner capacities to effectively shift our culture and results. It is often difficult to isolate and measure the effects of various interventions. Efforts are under way to define and test alternative measurement schemes to address burnout, resilience,[30,31] and work-life climate.[11] To expand on these efforts, we must take the opportunity to shift our mindsets regarding measurement to expand the aspects of moral resilience and ethical practice we wish to change. As with other strategies, focusing on measurement in this way means beginning with clarity about the values, ways of being, and collective commitments that will be reflected in the measures that are designed or adopted. It also invites a broader range of measurement strategies to capture what is realistically happening and the consequences, both quantitative and qualitative, on the people in all levels of the system, the people served, and the broader community. This is a fruitful area for further scientific and methodological innovation. Mindsets such as those represented by the Institute for Healthcare Improvement focus on rapid cycle improvements that are instigated, evaluated, and modified in real time[32,33] as well as frameworks for spreading, through which effective strategies in one setting are shared with other areas assuring impact and sustainability.[34] These offer a promising direction when the evidence base is developing and there is an urgent need for innovations to address the very real suffering of people at the front lines of clinical practice. New measurement methods, ongoing evaluation, and systems for monitoring progress and continuous improvement provide leaders and team members with vital information to guide design and demonstrate value.

It is vital to measure both positive and negative aspects—for instance, when moral resilience is present and when moral adversity or suffering is present, and when policies or practices undermine integrity and when integrity is supported. Most commonly, team and organizational measurement focuses on deviations from norms or standards rather than alignment with them. If we take for granted the instances where ethical behavior has been upheld and supported, we risk overlooking or minimizing the impact of *aligned* ethical behavior. Developing mechanisms for capturing both requires a shift in mindset and in the systems for capturing them. For example, a tool such as the Compassion in Action Review, a process that rests on non-negotiable ethical values of respect, inclusion, and integrity, involves a process of learning how to make sense out of what happened in situations that arise from moral adversity. Its goal is to acknowledge what happened, to identify the consequences (both constructive and negative), to generate alternative solutions based on reviewing and analyzing information about what happened and the assumptions that informed the decisions, and to support the team to self-correct and adapt. It provides a framework for learning from the gaps between what was intended and what happened, along with an action plan to address them. Within the process are opportunities to notice and embrace what went well and what can be amplified and leveraged in future events, which is vital for building not only individual moral resilience but also the collective moral resilience of the team. The process allows people to acknowledge their contributions amid perceived failure and to process seemingly contradictory perspectives and actions and create alternatives that serve both clinicians and patients. From this, patterns that have supported integrity and undermined it are identified and used to design solutions that the group commits to enact. Participants walk away with tangible next steps, insights about others and themselves, and engagement in their moral community. This process activates the growth mindset so vital to innovation into becoming an embodied experience.[35]

The Rushton Moral Resilience Scale (RMRS) is an example of an innovative measure to capture moral resilience at its core (see Chapter 9). The RMRS©™ was developed to measure moral resilience as conceptually defined through the domains of personal integrity, relational integrity, responses to moral adversity, and moral efficacy.[36] The RMRS can be used by organizations striving to measure the impact of interventions aimed at addressing the moral/ethical domain.[36] Efforts to measure aspects of organizational personnel health, including burnout and job satisfaction, are important to the generic work environment, but they fall short in capturing the impact of moral and ethical challenges and resultant moral suffering. Our initial research demonstrated that moral resilience is a distinct concept from generic resilience as measured using the Connor-Davidson resilience tool.[36] Measurement of moral suffering including moral distress and moral injury should include corollary measures that reflect the inherent strengths and capabilities of people in the system. Organizations may also measure moral resilience using specific subscales of the RMRS or the entire scale among clinicians and staff to understand baseline issues and promote programs and strategies to strengthen overall moral well-being and integrity. These data can be used to devise systemic solutions to address the patterns within the organization that create moral adversity and intervene to dismantle them or at least minimize their occurrence and impact. Instead of continuing to "admire the problem" by continuing to focus exclusively on it , exploration, and qualitative and quantitative measurement of the alternative way of being offers a more balanced approach and enhanced potential for sustainable change.[37]

Making sound decisions relies on accurate, timely, understandable, and coherent information. In our fast-paced healthcare environments, decisions are often made with incomplete or incorrect information. In our urgency to respond, we may seek data or information supporting those actions that cause the least disruption and are most economical or efficient rather than pausing long enough to ask new questions and discover new answers. It can lead to cutting corners in ways that undermine the healthcare enterprise and inadvertently create new and unexpected types of challenges and untoward consequences. The electronic medical record (EMR), for example, can become the driver of shortcuts that cause patient narratives to become muted when clinicians fail to revise or elaborate on their history as new information is discovered. Handoffs between team members may include opinions and personal judgments affected by implicit bias rather than facts and principled conclusions;[38] this can lead to labels being assigned to people or behaviors that are disrespectful or unjust.[39] Such practices affect the way patient preferences, goals, and understanding are communicated and acted upon, as well as undermining trust and endangering ethical practice. These patterns extend to the clinical team and can undermine relational integrity, teamwork, and collaboration.[40] Over-reliance on electronic communication can contribute to isolation, decreased empathy, and human connection. Without these relational capacities all aspects of the work environment and the people within it are degraded.[40,41]

As the uncertainty and complexity of the healthcare environment have intensified, we need information about national and local patterns and policies, cultural norms that impact health, and the systems providing services to differentiate those that empower from those that disempower. Misinformation, politicization, and polarization of healthcare decisions and services, such as anti-vaccine stances and legislation and executive actions aimed at members of the LGBTQIA+ community, present threats to clinician ethics and integrity.[42] Exposure to politics and political actions, particularly in an era of polarized politics, can be emotionally draining.[43,44] Clinicians might find themselves caught up in the magnetic force of identity and politics which could threaten interprofessional and clinician-patient relationships and undermine their relational integrity.

Within teams, the type of information that is collected, shared, reported, and acted upon arises from traditions passed on without reflection about whether they are relevant to current practice or the context of patient care. Individuals, teams, and organizations can lapse into patterns that reflect the mindset *"We've always done it this way"* instead of asking whether what is currently being done is useful, effective, or ethically justified.

In many cases, we expend a great deal of energy to collect data that are neither used nor are relevant to the results we desire.[45,46] Making decisions based on efficiency measures alone, for example, fails to account for the processes that create the conditions for healing, namely, "interpersonal trust, social relationships, respectful interactions, emotional engagement, mindfulness (reflective thinking), compassion, and human touch."[47] Clearly, such elements are difficult to isolate without new measurement mindsets.[48] Creative new methods that capture the processes and outcomes of innovation are needed to transform the clinical environment. Arguably, if the relational and ethical aspects are aligned, the desired results will follow. Building a new vision for clinical practice requires complexity-based, developmental evaluation methodologies that produce data useful in fostering social innovation. These methodologies involve iterative and responsive learning feedback loops, alignment of purpose and values, and the development of measures as the process evolves, as well as a priori evaluation methods designed to capture system dynamics and complexities.[47,49] Novel evaluation methods increase the likelihood that system design will facilitate acting with integrity and producing outcomes of value to patients, families, clinicians, organizations, and the broader community.[37]

To make principled, ethically grounded decisions, we need access to complete and accurate information. Initiatives to address moral adversity need to leverage coherent, understandable, and actionable information about the patterns that create the conditions for moral resilience and ethical practice. Mary Ann Beil, vice president for corporate ethics at Memorial Health in Savannah, Georgia, developed a bioethics performance improvement team to examine the patterns that were creating moral adversity for clinicians.[50] The purpose of the initiative was to align corporate and clinician values surrounding quality care for the people they were serving by addressing a gap identified by clinicians as undermining their ability to do so. Information collected by the team identified practice patterns that caused moral disagreement, conflict, or distress. From these patterns, interprofessional teams worked within clinical specialties to develop unique evidence-based triggers for ethics consultation to facilitate proactive identification and system responsiveness. Systemic structures within clinical specialties resulted in weekly transdisciplinary ethics rounds where cases identified based on the ethics triggers are routinely addressed. In recognition of the role nurses play at the point of care and to facilitate the process of identifying high-risk cases, nursing ethics liaisons on specialty specific units are trained to apply the criteria and empowered to routinely bring forward cases at risk for ethical concerns or conflict to a weekly transdisciplinary ethics meeting. Rather than waiting until moral/ethical conflict has solidified, a routine review such as this makes possible early identification of risk factors and moral/ethical disagreements and conflicts.[51,52] Mechanisms such as these to proactively identify ethical complexity and conflict are important in shifting the patterns of individual and collective communication and decision-making.[53,54,55]

Maintaining transparency and using the information flow to leverage change are important dimensions of a CFSR. Who does and does not have access to what kinds of information is a vital leverage point in creating a culture of ethical practice. Most frontline clinicians are generally not privy to institutional criteria that guide decision-making in healthcare organizations. Leaders who are committed to creating a culture of ethical practice recognize that transparency in decision-making is necessary for integrity at all levels of the organization.[56] A culture of ethical practice that fosters moral resilience in every member of the organization creates communication patterns that empower people to be their best, even when difficult decisions must be made. Humans seek to resolve uncertainty and dissonance by creating narratives that complete the details that are left unsaid or omitted. This human tendency can allow healthcare professionals and leaders to create explanations that may not be accurate. All involved in complex decision-making may employ confirmatory biases to justify their point of view or position.[57,58] In contrast, when there is transparency, information flows in ways that leverage moral resilience and ethical practice; people explain the reasons for what they do and take responsibility for their decisions and actions. This becomes the norm rather than the exception; with it, trust is fostered rather than broken.[1,59,60]

One strategy for enhancing information flow regarding ethical practice in healthcare organizations is the accountability of ethics committees and consultation services to report to leadership about the ethical concerns of the organizational community. Importantly, the reporting structure influences the degree of impact that such data can have on organizational behavior and decision-making. Having mechanisms in place for individuals and groups to give voice to ethical issues and concerns contributes to shifting the culture in ways that are aligned with ethical practice. Many ethics committees, for example, engage in routine case review as part of their quality improvement process to identify themes, evaluate the effectiveness of the consultation process, inform policy development, and guide education. Others, based on their inclusion in the hospital's committee leadership structure, have membership on the administrative committee of the organization. From this vantage point, there are regular opportunities to share trends and the volume and content of ethics consultations; participate in proactive and ongoing review of hospital policies and processes; and highlight ethical concerns that may be unrecognized or overlooked. This can contribute to seeing ethics as integrated into the fabric of the organization.[61,62]

Although not designed using a CFSR approach, the Veterans Health Administration (VHA) is the largest integrated healthcare system in the United States. Nine million enrolled veterans receive care from over 370,000 staff at 171 medical centers and 1,298 outpatient sites of care.[63]

Veterans Affairs' National Center for Ethics in Health Care (NCEHC) is VHA's primary healthcare ethics resource, addressing complex ethical questions in all aspects of care, including clinical, professional, and organizational issues, business, and research. NCEHC uses a hub and spoke model to provide tertiary ethics consultation to VHA facility healthcare ethics staff.[64,65] VHA's healthcare ethics resources have focused on ethical leadership, program implementation, ethics quality, learning needs, performance, areas of improvement, staff perception, and, importantly, ethics consultants' skills, knowledge, and proficiency. VHA's healthcare ethics consultation "IEWeb" database yields data that point to many of the root causes of moral adversity and suffering, and highlight the importance of simultaneously intervening at multiple levels to create the synergy and momentum for change.[63,64,65]

The features of an enabling environment include professional culture, institutional culture, workforce policy, and financing policy, among others. An enabling environment should engage the individual capacities described in Chapter 7, including the attitudes/perceptions, knowledge, skills, and behaviors needed for integrity-preserving action, together with the collective strategies discussed in Chapter 10 on the institutional and system levels that support individual health and well-being, governance, organizational change, employee experience, workforce, patient/family outcomes, and so on. Aligning individual integrity with systemic integrity-preserving design harnesses the energy and creativity of a critical mass to propel lasting change. When healthcare organizations are seriously engaged in creating a culture that supports ethical practice, they feel the urgency for renewal and increased effectiveness. The mutually reinforcing objectives of moral resilience and ethical practice include grassroots engagement parallel with a strategy for engaging senior leadership that creates bottom-up and top-down inspiration and innovation and contributes to shared governance. Frameworks such as the Standards for Establishing and Sustaining Healthy Work Environments[21] and the Healing Healthcare Initiative of the Schwartz Center for Compassionate Care offer critical elements and evidence-based solutions that can be leveraged using a CFSR.[66] The Healing Healthcare Initiative, currently in the pilot stage with leaders from six healthcare organizations, is a year-long, practical and applied educational program aligned around the core values of psychological and physical safety; trust and trustworthiness; diversity and equity; inclusion, voice, and choice; team cohesiveness and collaboration; mental health and well-being. This pilot will support the six participating organizations to develop sustainable roadmaps designed to assure that healthcare professionals and those in their care can thrive.[67]

Initiatives such as MEPRA engage nurses at the point of care in cultivating the skills and attitudes needed to engage with their leaders and constructively communicate their perspectives, offer solutions, and harness their dedication to enact changes within their scope of influence.[15,16] Simultaneously, nursing leaders are engaged in developing parallel skills that are needed to align and support the efforts of their colleagues. Such efforts must be expanded to include all members of the interprofessional team and senior leadership. For example, the American Organization of Nurse Leaders (AONL) has created a comprehensive program meant to promote nurse leaders' self-care practices through a community of practice and learning. In this program, participants engage in learning activities and a community of sharing to promote self-care through physical and mental activities.[68] The program helps to promote resilience among leaders, who can then provide compassionate caring leadership to staff, thus promulgating nourishing work environments for all staff. Such programs could be expanded to specifically include content related to values alignment, moral resilience, and ethical leadership. Meaningful engagement of clinicians will require leadership models that (1) provide leaders with incentives to seek sustainable solutions that generate immediate as well as longer-term results, rather than just short-term gains, and (2) align essential ethical values with organizational values that drive safe, high-quality patient care, and respect and honor everyone's contributions to the results produced.

Leveraging a CFSR requires engaging in a dynamic process to simultaneously address laws, regulations, and policies, including healthcare financing (e.g., insurance reform), so that clinicians can practice ethically and serve those they are responsible for benefiting. Systematically discovering and documenting the factors that contribute to or undermine the care of individual or collective patients, the integrity of clinicians, or the organizational mission informs the specific actions that are needed to shift them.[69] Consider a cardiology fellow caring for a patient with end-stage cardiomyopathy who meets the medical criteria for a heart transplant but is denied because of insufficient financial and social resources. Recognizing the ethical obligation of promoting social justice, clinicians can name the sources of their moral adversity and engage in individual and collective advocacy within their professional organizations and institutions, thereby giving voice to the impact of such policies on patients, families, and clinicians themselves. Engaging with groups focused on healthcare reform, access and allocation of healthcare resources, reimbursement models, and sharing the lived experience of people who are directly impacted by local, state, and federal policies can create a leverage point for change.[70] These efforts can be intensified when interprofessional initiatives are aligned. The initiative by several critical care societies to address burnout is an example of the kind of collaborative alignment that is needed.[71] Healthcare leaders must use their broader platform based on organizational reputation and spheres of influence to articulate and communicate their commitment to these issues and to participate in developing alternative solutions with organizations such as the American Hospital Association, the Joint Commission, and the Institute for Healthcare Improvement, among others.[72] Institutions such as the National Academies of Science, Medicine & Engineering and the US Surgeon General are ideally situated to bring together diverse stakeholders to examine issues such as their initiative focusing on clinician well-being to develop an agenda for addressing the myriad factors that undermine it.[27,73,74,75]

At the organizational level, policies provide guidance that can be useful in ambiguous situations or where ethical conflict is present. For example, a provision in Maryland's Health Decisions Act acknowledges that on some occasions medical treatment is ineffective and, in those situations, clinicians are not obligated to continue treatment that will have no effect on longevity or quality of life.[76,77] Physicians interpreted this provision, reflected in a hospital policy, more broadly, and orders were written to limit treatment for a seriously ill patient with a poor prognosis. A nurse who provided day-to-day care for a critically ill patient for several weeks asserted that the order exceeded the provisions of the statute. She had the courage, support, and moral resilience to challenge the interpretation of the statute and the hospital policy because she did not believe that the patient's condition met the criteria outlined in the policy. This instigated an ethics consultation where there was an opportunity to clarify the intent and process for invoking the policy. Through the process, it was possible to understand the reasoning and interpretation of the policy and the perspectives of diverse stakeholders; ultimately, the decision was reversed, and treatment continued.

Interorganizational methods for raising awareness, shifting the narrative, and identifying promising solutions create an enabling environment for change. This was the case with the Symposium on Transforming Moral

Distress to Moral Resilience convened in 2016 by the *American Journal of Nursing*, the *Journal of Christian Nursing*, and Johns Hopkins University School of Nursing and Berman Institute of Bioethics.[78] A key lever for change is to shift the dialogue about possible solutions to a long-standing, entrenched problem. To this end, the symposium first acknowledged the fine work that had been done for three decades focusing on moral distress and its incidence, sources, and consequences. The organizers then engaged others in creating and implementing an agenda to mitigate the detrimental effects of moral distress by shifting the dialogue to examine the role moral resilience might play in addressing it. Recommendations for practice, education, policy, and research were generated and disseminated.[79] Since the symposium, the American Nurses Association convened a professional issues panel on the subject with a subsequent Call to Action for individual nurses, nurse leaders, and organizations;[79] toolkits to recognize and address moral distress and professional association position statements on this occupational challenge are available.[80] These organizationally focused national initiatives are also reflected in interprofessional efforts such as the critical care societies' collaborative work focusing on burnout that identified moral distress as a key driver.[71] A follow-up study to the 2016 symposium indicated that ethics education, scholarship, fostering ethical practice environments, and developing new initiatives in nursing ethics promoted ethical practice and skillful responses to issues nurses encounter in practice.[81] These are examples of leverage points that can be aligned toward addressing the underlying factors that contribute to moral suffering and distress. Similar activities, such as the National Academies Action Collaborative focusing on Clinician Well-being brings together diverse stakeholders to create learning communities to share resources and synergize interventions.[82]

Supporting Principled Change-Makers and Risk-Takers

Clinicians who are morally resilient and routinely engage in ethical practice are emerging from the bedside to the boardroom. Largely unnoticed, they continue serving from their inner capacities and universal values, not seeking fame or recognition for their contributions. They invest in their own learning and growth; they proactively inform themselves about the culture at work and see patterns that promote an ethical culture. They have the courage to take on difficult issues. These clinicians need to be supported to establish new norms and behaviors that are congruent with values, intentions, and commitment and established ethical standards. This is not to suggest that the norm that is created is one of heroic bravery; rather, it is a humble and disciplined engagement with courage, clear boundaries, and shared responsibility with the organizations where they practice. When individuals act courageously to embody their commitments, they invite others to do the same; and simultaneously, people consciously collaborating within the system need to respond to the dynamic interplay of organizational and societal drivers and constraints—they co-create the ethical culture.

A culture of ethical practice requires us to proactively support those who are practicing at the point of care as well as leaders who are willing to take risks and pursue action in the face of resistance or rejection. We need to develop reliable and safe spaces and processes for ethical concerns to be voiced and examined. If these are not present, the likelihood is that the range of ethical violations will be ignored or normalized. Consider the following incident. In a large academic medical center, a nurse observed an egregious ethical infraction. She informed her nurse manager and the risk manager for the hospital, even though she was afraid of the consequences for herself, the clinician whose behavior violated core ethical values, and the reputation of the institution. The risk manager, a senior leader within the organization, proactively supported the nurse's principled actions and ensured that no retaliation or other harmful steps were taken. The process was respectful, supportive, and aligned with the values espoused by the organization. Norms of confidentiality were upheld, and the issue of concern was investigated, revealing that her concerns were legitimate and serious. Action was taken to swiftly address the significant breach of the organizational and professional ethical norms. Ultimately, the incident led to a board of trustees' request for an action plan to redress the root factors that led to the breach and to intensify accountability of all members of the team and organization to address such lapses. The risk manager's diligence in understanding the concerns of the person reporting, the comprehensive exploration of the root factors, and the development of a remedial action plan drew on a commitment to do the right thing despite resistance, fear, or external pressure.

We need more such courageous clinicians and leaders to begin to shift the culture from fear and silence to courage and speaking up about such infractions. As illustrated, such efforts require a strong web of interconnected people and mechanisms to leverage when situations arise. It cannot be the responsibility of just a few people; rather, it should involve people at all levels of the organization who are committed to supporting each other's efforts, particularly when the stakes are high. Some organizations have created rapid response mechanisms to address urgent matters, including those that involve threats or violations of ethical standards, along with reporting mechanisms for breaches of quality and safety.[83,84] Such mechanisms could be expanded to include systematic inquiry about current or potential ethical issues or lapses in ethical behavior.

Ethics consultation, when done effectively, is another mechanism for supporting ethical practice of principled risk-takers whose actions are based on compassionate, respectful care, even though there may be differing opinions or reasoning about the proper course to pursue. Processes such as ethics consultation can offer support to members of the clinical team whose concerns have been dismissed or disregarded by giving them access to resources outside of the clinical team.[85,86] Policies that give all members of the clinical team access to ethics consultants without approval from the medical or administrative leadership help to create a safe space where all perspectives can be heard, understood, and considered.[87] Such strategies provide space and process for new insights, conflict mediation, and recommending actions that support integrity. Ensuring that the membership of institutional ethics committees is balanced, proportional, and representative of all relevant stakeholders in the community is an important way to assure marginalized voices can be heard, understood, and honored and for power dynamics to be acknowledged and mitigated. Transdisciplinary representation in the consultation team sends an important message to those with the least authority to see that their discipline is included, respected, and meaningfully engaged in the discussion.

Ethics consultants must also be willing and able to take risks themselves to offer additional protection and support to members of the community who express fears of retaliation by simply requesting ethics consultation. Non-physician team members, for example, may share their concerns about exercising the option of requesting consultation because of fears of retaliation. In a case involving a critically ill patient who was unrepresented,[88] a nurse caring for her requested ethics consultation because of concerns that the patient's interests were not being fully protected and decisions were being made that would result in irreversible consequences. She had already brought the issue to the physicians involved and her concerns were dismissed as misguided. She persisted and with the support of her nurse manager called the ethics team for assistance, although she was concerned about retaliation. The ethics consultant, after speaking with the various stakeholders, led a discussion with the interprofessional team, taking care to have the nurse who was worried about retaliation to sit nearby for additional support. It was clear that there were widely divergent views about the patient's condition and outcome, and the process for decision-making. There were also strong emotions associated with the various points of view and tension between members of the team. After the physician shared his perspective on the patient's condition, the consultant turned to the nurse and asked her to share her perspective. It sharply contrasted with what the physician had conveyed and suggested a level of functioning that was different from his assessment. The nurse gave recent evidence to support her claims, highlighted concerns about who was speaking on behalf of the patient, and expressed worries that decisions to limit certain therapies could be premature. The physician disputed the claim, saying it was likely that the patient would eventually die anyway. The ethics consultant clarified the boundaries of ethical permissibility, interpreted the hospital policies and state laws that were relevant to the case, and suggested that further procedural safeguards were necessary. It was not a suggestion that was popular with some members of the clinical team, but the consultant made clear that bringing the issue forward was the correct path to pursue—regardless of what the ultimate decisions were. As is often the case, ethics consultants must weigh the risks of taking an unpopular stand with the impact on the functioning of the service in the long term. In the end, connecting back to core values and sourcing actions from a place of groundedness and clarity can provide ethics consultants with the courage needed to recalibrate when power gradients create barriers to inclusion and respectful engagement.

Transformational Design for Sustainable Results

How do we make a culture of ethical practice a reality? What platforms do we create and what methods and techniques do we use to embody the values and principles that underpin integrity and compassion while formulating and enforcing social instruments to uphold rights and realize the full potential of interprofessional clinicians? Most important, how do we begin our work? We begin by looking within—to our attitudes, our worldviews, and the spirit that informs our decisions even in the face of opposition. We ask ourselves, *"Who am I? Do I embody the values that underpin a culture of ethical practice?"*

Results are essential in designing sustainable and meaningful initiatives. Generally, when developing strategic plans, most conventional programs, projects, and institutions create vision statements and articulate the impact and outcomes they wish to produce. Core or essential ethical values that form the basis of strategy and action are articulated. Yet most ultimately focus on outputs—production of goods and services, investments in infrastructure, and selected social and economic aspects such as health, education, income, and benefits. Transformational leaders who are committed to creating a culture of ethical practice know that although outputs and outcomes are important, they do not provide a true measure of human potential and well-being. These leaders also hold with more ease the seeming paradox of accountability and results along with the unpredictability of emergence. This is particularly challenging in chaotic and uncertain healthcare environments.

Healthcare organizations and staff spend enormous amounts of time developing plans to translate policies into programs and projects to achieve stated goals. They use a plethora of tools and techniques for analysis, strategic planning, implementation, measurement, and results-based management. For example, SMART goals (Specific, Measurable, Agreed upon, Realistic/relevant, Time-based)[89,90] and SWOT (Strengths, Weaknesses, Opportunities, Threats) analyses, which are common, conventional methods for logical planning, may be useful, they but are limited for some types of issues.[91,92] Logical frameworks and brilliant analyses are necessary but not sufficient to produce sustainable and meaningful change. We must consider whether these tools and techniques are adequate to deal with the urgency and complexity of issues facing healthcare today. *Do they leverage the inner capacities of individuals, teams, and leaders to shift the patterns that keep the current paradigm in place? Will they help us translate our mission and vision into reality so that it is visible in moment-to-moment decisions, actions, and communications?* These and other questions help us to align our efforts in ways that unleash new potential and meaningful and sustainable results.

Measuring organizational success requires that healthcare entities think beyond operational aspects alone. The US Surgeon General's Framework for Workplace Mental Health & Well-Being offers a useful blueprint for determining organizational outcomes.[93] Measuring employee perceptions and experiences, such as workplace connections, employee engagement, sense of belonging, organizational trust, ethical enrichment, and organizational mission/behavior congruence could give organizations indicators for their performance as an overall ethical workplace. Coupling these measures with employee moral resilience, such as by using the RMRS-16©™ or one of the subscales, can paint a vivid picture of the way an organization's behaviors and values effect the overall level of ethical integrity among staff and stand as a clear sign the organization values ethics along with operations and other business-oriented metrics. Our research suggests that enhancing moral resilience can be a moderator of the impact of moral adversity and when combined with organizational effectiveness has the greatest potential to reduce the detrimental impact of moral suffering.[94]

Some think that working with inner capacities to solve problems is simple, or that all we need are technological solutions. Transformational power is created when we weave technological results, system-level shifts, and the embodiment of our deepest self together synergistically. Transformational techniques and methods are sophisticated yet simple and accessible. They center on doing what we are already doing with mindful awareness, intentional design, curiosity, and principled action. Inevitable obstacles and obstructions become opportunities for growth, and for revising strategies and tactics without compromising values and principles. This requires sustained and disciplined practice to return over and over to the same questions: "Who am I? What needs to be understood? What actions reflect integrity and alignment of essential values?" As discussed in Chapter 7, the exploration of the interplay among individual integrity, relational integrity, and the broader moral community is an ongoing, synergistic process.

Transformational results can be achieved if the way people work and the processes organizations already use are leveraged to implement transformational practices and co-create responses that work for all instead of a few. "Insanity is doing the same thing over and over again and expecting different results."[95] This is not about introducing new tools, implementing the latest management "flavor of the month" intervention, or tinkering at the margins. It is about creating the culture of transformation, where people embrace change leading to results rather than fear it. At a time of unprecedented uncertainty and instability, leaders and point of care clinicians are reeling with the pace of change in healthcare and in society. Complex healthcare organizations employ a variety of procedures, processes, tools, and techniques and are often unwilling to embark on

Table 11.1. Key Elements of Transformational Design and Action©2018

- Use practices, techniques, and methods that draw from inner capacity in every step of planning and implementation.
- Embody the values that underpin the vision and mission that are articulated in the initiatives.
- Co-create new patterns, new rules of the game, new systems for sustainable change.
- Transcend disempowering patterns in teams and organizations.
- Create a new narrative.

vital, radical transformation. Instead of embracing efforts to substantially shift the patterns that create moral adversity and suffering, most of the effort is spent on preserving the status quo. Rather than adding more to an already overflowing plate, transformational processes are aimed at doing what we are already doing differently, not adding more burden to already beleaguered clinicians and leaders.

What is different in the way we design, plan, and implement our change initiatives using transformational design? The foundational change is that every step sources our inner capacities and our wisdom and is based on embodying universal values such as dignity, compassion, fairness, and courage to create strategic action. Table 11.1 reflects key elements of transformational design.

These transformational approaches have generated just and sustainable results worldwide.[1] If we cannot or do not transform the way we plan and implement large-scale or small initiatives to cultivate moral resilience and a culture of ethical practice, we will not produce the results needed for the future we want to create.

Use Practices, Techniques, and Methods that Source Our Inner Capacity in Every Step of Planning and Implementation

This is a radical shift in orientation for clinicians engaged in systems change to address the root factors that instigate moral adversity and suffering while remaining deeply aligned with their own inner being. In the implementation of the program Toward a Culture of Ethical Practice (TCEP) using the CFSR model, a group of nurse leaders used the CFSR process to design an initiative to cultivate a healthy workplace. An exploration of individual values, purpose, and intention was aligned to articulate the shared values that would underlie the initiative. These became the touchstone for all subsequent decisions. Doing so takes discipline to overcome the tendency to go straight to tactics or "quick fixes." This is especially challenging in fast-paced clinical environments where the expectation of a "quick fix" is prevalent and there is little tolerance for process or missteps. The design team developed norms of engagement and relationship that they would hold themselves accountable for, articulated the shifts they wished to cultivate, and began to develop specific methods to achieve the desired results. Design in this way requires a commitment to a vision that generates results now and in the longer term with clear strategies, benchmarks, a measurement dashboard, sustained investment, and leadership. Simultaneously, senior leadership must be engaged to enable the newly developed skills and patterns to take hold and to thrive by embodying the values, processes, and norms that have been agreed upon by all.

Embody the Values that Underpin the Vision and Mission We Articulate in Our Initiatives

The values underpinning a system guide strategic action. At the system level, we formulate ethical norms and enact policies, regulations, and policies to promote safe care and advocate social justice. In healthcare, we establish rules and systems for financing, resource allocation, quality and safety, education, human resources, decision-making, and so on. Much of what we have done in these areas so far has benefited a few while depriving many. Some of us can see the unworkable systems and connect them to how we set the rules of the game. When clinicians work together, they intentionally or unintentionally create informal organizational norms that are reflected in practice patterns, some of which may produce detrimental results. The more invisible and unexamined the norms may be, the more difficult it is to shift the patterns they produce. For example, we have policies and laws to essentially promote human well-being, yet well-being and justice are often not attained. A common example in healthcare organizations is reflected in practice patterns that deny the basic needs of clinicians at the point of care. We know that when our basic needs are unmet, we are more vulnerable to lapses in integrity, quality, and safety. Yet little attention has been given to understanding the factors that underlie such lapses, such as failing to take breaks for renewal and nourishment, in patterns that become normalized and taken for granted. We "talk about values" rather than "embody values." Many healthcare organizations profess their commitment to the people who serve in them, but there are gaps in how such values are manifested in day-to-day practice. For instance, a hospital may fail to invest in healthy food options for those who work off-shifts and weekends in favor of savings that are divorced from the impact of the decisions on the people providing direct services. Few hospitals measure the impact of the quality of their staff food offerings on the health of the workforce but framing such decisions as ethical rather than managerial offers the potential for new insights to emerge. Linking how physiologic balance impacts cognitive, emotional, and relational skills, judgment, flexibility, and ultimately patient care and the workforce shifts the dialogue to account for the human dimensions.

Transformational design provides a template to translate values-based rhetoric into reality in terms of moment-to-moment behaviors, choices, and action. This means putting in place shared accountabilities for upholding our collective values. Questions such as *"What would need to be in place for a shift from X to Y to be a leverage point for culture change?"* can help to identify opportunities. These kinds of questions can be included in regular performance dashboards and embedded into unit-based and organizational priority setting.

Similarly, there are patterns where disrespectful, disruptive, and potentially abusive behaviors are allowed to become normative. These issues were prevalent before the COVID-19 pandemic but have become more common, especially when people are exhausted and empathy is depleted.[96,97] Leaders may themselves fall into patterns of dismissing, disrespecting, or systematically undermining the efforts of some targeted individuals. For some senior leaders who are replaced when new leadership is hired or situations become untenable, "gag clauses" are included as part of their severance package. Such practices not only silence those whose perspectives are needed if patterns are to be identified and solutions designed, but also create cynicism and mistrust among those who may consider leadership positions in the future. Anecdotal reports suggest that this pattern has intensified in the aftermath of the COVID-19 pandemic.[96,97] Systemic work is needed to address the behaviors of organizational leaders who exhibit behaviors contrary to accepted norms,[98] and to develop reporting systems that identify deviations from professional and interpersonal norms and enable new patterns.

The key is practice—practice to embody our values while in action, to have the courage to create, to speak truth to those with power, to take strategic action, and to produce results. This is one of the most important aspects of the CFSR model. Unlike other models, it focuses on ongoing practice to continue to align and synergize one's personal transformation process with a broader change initiative—whether it focus on the team, the organization, or the system. Participants in the TCEP program regularly introduced themselves using the simple, but profound template: "My name is . . . I stand for . . ." Not only was saying it a reminder of what grounds each person's life and work, but it offers others an opportunity to remember their values and connect to them too. Repeating these practices begins to weave together shared and unique values into a cohesive whole and creates new norms to support their emergence. When an organization professes their commitment to values such as compassion and its members see visible evidence of it in the way people relate to one another, how decisions are made and communicated, and how conflicts and mistakes are addressed, confidence and trust begin to take hold. Using frameworks such as "Compassionomics" to embrace values such as compassion as a financial driver within healthcare organizations has the potential to shift from seeing compassion as aspirational to using its power to produce results and healthy workplaces.[99]

People within healthcare systems need space and infrastructure to refresh and support their emerging capacities in moral resilience, or their newly learned skills can be dampened or extinguished. Yet even simple practices take leadership and sustained commitment to become normative. Clinicians with newly developed mindfulness skills returning to an environment where managerial support is lacking require additional effort to preserve those skills. Creating system processes that cause clinicians to pause, breathe, and recall their intentions for their profession during a busy day can support skills such as mindfulness.[100] A mindful pause at the beginning of a meeting allows people to arrive and release the remnants of the prior meeting or encounter. When repeated over time, such practices become normative. Systematic mechanisms embedded in the performance appraisal process can invite clinicians to identify their mindfulness practice as a professional goal aimed at enhancing their clinical performance; these mechanisms can reinforce and reward actions that are aligned with individual team and organizational goals. At the organizational level, new management dashboards can measure behaviors that reflect ethical practice, moral adversity, and its consequences and responses, or resolution of troubling ethical situations; additions such as these are needed to bring the values and behaviors of individuals, teams, and leaders into alignment. Factors such as the results of weekly ethics rounds, tracking of key indicators within the electronic medical record, and the number and focus of ethics consultations are promising directions.[51] Making these data a regular part of reports to organizational leaders with shared accountability for addressing them helps to advance a new paradigm.

Often these dimensions are siloed, making them appear as separate efforts. Creating new patterns within ourselves and aligning them with our broader change efforts unleashes unacknowledged potential and energy. No longer is our attention dispersed or distracted; rather, it is focused on what matters most. An opportunity to focus on what matters most in healthcare organizations resides in the prevailing and nearly universal commitment of clinicians to the well-being and benefit of those they serve. Keeping this focus as the core of their values provides an opportunity to align this shared value amid confusion, uncertainty, or conflict. We can practice orienting ourselves toward these shared values in the processes and systems we use to engage in exploring the challenges, issues, and solutions. Mechanisms such as G.R.A.C.E. offer a simple mnemonic to help clinicians cultivate the conditions for compassion to arise and to orient in this direction during their clinical duties.[101] This often requires transformational design to develop the new patterns of communication, decision-making, and conflict resolution. Adopting new patterns such as a process for engaging in an "ethics conversation" is a mechanism for intentionally engaging shared values, exploring their alignment, and leveraging their strength to devise solutions that support rather than undermine the integrity of all.[102] The emerging role of Chief Wellness Officers within healthcare systems has the potential to support the emergence of new patterns and synergies within organizations. Strategies to align efforts to address moral suffering from an organizational perspective focus on removing impediments to high-quality, safe clinical care, reformulating institutional policies and processes, addressing inequities, harnessing the creativity of "workarounds, and creating community."[103]

Co-create New Patterns, Developing New Rules of the Game and New Systems for Sustainable Change

In today's interdependent yet fragmented world, intrinsic human capabilities need to be sourced for sustainable change. A system delivers what it is designed to deliver. The rules of the game—the formal rules that determine who gets to play, where, and how; or the informal norms in culture and society—determine what happens to people and the planet. In every part of the world, the thinking on policies, rules, and regulations is done by a few for the many, with the assumption and justification that people and citizens do not have the expertise to influence policy or the ability to think critically.[5]

The same is true in healthcare. Systems design does not routinely include robust processes of co-creation with people at the front lines. Often leaders are legislating decisions without meaningful and authentic engagement or leveraging shared ethical values and commitments. Under stress, systems adapt by reducing opportunities for engaging the clinicians and other healthcare workers and implementing top-down control and decision-making. Solutions are often designed without the participation of those most intimately affected by the problem. As described in Chapter 10 partial solutions can address a dimension of the problem, but without engagement of point of care personnel, sustainable and meaningful solutions are likely to continue to be elusive. Intentionally involving clinicians in co-creating solutions by acknowledging their knowledge, skills, and wisdom builds trust and enhances their engagement in deploying needed changes. Creating learning communities, where all stakeholders have a responsibility for the result, leverages the social capital embedded in complex organizations in a fresh way.

Acknowledging that sufficient resources exist and must be radically redistributed within a healthcare enterprise can neutralize the perceptions arising from competition and fear. A scarcity paradigm stifles creativity and undermines authentic connections among patients, families, clinicians, and organizational leaders. Methods to reallocate resources based on alignment with core values are needed. This means that hard choices can and must be made when examining programs and practices that have heretofore been "sacred cows" within an organization. For example, is it just or advisable for *all* tertiary medical centers to engage in *all* cutting-edge treatments, programs, or practices? If one relies exclusively on a utilitarian framework, an argument for doing so results in the greatest good for the greatest number. But does it hold when doing so diffuses the human and material resources of an organization to the point that clinical personnel bear the brunt of implementing the decision because the cumulative human costs go unaccounted for? Pediatric intensive care units, for example, are reporting unprecedented levels of moral distress, in part related to shifts in the patient population to more chronically critically ill patients as the boundaries of innovation become blurred or exaggerated.[104,105] Current practices can be reevaluated, and those that are not aligned with essential moral/ethical values and commitments, those that are not grounded in evidence, or those that have marginal demonstrated benefit should be abandoned. This shift in paradigms can take us from scarcity to abundance. Realigned with abundance, there is possibility and flexibility, and a new narrative about the delivery of clinical care is possible.

Transcend Disempowering Patterns in Teams and Organizations

Individual moral resilience alone will not shift the organizational decisions, structures, and processes that contribute to imperiled integrity. Yet, because organizations are composed of individuals, there is the possibility that reaching a critical threshold of morally resilient individuals within organizations will begin to produce results toward a broader goal of culture change. Building unit-based capacity by enrolling nurses in the foundational MEPRA program, for example, resulted in the development of a critical mass of people who shared the same foundation, vocabulary, and skills.[15,16] They became ambassadors and unit-based leaders in identifying and addressing ethical issues and integrating MEPRA practices into their roles as point of care clinicians, preceptors, and mentors.[15,16] In addition to understanding the individual, team, and organizational shifts that are necessary for integrity-preserving workplaces (see Chapter 10), it is important to understand the interplay between individuals, the work environment, societal expectations, and formal practice policies that impinge on integrity. Research has demonstrated that it is the combination of individual moral resilience and organizational effectiveness that has the greatest potential to reduce moral suffering.[106] Today's healthcare environment is rife with ethical tensions, dissonance, conflict, and confusion. In a broader sense, clinicians and leaders of healthcare organizations must design specific strategies to begin to address some of the more vexing challenges using the same CFSR process.

A necessary shift to align individual moral resilience with a culture of ethical practice is a shift from authoritarian, insensitive hierarchy to synergistic responsible alliances.[107] Authoritarian, competitive, and divisive paradigms promote inequality within the healthcare team. When such patterns are present and go unaddressed, entrenched patterns of communication, decision-making, or conflict resolution become normative and contribute to interprofessional conflict and moral distress.[51,108] Such realities do not mean that change is impossible, but they must be recognized and systematically addressed.

Disparities in role accountability, different knowledge paradigms, and divergent views of treatment planning fuel conflict among interprofessional teams.[109,110] They breed patterns where certain types of knowledge are privileged even when not applicable to the clinical problem, while other types are dismissed even when applicable.[40,111] Clinicians begin to focus on tensions in the nurse–physician or team–family relationship rather than what is best for the patient.[111] When conflicts are internalized rather than openly addressed, each profession suffers and patient care is compromised. In the absence of interprofessional models for functioning optimally within a team, this paradigm can lead to dysfunctional teams and undermine quality, safety, and ethical practice.[40,111,112]

Consider a decision about the timing of discharge for a patient hospitalized for several weeks because of complications following a routine abdominal surgery. Such decisions are often complex, requiring consideration of multi-factorial conditions outside of the patient's physical status. The ultimate decision resides with the physician, yet input from other members of the healthcare team such as nurses and physical, occupational, or respiratory therapists is necessary for the patient to make a safe transition out of the hospital. When healthcare teams are operating from unexamined patterns, the views of certain members of the team may be dismissed or viewed as barriers to achieving a timely discharge instead of a legitimate concern that requires investigation. Requests for additional discharge training, for example, may be met with resistance or disregard in response to throughput or efficiency pressures. Factors necessary for a successful transition such as training in how to administer medications, complete postoperative procedures, strengthen atrophied muscles, and the like may be overlooked or their importance minimized. When clinicians can reorient toward their service to the patient, create a space where various types of knowledge are visible and open for examination, and contributions to the goal of a safe discharge are honored, considered, and aligned, new patterns can emerge. Shared decision-making respects the role and worldview of each team member, including distinctive core goals, unique knowledge, context, and moral/ethical values.[113] Skillful communication can counteract background conversations that reinforce competition, either/or thinking, or negative assumptions, thereby enhancing and building upon the contributions of all team members.[1] Cooperative, transparent decision-making fosters processes that remediate high-risk situations, build trust, and foster relational integrity.

At the organizational level, similar patterns of unexamined assumptions, biases, and relationships can emerge. Clinical leaders, for example, may find their communication and decision-making with leaders in finance, human resources, or law led to perpetration of assumptions about the impact of decisions on the care of patients and families. Likewise, colleagues in finance, for example, may see expenditures for services to provide care to a population of patients or expensive line items as excessive or optional. Without a common vocabulary, process, and framework for addressing complex issues, similar resistant patterns can develop. Yet when we can notice and address these patterns from a value-based intention, new possibilities emerge.

Competition among members of the interdisciplinary team is another pattern that may contribute to moral adversity. It often emerges from fear. The assumption that, if someone succeeds, there is less opportunity for others contributes to a pattern of framing issues as black or white, good or bad, win or lose. Competition can become the unconscious motivation for some clinicians and organizational leaders. Leveraging power and authority for a desired outcome, regardless of its impact on others, creates an environment corrosive to teamwork and the goals of clinical care.[40,114,115,116,117] This competitive culture that is focused on short-term gains reinforces individual achievement and productivity rather than basing professional advancement, recognition, or institutional reputation on the contributions of the entire team.[118,119] Competition and the perception of scarcity thrive in an environment of fear. When fear is present, possibilities narrow, and creativity is lost. Reinforced by the constant refrain on the part of individuals and organizations that there are not enough people, time, energy, or money, the paradigm of scarcity contributes to a detached, procedure-oriented, numbers focused culture. As healthcare has become a commodity, relying exclusively on throughput and productivity-focused metrics risks diverting attention from the core task of providing engaged care for people who need healthcare services to an endless array of tasks aimed at meeting metrics designed by individuals who do not provide direct care or may not share similar values or priorities. Such disconnects add to the moral and ethical adversity that many clinicians experience and explain in part the burgeoning problem of burnout and moral distress or suffering among clinicians.[40,120,121,122,123]

Clinicians and leaders who are cultivating a culture of ethical practice are making new patterns, not only solving problems.[1] They are able to recognize, distinguish, and address what is not working and create alternatives. In complex multidisciplinary healthcare environments, this involves identifying, designing, and implementing new ways to respond to ethically challenging issues and situations. It requires the ability to understand the sources of action (or inaction), whether they are readily observable or hidden, and the attitudes that shape them. In addition, it demands an ability to understand the cultural norms that inhibit or enhance progress and the forces that legitimize structures and systems.[5] In essence, this requires going beyond the surface level of challenging problems to discover their deeper dimensions and on from there to design and implement new programs that address them. As discussed in Chapter 10, this approach involves actively seeking to identify the patterns that must be shifted to support ethical practice and create the outcomes desired. Understanding the patterns that maintain the status quo provides the foundation for designing the new patterns needed to shift to a new reality.

When clinicians and leaders know and use transformational processes, the way that business is transacted and routine activities are performed becomes a continuous opportunity for extraordinary change. Everyday ethics leverages paradigm shifts. Shifting from viewing ethical dilemmas as the defining feature of ethical practice to seeing ethics as embedded in every moment enables clinicians and leaders to reframe their work through the lens of integrity. Moral resilience and a culture of ethical practice require clinicians to have the power to transcend paradigms that do not serve the people they care for or humanity at large. The mindset or paradigm out of which the system—its goals, structure, rules, delays, and parameters—arises must be aligned with deeper purpose and ways of being. For example, paradigms of ethical practice can begin to shift when clinicians or leaders begin to manifest an alternative approach to everyday ethical issues.

We have many opportunities to influence change through policies, day-to-day activities, routine meetings, reports, planning sessions, and so forth. *Do we know how to make these everyday activities spaces where transformation can naturally emerge?* These opportunities present themselves regularly and frequently in every organization, in all human endeavors, but they remain largely unutilized. The pace of transformational results would accelerate exponentially if we could harness the transformative potential of the numerous routine activities toward meaningful and sustainable results. Likewise, we can harness the power of peer-to-peer social engagement to create momentum and engagement, not by mandating change but by engaging people in co-creating the conditions for the desired changes to take hold and flourish.

Beyond team and organizational patterns, it is also vital to engage the public in transforming the patterns reflected in community and societal values, worldviews, cultural norms, and so on that impact the way healthcare (and health more generally) is understood, the expectations that accompany it, and the assumptions that are operating.[87,124,125] Work within the palliative care field to engage the public in considering their preferences for care at the end of life or advocacy efforts to reduce healthcare disparities for specific populations or diagnoses is an example.[126,127,128,129] During the COVID-19 pandemic, the divide between clinicians and the public widened as discord among people escalated around approaches to managing the pandemic.[130] Efforts to engage the public in understanding the dual responsibility of clinicians and the public called for a recalibration of the social contract.[130] Methods such as performances using Greek tragedies to illustrate the current and historical context of healthcare offers clinicians and the public a rare opportunity to understand complexity of healthcare delivery.[126,131] Within the context of moral resilience and ethical practice, leading organizations such as the American Society for Bioethics and Humanities, medical and nursing professional organizations, healthcare-focused societies, advocacy and policy institutes, and philanthropic foundations that impact healthcare policy will continue to be vital in creating the kinds of shifts that are necessary.[27,80,82,86,132,133,134] The time is ripe for new methods for engaging the providers and recipients of healthcare in a new, transformative dialogue.

Creating the New Narrative

Our narratives reflect the details and interpretation of the events of our lives. They are vital in understanding others and ourselves and contribute to our identities, memories, and meaning making. In healthcare, the predominant collective narrative surrounding moral distress is punctuated by themes of powerlessness, feelings of victimization, and despair. If we continue with the current narrative, it will likely become a self-fulfilling prophecy. To shift toward moral resilience and a culture of ethical practice, new narratives will be necessary. This will require seeing the situations and contexts that ignite moral distress differently. We can notice the extraordinary integrity-preserving results produced by other clinicians when we ourselves have worldviews and mental maps that allow us to see these extraordinary results. This will initially involve shifting our own vision to locate the elements of these complex ethical situations that indicate moral conscientiousness and integrity despite the obstacles that are present. Until we can see things clearly ourselves, we will be unable to see moments of integrity in others. In Chapter 2, we described how individual narratives can relate and perpetuate moral distress, and in Chapters 7 and 8 how they can be reshaped to repair moral integrity and restore moral resilience in individuals. Table 11.2 offers guidance for creating a new narrative.

Intentionally documenting what and how clinicians who embody ethical practice and moral resilience are *being* in action begins to shift the current paradigm and create a new future that fosters moral resilience and a culture of ethical practice. Likewise, such acknowledgment contributes

Table 11.2. Guidance for Creating a New Narrative©2018

- Begin by expanding heart space and inner potential.
- Adopt personal reflection and insight as the pathway to concise, clear expression.
- Be bold; behold possibility.
- Invite engagement without competition.
- Name the shift you want to see and be it.
- Inspire yourself and others.
- Connect your initiatives with a shift to a larger purpose.
- Let go of limiting beliefs and assumptions.
- Help others see their own possibilities for co-creation.
- Make the invisible visible without polarizing.
- Celebrate and embrace what is working.
- Transcend seeming dichotomies by embodying ethical values and actions.
- Break the "hero" archetype of today and build the archetypes required for a paradigm shift.
- Choose words with intention and care. Language must authentically reflect the new paradigm.
- Connect local courageous actions to the differences they make in the world.
- Foster full potential for action now, not later.
- Open and foster space for synergy to emerge.
- Focus on and magnify your connection to what you stand for in life and work.
- Enable risk in connecting to your moral compass.
- Disrupt patterns that no longer serve a useful purpose.

significantly to generating a new narrative that reflects the potential of moral adversity to serve as a catalyst for moral and ethical progress and to fuel efforts aligned with moral resilience and ethical practice instead of undermining integrity. For example, the Daisy Foundation and the American Nurses Association Ethics Advisory Board created two new categories of acknowledgment focusing on exemplary ethical practice by nurse leaders and nurses at the point of care.[135] These systemic mechanisms can be instrumental in helping everyone recognize and honor examples of ethical practice and leadership. Using the CFSR requires that we pay attention to how we are being in each moment. Questions such as: "*When am I able to ground myself in who I most essentially am?*" "*Do I source the qualities that manifest my essence in the world?*" and "*Am I able to source the inner capacities that are uniquely mine in service of individuals and the collective?*" These ongoing practices require both individual and collective awareness of the process and content of our communications and behaviors.

Clinicians who are morally resilient can distinguish how their current stories about ethical practice and moral distress are told from narratives that generate paradigm shifts. Such clinicians can have conversations with people about what they are doing and connect them to outcomes and impact. They deepen the inquiry by focusing on what really matters to people—the outcomes and impacts they want to produce—and drawing them to a broader view and context. They create the space for people to access their own power to go beyond the more mundane to leverage their basic goodness for the benefit of others. Questions such as "*What do you fundamentally care about?*" "*When ethical conflicts arise, what values will guide your actions?*" invite others to connect to and acknowledge their deeper commitments behind their actions. Leaders in organizations can engage colleagues and staff in manifesting a new paradigm by using these same approaches.

We may not notice our new patterns or embrace our moment-to-moment contributions. As clinicians or leaders, we tend to overlook the actions we do each day that make a difference in the lives of others. Many of us will say, "I'm *just* doing my job." Though true, this may lead us to ignore the impact that doing our job well has on the lives of the people we serve. Learning to notice these patterns paves the way for noticing ongoing shifts that are occurring. When we can notice emergent and unpredictable events and use the CFSR response to gauge what is emerging, it fosters new insights and possibilities. It leads to questions such as "*How can*

I translate this new way of seeing the context and nuances into policies, practices, and program design?" "How will I ensure coherence with this approach while I am communicating about what is happening in the process of creating a culture that supports moral resilience and ethical practice?" Linking the broader impact, outcomes, and outputs is essential to specify and clarify the contribution of a new paradigm to desired results.

It is essential to note the system shifts and new conversations that *are* emerging within the professions, among healthcare providers, the public, and healthcare organizations.[80,82,133,134] As healthcare delivery in the United States is restructured, there will be important opportunities and incentives for clinicians to engage with patients and their families to examine heretofore taboo topics such as a more robust understanding of the trade-offs associated with treatment options by expanding our understanding of what constitutes cost or burden to those receiving treatment. It is likely that access to healthcare will continue to be a hotly debated topic that offers the potential for clinicians, patients, families, and other stakeholders to create a new narrative that more fully reflects fundamental values of respect, compassion, and equity. Opportunities also emerged during the COVID-19 pandemic for clinicians to share a more realistic narrative of their work and the impact of a broken healthcare system on their patients and their own wellbeing.[136,137,138] It unleashed pent up emotions and unheard accounts of how the patterns of greed, inequities, and unhealthy hierarchy were driving a wedge between the core values of the professions and the healthcare organizations where they practice.[139] We must skillfully and constructively employ communication methods, including social media, to modulate the tenor of change that is necessary and justified. This will require shifts in thinking about the various communication vehicles, such as storytelling, to enroll others in the vision and change process and to leverage their commitments to produce results.

Communicating differently by creating spaces for individual clinicians, patients, families, and healthcare executives to explore their commitment to ethical practice and moral resilience, as "intention in action," will be vital in shifting the heretofore predominantly negative narrative surrounding ethically complex cases and the moral residue that often accompanies them. Communications that focus on telling others what to think or do will be ineffective in shifting the narrative in ways that are sufficient to ignite and sustain changes in solidified patterns or address resistance. Shifting to a new narrative will also require communicating concrete strategies for sustainable results using the CFSR succinctly without making the complex, interdependent issues confusing. For example, novel work to rehabilitate our relationship with moral distress and foster a culture of ethical practice could be distilled to three powerful points: (1) solve problems to support integrity, (2) shift patterns that undermine moral resilience and ethical practice, and (3) draw on the inner potential of all members of the healthcare team and organization to produce meaningful and sustainable results that benefit all. Such communication can inspire others to see and document the new narrative themselves. Instead of attributing changes to a few, new patterns that highlight the unique and cumulative contributions of all members of the team will create new spaces to celebrate and honor the collective effort of everyone.

Emphasizing the different responses that arise using the CFSR is essential for differentiating the partial responses of the past from new ways of being and working together. By creating a new narrative, we can acknowledge the contribution of various efforts and highlight the absence of the sustainable results we desire. Using new perspectives to identify, name, and address the patterns that have stalled progress in the past and offering a robust alternative offers fuel for progress. Similarly, new forms of expression such as stories, poetry, song, visual art, and films are important vehicles to engage and inspire others.[131,140] Recognizing the tendency of clinicians and healthcare organizations to divorce themselves from these forms of expression and understanding offers opportunities to engage previously unengaged parts of ourselves to nourish the changes we desire. Multi-pronged efforts will be needed to "meet people where they are" and to enroll them in being part of the solution.

Healthcare leaders and organizations must join with clinicians to leverage their shared commitment to ethical practice to make meaningful and sustainable change possible. Without a shared vision and common resolve, the patterns of the past are likely to continue, and real progress in addressing the sources of moral adversity, mitigating the detrimental effects of moral suffering, and designing healthy workplaces will remain elusive. Models such as those created by Pavlish et al.[52,53,141] offer direction for leaders to address the moral concerns and distress of clinicians. Ethics nurse liaison programs can support clinicians to shift out of powerlessness related to moral suffering into ethical competence and moral agency and thereby contribute to enabling an ethical practice environment.[2,54] The question for all stakeholders is not whether we have enough data to justify attention to this issue. Rather, the question is whether we have the moral investment, courage, and resolve to begin first with ourselves and then with others to bring about a paradigm shift in our behaviors, choices, and actions. When leaders in healthcare organizations join with clinicians at the point of care to design the architecture for ethical practice, meaningful and sustainable change is possible. Leveraging top-down and grassroots engagement and design is fundamental to a CFSR. With a dedicated commitment to the world, clinicians and leaders in healthcare have an unprecedented opportunity to create a new reality for the future.

References

1. Sharma M. Radical transformational leadership: strategic action for change agents. San Francisco, CA: North Atlantic Books; 2017.
2. Fitzgerald H, Rushton C. Designing a culture of ethical practice in health care: a new paradigm. In Deem MJ, Hagerty Lingler J, editors, Nursing ethics: normative foundations, advanced concepts, and emerging issues. In press.
3. James TA. Teamwork as a core value in health care. Published August 6, 2021. Accessed May 29, 2023. https://postgraduateeducation.hms.harvard.edu/trends-medicine/teamwork-core-value-health-care.
4. Gentile MC. Giving voice to values: how to speak your mind when you know what's right. New Haven, CT: Yale University Press; 2010.
5. Hawkins B, Rosenberg M. Building a compassionate healthcare system through creativity, communication and connection. In The Inaugural Compassion in Action Healthcare Conference. Boston, MA, June 2017. http://compassioninactionconference.org/media/Compassion-in-Action-Healthcare-Conference-Program-Book.pdf.
6. Losty LS, Bailey KD. Leading through chaos: perspectives from nurse executives. Nurs Adm Q. 2021;Apr–Jun 2001;45(2):118–125.
7. Chipps E, Kelley MM, Monturo C, et al. Reflections from the middle: exploring the experience of nurse managers across the United States during the COVID-19 pandemic. J Nurs Adm. Jun 1, 2022;52(6):345–351.
8. Brewer K, Horning M, Walker M, et al. Analyzing the effects of family presence and visitation restrictions during the COVID-19 pandemic among nurse leaders and non-nurse leaders. J Nurs Adm. 2023;53(3):132–137.
9. Standiford TC, Davuluri K, Trupiano N, et al. Physician leadership during the COVID-19 pandemic: an emphasis on the team, well-being and leadership reasoning. BMJ Leader. 2021;5:20–25.
10. Hertelendy AJ, Gutberg J, Mitchell C, et al. Mitigating moral distress in leaders of healthcare organizations: a scoping review. J Healthc Manag. 2022;67(5):380–402.
11. Institute of Medicine. Building a resilient workforce: opportunities for the Department of Homeland Security: workshop summary. Washington, DC: National Academies Press; 2012.

12. Ramachandran S, Balasubramanian S, James WF, et al. Whither compassionate leadership? a systematic review. Manag Rev Q. 2023;online ahead of print.
13. West MA. Compassionate leadership: sustaining wisdom, humanity and presence in health and social care. Sligo, Ireland: Swirling Leaf Press; 2021.
14. Mullan F. Avedis Donabedian: a founder of quality assessment encounters a troubled system firsthand: interview. Health Aff. 2001;20(1):137–141.
15. Rushton CH, Swoboda SM, Reller N, et al. Mindful Ethical Practice and Resilience Academy: Equipping nurses to address ethical challenges. Am J Crit Care. 2021;30(1):e1–e11.
16. Rushton C, Swoboda S, Reimer T, et al. Boyce, D., Hansen, G. The Mindful Ethical Practice & Resilience Academy (MEPRA): Sustainability of impact. Am J Crit Care. 2023;32(3):184–194.
17. American Nurses Association. Pulse on the nation's nurses survey series: annual assessment survey. Published November 2022. Accessed March 7, 2023. https://www.nursingworld.org/practice-policy/work-environment/health-safety/disaster-preparedness/coronavirus/what-you-need-to-know/annual-survey--third-year/.
18. Bellora-Bienengraber L, Radtke RR, Widener SK. Counterproductive work behaviors and work climate: the role of an ethically focused management control system and peers' self-focused behavior. Account Organ Soc. 2022;96:101275.
19. Kuenzi M, Mayer DM, Greenbaum RL. Creating an ethical organizational environment: the relationship between ethical leadership, ethical organizational climate, and unethical behavior. Pers Psychol. 2020;73(1):43–71.
20. Pauly B, Varcoe C, Storch J, Newton L. Registered nurses' perceptions of moral distress and ethical climate. Nurs Ethics. 2009;16(5):561–573.
21. American Association of Critical-Care Nurses. AACN standards for establishing and sustaining healthy work environments. 2nd ed. Aliso Viejo, CA: AACN; 2016.
22. Johns Hopkins University School of Nursing. R^3 – the Renewal, Resilience and Retention of Maryland Nurses Initiative. 2023. Accessed May 26, 2023. https://nursing.jhu.edu/faculty_research/research/centers/R3/.
23. R^3—the Renewal, Resilience and Retention of Maryland Nurses Initiative, Mind the Gap: preparing nurses to practice with resilience and integrity. 2021, 1–30. Wikiwisdom Forum.
24. Johnson, B. Polarity management: identifying and managing unsolvable problems. Amherst, MA: HRD Press; 1996.
25. Giordano LA, Elliott MN, Goldstein E, Lehrman WG, Spencer PA. Development, implementation, and public reporting of the HCAHPS survey. Med Care Res Rev. 2010;67(1):27–37.
26. Scoville R, Little K, Rakover J, et al. *Sustaining improvement: IHI white paper.* Cambridge, MA: Institute for Healthcare Improvement; 2016.
27. Perlo J, Balik B, Swensen S, et al. *IHI framework for improving joy in work: IHI white paper.* Cambridge, MA: Institute for Healthcare Improvement; 2017.

28. IHI Team. Joy in work: more than the absence of burnout. Institute for Healthcare Improvement. Published August 1, 2017. Accessed May 29, 2023. https://www.ihi.org/communities/blogs/joy-in-work-more-than-the-absence-of-burnout.
29. IHI Multimedia Team. How a joy in work team advanced culture change. Institute for Healthcare Improvement. Published June 1, 2018. Accessed May 29, 2023. https://www.ihi.org/communities/blogs/how-a-joy-in-work-team-advanced-culture-change.
30. National Academies of Sciences, Engineering, and Medicine. Taking action against clinician burnout: a systems approach to professional well-being. Washington, DC: National Academies Press; 2019.
31. Sexton JD, Pennebaker JW, Holzmueller CG, Wu AW, Berenholtz SM, Swoboda SM, et al. Care for the caregiver: benefits of expressive writing for nurses in the United States. Prog Palliat Care. 2009;17(6):307–312.
32. Berwick D, Loehrer S, Gunther-Murphy C. Breaking the rules for better care. JAMA. 2017;317(21):2161–2162.
33. Wagner EH, Glasgow RE, Davis C, Bonomi AE, Provost L, McCulloch D, et al. Quality improvement in chronic illness care: a collaborative approach. Jt Comm J Qual Improv. 2001;27(2):63–80.
34. Massoud MR, Nielsen GA, Nolan K, et al. A framework for spread: from local improvements to system-wide change: IHI innovation series white paper. Cambridge, MA: Institute for Healthcare Improvement; 2006.
35. Weintraub P, McKee M. Leadership for innovation in healthcare: an exploration. Int J Health Policy Manag. 2019;8(3):138–144.
36. Heinze KE, Hanson G, Holtz, H, et al. Measuring health care professionals' moral resilience: validation of the Rushton Moral Resilience Scale. J Palliat Med. 2021;24(6):865–872.
37. Nelson KE, Hanson GC, Boyce, D, et al. Organizational impact on health care workers' moral injury during COVID-19: a mixed-methods analysis. J Nurs Adm. 2022;52(1):57–66.
38. FitzGerald C, Hurst S. Implicit bias in healthcare professionals: a systematic review. BMC Med Ethics. 2017;18(1):19.
39. Goddu AP, O'Connor KJ, Lanzkron S, et al. Do words matter? Stigmatizing language and the transmission of bias in the medical record. J Gen Intern Med. 2018;33(5): 685–691.
40. Rushton CH, Manbauman C. A web of interconnection: relational integrity in critical care nursing. 2023 AACN Adv Crit Care. In press.
41. McBride S, Alexander GL, Baernholdt M, et al. Scoping review: Positive and negative impact of technology on clinicians. Nurs Outlook. 2023;71(2):101918.
42. Hendrix JM, Sharp CD, Page SL, Popovich M. The disinformation and politicization of health care. ASA Monitor. 2023;87:40–42.

43. Ford BQ, Feinberg M, Lassetter B, et al. (2023). The political is personal: The costs of daily politics. J Pers Soc Psychol. 2023;125(1):1–28.
44. Webster SW, Albertson B. Emotion and politics: Noncognitive psychological biases in public opinion. Annu Rev Political Sci. 2022;25(1):401–418.
45. Cutler D, Wikler E, Basch P. Reducing administrative costs and improving the health care system. N Engl J Med. 2012;367(20):1875–1878.
46. Berwick DM, Hackbarth AD. Eliminating waste in US health care. JAMA. 2012;307(14):1513–1516.
47. Stichler JF. Healthy, healthful, and healing environments: a nursing imperative. Crit Care Nurs Q. 2009;32(3):176–188.
48. Quinn M. Evaluation for the way we work. Nonprofit Q. Published 2006. Accessed February 12, 2018. http://nonprofitquarterly.org/2006/03/21/evaluation-for-the-way-we-work/.
49. Campbell CA. Reflections on leadership. Perspect Health Inf Manag. 2013;10:1b.
50. Sofer D. Panel discussion 2: promising system and environmental strategies for addressing moral distress and building moral resilience. Am J Nurs. 2017;117(2):S18–S20.
51. Anderson-Shaw L, Ahrens W, Fetzer M. Ethics consultation in the emergency department. JONAS Healthc Law Ethics Regul. 2007;9(1):32–35.
52. Pavlish C, Brown-Saltzman K, Hersh M, Shirk M, Nudelman O. Early indicators and risk factors for ethical issues in clinical practice. J Nurs Scholarsh. 2011;43(1):13–21.
53. Pavlish C, Brown-Saltzman K, Fine A, Jakel P. Making the call: a proactive ethics framework. HEC Forum. 2013;25(3):269–283.
54. Trotochaud K, Fitzgerald H, Knackstedt A. Ethics champion programs: a promising practice to promote moral agency in healthcare settings. Am J Nurs. In press.
55. McAndrew NS, Leske JS, Garcia A. Influence of moral distress on the professional practice environment during prognostic conflict in critical care. J Trauma Nurs. 2011;18(4):221–230.
56. Brenner MJ, Hickson GB, Boothman, JD, et al. Honesty and transparency, indispensable to the clinical mission—Part III: How leaders can prevent burnout, foster wellness and recovery, and instill resilience. Otolaryngol Clin North Am. 2022;55(1):83–103.
57. Mercier H. Confirmation bias—my side bias. In Pohl RF, editor, Cognitive illusions: intriguing phenomena in judgement, thinking and memory. London: Taylor and Francis; 2016: 99–114.
58. Nickerson RS. Confirmation bias: a ubiquitous phenomenon in many guises. *Rev Gen Psychol.* 1998;2(2):175–220.
59. Reina ML, Reina DS, Rushton CH. Trust: the foundation for team collaboration and healthy work environments. AACN Adv Crit Care. 2007;18(2):103–108.

60. Rushton CH, Wood LJ, Grimley K, et al. Rebuilding a foundation of trust: A call to action in creating a safe environment for everyone. PXJ. 2021;8(3):5–12.
61. Danis M, Fox E, Tarzian A, et al. Health care ethics programs in U.S. hospitals: results from a national survey. BMC Med Ethics. 2021;22(1):107.
62. Nelson WA, Taylor E, Walsh T. Building an ethical culture. Health Care Manag. 2020;39(4):168–174.
63. US Department of Veterans Affairs. About Veterans Health Administration. Updated June 30, 2023. Accessed June 2, 2023. https://www.va.gov/health/aboutvha.asp.
64. Tarzian AJ, Berkowitz KA, Geppert CMA. Tertiary healthcare ethics consultation: enhancing access to expertise. J Clin Ethics. 2022;33(4):314–322.
65. Geppert CM, Berkowitz KA, Schonfeld T, Tarzian AJ. COVID-19 ethics debrief: pearls and pitfalls of a hub and spoke model. J Clin Ethics. 2022;33(1):63–68.
66. Schwartz Center for Compassionate Healthcare. Healing Healthcare Initiative. Updated 2023. Accessed December 15, 2022. https://www.theschwartzcenter.org/hhi/.
67. Schwartz Center for Compassionate Healthcare. Six pilot health organizations selected for Schwartz Center's inaugural Healing Healthcare Initiative. Published January 24, 2023. Accessed June 2, 2023. https://www.theschwartzcenter.org/press/six-pilot-health-organizations-selected-for-schwartz-centers-inaugural-healing-healthcare-initiative/.
68. American Organization for Nursing Leadership. Personal resilience for leaders. Accessed March 25, 2023. https://www.aonl.org/education/Personal-Resilience-for-Leaders.
69. Ulrich B, Cassidy L, Barden C, et al. National nurse work environments—October 2021: a status report. Crit Care Nurse. 2022;42(5):58–70.
70. Institute of Medicine. Primary care and public health: exploring integration to improve population health. Washington, DC: National Academies Press; 2012.
71. Moss M, Good VS, Gozal D, et al. An official critical care societies collaborative statement: burnout syndrome in critical care healthcare professionals: a call for action. Crit Care Med. 2016;44(7):1414–1421.
72. American Nurses Association. Exploring moral resilience toward a culture of ethical practice. Silver Spring, MD: ANA; 2017. Accessed February 12, 2018. www.nursingworld.org/MainMenuCategories/Policy- Advocacy/Professional-Issues-Panels/Moral-Resilience-Panel/ExploringMoralResilience.pdf.
73. National Academy of Medicine. Action collaborative on clinician well-being and resilience. Washington DC: NAM; n.d. Accessed February 12, 2018. http://nam.edu/initiatives/clinician-resilience-and-well-being/.
74. US Department of Health and Human Services. Addressing health worker burnout: The U.S. Surgeon General's advisory on building a thriving health

workforce. Published 2022. Accessed February 24, 2023. https://www.hhs.gov/surgeongeneral/priorities/health-worker-burnout/index.html

75. US Department of Health and Human Services. Current priorities of the U.S. Surgeon General. Published 2022. Accessed March 7, 2023. https://www.hhs.gov/sites/default/files/workplace-mental-health-well-being.pdf.
76. Rushton CH, Schwartz J. A legislatively mandated council: a model for palliative care policy integration. J Palliat Med. 2011;14(11):1240–1245.
77. Maryland Health Care Decisions Act of 1993. Md. Code Ann., Health-Gen. Sections 5.601-S.618; 1994.
78. Rushton CH, Schoonover-Shoffner K, Kennedy MS. Executive summary: transforming moral distress into moral resilience in nursing. Am J Nurs. 2017;117(2):52–56.
79. Rushton CH. Cultivating Moral Resilience. *Amer J Nur.* 2017;117(2–S1):S11–S15.
80. American Nurses Association Professional Issues Panel on Moral Resilience. Exploring moral resilience toward a culture of ethical practice. Silver Spring, MD: ANA; 2017. Accessed June 14, 2023. www.nursingworld.org/MainMenuCategories/Policy-Advocacy/Professional-Issues-Panels/Moral-Resilience-Panel/ExploringMoralResilience.pdf.
81. Koirala B, Davidson PM, Rushton, CH. Ethics in nursing: progress on national nursing ethics summit. Nurs Outlook. 2022;70(1):154–165.
82. National Academy of Medicine. National plan for health workforce well-being. Washington, DC: National Academies Press; 2022. Accessed May 29, 2023.
83. Pitts SI, Maruthur NM, Luu N, Curreri K, Grimes R, Nigrin C, et al. Implementing the comprehensive unit-based safety program (CUSP) to improve patient safety in an academic primary care practice. Jt Comm J Qual Patient Saf. 2017;43(11):591–597.
84. Pottenger BC, Davis RO, Miller J, Allen L, Sawyer M, Pronovost PJ. Comprehensive unit-based safety program (CUSP) to improve patient experience: how a hospital enhanced care transitions and discharge processes. Qual Manag Health Care. 2016;25(4):197–202.
85. Carrese JA. Members of the American Society for Bioethics and Humanities Clinical Ethics Consultation Affairs Standing Committee. HCEC pearls and pitfalls: suggested do's and don'ts for healthcare ethics consultants. J Clin Ethics. 2012;23(3):234–240.
86. Tarzian AJ. ASHB Core Competencies Update Task Force. Health care ethics consultation: an update on core competencies and emerging standards from the American Society for Bioethics and Humanities' Core Competencies Update Task Force. Am J Bioethics 2013;13(2):3–13.
87. Rushton CH. Creating a culture of ethical practice in health care delivery systems. Hastings Cent Rep. 2016;46(S1):S28–S31.
88. Ozar D. Who are "unrepresented" patients and what count as "important" medical decisions for them? AMA J Ethics. 2019;21(7):E611–616.

89. De Korne DF, Sol KJ, van Wijngaarden JD, van Vliet EJ, Custers T, Cubbon M, et al. Evaluation of an international benchmarking initiative in nine eye hospitals. Health Care Manage Rev. 2010;35(1):23–35.
90. Doran GT. There's a S.M.A.R.T. way to write management's goals and objectives. Manag Rev. 1981;70(11):35–36.
91. Fine LG. The SWOT analysis: using your strength to overcome weaknesses, using opportunities to overcome threats. Kick It, LLC; 2010.
92. Humphrey AS. SWOT analysis for management consulting. SRI Alumni Association Newsletter. Dec 2005. http://www.sri.com/sites/default/files/brochures/dec-05.pdf.
93. Office of the Surgeon General, Framework for Workplace Mental Health&Wellbeing, 2022, accessed August 2, 2023, https://www.hhs.gov/surgeongeneral/priorities/workplace-well-being/index.html.
94. Rushton CH, Thomas TA, Antonsdottir IM, et al. Moral injury and moral resilience in health care workers during COVID-19 pandemic. J Palliat Med. 2022;25(5):712–719.
95. Goltz J. You're the boss; insanity redefined. New York Times, July 21, 2011.
96. Serafin L, Kusiak A, Czarkowska-Pączek B. The COVID-19 pandemic increased burnout and bullying among newly graduated nurses but did not impact the relationship between burnout and bullying and self-labelled subjective feeling of being bullied: a cross-sectional, comparative study. Int J Environ Res Public Health. Feb 2, 2022;19(3):1730.
97. Lewis C. The impact of interprofessional incivility on medical performance, service, and patient care: a systematic review. Future Healthc J. 2023;10(1):1–9.
98. Hickson GB, Pichert JW, Webb LE, Gabbe S. A complementary approach to promoting professionalism: identifying, measuring, and addressing unprofessional behaviors. Acad Med. 2007;82(11):1040–1048.
99. Trzeciak S, Mazzarelli A. Compassionomics: the revolutionary scientific evidence that caring makes a difference. Studer Group; 2019.
100. Chmielewski J, Łoś K, Łuczyński W. Mindfulness in healthcare professionals and medical education. Int J Occup Med Environ Health. 2021;34(1):1–14.
101. Halifax J. G.R.A.C.E. for nurses: cultivating compassion in nurse/patient interactions. J Nurs Educ Pract. 2014;4(1):121–128.
102. Helft PR, Bledsoe PD, Hancock M, Wocial LD. An evaluation of unit-based ethics conversations. JONAS Healthc Law Ethics Regul. 2010;12(2):48–54.
103. Buchbinder M, Berlinger N, Browne A, Buchbinder L, Jenkins T. Responding to moral stress in hospital based clinical practice. Summary and key recommendations from STEPPS (2023). https://www.steppsmed.com/summary.
104. Henderson CM, Williams EP, Shapiro MC, Hahn E, Wright-Sexton L, Hutton N, et al. "Stuck in the ICU": caring for children with chronic critical illness. Pediatr Crit Care Med. 2017;18(11):e561–e568.

105. Shapiro MC, Henderson CM, Hutton N, Boss RD. Defining pediatric chronic critical illness for clinical care, research, and policy. Hosp Pediatr. 2017;7(4):236–244.
106. Rushton C, Nelson K, Antonsdottir I, et al. Perceived organizational effectiveness, moral injury, and moral resilience among nurses during the COVID-19 pandemic: secondary analysis. Nurs Manage. 2022;53(7):12–22.
107. Zajac S, Woods A, Tannenbaum S, et al. Overcoming challenges to teamwork in healthcare: a team effectiveness framework and evidence-based guidance. Front Commun. 2021;6:606445.
108. Whitehead PB, Herbertson RK, Hamric AB, Epstein EG, Fisher JM. Moral distress among healthcare professionals: report of an institution-wide survey. J Nurs Scholarsh. 2015;47(2):117–125.
109. Stein-Parbury J, Liaschenko J. Understanding collaboration between nurses and physicians as knowledge at work. Am J Crit Care. 2007;16(5):470–477.
110. Cullati S, Bochatay N, Maître F, et al. When team conflicts threaten quality of care: a study of health care professionals' experiences and perceptions. MCP:IQ&O. 2019;3(1):43–51.
111. Azoulay E, Timsit J, Sprung CL, Soares M, Rusinová K, Lafabrie A, et al. Prevalence and factors of intensive care unit conflicts: the Conflicus study. Am J Respir Crit Care Med. 2009;180(9):853–860.
112. Kaissi A. Manager-physician relationships: an organizational theory perspective. Health Care Manag. 2005;24(2):165–176.
113. Hsiao CH, Wu JC, Lin PC, et al. Effectiveness of interprofessional shared decision-making training: a mixed-method study. Patient Educ Couns. 2022;105(11):3287–3297.
114. Bedwell WL, Wildman JL, DiazGranados D, Salazar M, Kramer WS, Salas E. Collaboration at work: an integrative multilevel conceptualization. Hum Resour Manage Rev. 2012;22(2):128–145.
115. Weller J, Boyd M, Cumin D. Teams, tribes and patient safety: overcoming barriers to effective teamwork in healthcare. Postgrad Med J. 2014;90(1061):149–154.
116. Samai C, Campbell R. Culture, teamwork and engagement: 40 years of finding the right ingredients. Curr Opin Cardiol. 2021 Jan;36(1):105–109.
117. Bailey KD, Cardin S. Engagement in nursing: One organization's success. Nurs Adm Q. 2018;42(3):223–230.
118. Dietz AS, Pronovost PJ, Mendez-Tellez PA, et al. A systematic review of teamwork in the intensive care unit: what do we know about teamwork, team tasks, and improvement strategies? J Crit Care. 2017;29(6):908–914.
119. Frankel A, Haraden C, Federico F, Lenoci-Edwards J. A framework for safe, reliable, and effective care. Cambridge, MA: Institute for Healthcare Improvement; 2017. Accessed February 12, 2018. http://www.ihi.org/resources/Pages/IHIWhitePapers/Framework-Safe-Reliable-Effective-Care.aspx.

120. Silverman H, Wilson T, Tisherman S, et al. Ethical decision-making climate, moral distress, and intention to leave among ICU professionals in a tertiary academic hospital center. BMC Med Ethics. Apr 19, 2022;23(1):45.
121. Schlak AE, Rosa WE, Rushton CH, et al. An expanded institutional and national-level blueprint to address nurse burnout and moral suffering. Nurs Manage. 2022;53(1):16–27.
122. Houston S, Casanova MA, Leveille M, Schmidt KL, Barnes SA, Trungale KR, et al. The intensity and frequency of moral distress among different healthcare disciplines. J Clin Ethics. 2013;24(2):98–112.
123. Oh Y, Gastmans C. Moral distress experienced by nurses: a quantitative literature review. Nurs Ethics. 2015;22(1):15–31.
124. Meth N, Lawless B, Hawryluck L. Conflicts in the ICU: perspectives of administrators and clinicians. Intensive Care Med. 2009;35(12):2068–2077.
125. Fry-Bowers E, Rushton C. Reimagining nursing's social contract with the public. Am Nur J. 18(9), 3-8.
126. Institute of Medicine. Dying in America: improving quality and honoring individual preferences near the end of life. Washington, DC: National Academies Press; 2015.
127. Coalition to Transform Advanced Care. Coalition to transform advanced care: about Internet. Washington, DC: C-TAC; 2017. http://www.thectac.org/about/.
128. Back AL, Grant MS, McCabe PJ. Public messaging for serious illness care in the age of Coronavirus disease: cutting through misconceptions, mixed feelings, and distrust. J Palliat Med. 2021;24(6):816–819.
129. Findling MG, Blendon RJ, Benson JM. Polarized public opinion about public health during the COVID-19 pandemic: political divides and future implications. JAMA Health Forum. 2022;3(3):e220016.
130. Fry-Bowers E, Rushton C. Who will be there to care if there are no more nurses? Hastings Center Bioethics Forum. Published September 23, 2021. Accessed March 26, 2023. https://www.thehastingscenter.org/who-will-be-there-to-care-if-there-are-no-more-nurses/.
131. Rushton C, Doerries B, Greene J, Geller G. In the tragedy of this pandemic, dramatic interventions can heal moral suffering. The Lancet. Published July 23, 2020. Accessed March 26, 2023. https://www.thelancet.com/journals/lancet/article/PIIS0140-6736(20)31641-X/fulltext.
132. Dyrbye LN, Shanafelt TD, Sinsky CA, et al. Burnout among health care professionals: a call to explore and address this underrecognized threat to safe, high-quality care. NAM Perspectives. Washington, DC: National Academy of Medicine; 2017. http://nam.edu/wp-content/uploads/2017/07/Burnout-Among-Health-Care-Professionals-A-Call-to-Explore-and-Address-This-Underrecognized-Threat.pdf

133. CEO Coalition. Updated 2023. Accessed December 27, 2022. https://www.ceocoalition.com.
134. American Medical Association. AMA STEPS Forward Program. Updated 2023. Accessed March 23, 2023. https://www.ama-assn.org/practice-management/ama-steps-forward.
135. The Daisy Foundation. The DAISY award for nursing ethics. Accessed March 24, 2023. https://www.daisyfoundation.org/nursing-ethics.
136. Butler CR, Wong SPY, Wightman AG, O'Hare AM. US clinicians' experiences and perspectives on resource limitation and patient care during the COVID-19 pandemic. JAMA Netw Open. 2020;3(11):e2027315.
137. Gonzalez CM, Hossain O, Peek ME. Frontline physician perspectives on their experiences working during the first wave of the COVID-19 pandemic. J Gen Intern Med. 2022;37:4233–4240.
138. Butler CR, Wong SPY, Vig EK, et al. Professional roles and relationships during the COVID-19 pandemic: a qualitative study among US clinicians. BMJ Open. 2021;11:e047782.
139. Berwick DM. *Salve Lucrum*: the existential threat of greed in US health care. JAMA. 2023;329(8):629–630.
140. Rynders T. How the arts help us hold grief and maintain collective care. JAMA Ethics. 2022;24(7):E681–684.
141. Pavlish C, Brown-Saltzman K, So L, Wong J. Support: an evidence-based model for leaders addressing moral distress. J Nurs Adm. 2016;46(6):313–320.

Afterword

A VISION FOR THE FUTURE

Cynda Hylton Rushton

IMAGINE A HEALTHCARE system where clinicians and leaders cultivated and embodied their moral resilience and practiced within a culture where ethical practice was normative, systems were in place that reflected essential shared values, and leaders demonstrated their essence in communication, decisions, priorities, and investments. Imagine a new paradigm as well where communities collaborated with clinicians and healthcare organizations to design systems with purpose, transparency, shared values, and a results orientation; where the expectations of those we serve and the greater society are realistically aligned with what is possible within the limits of biological and scientific understanding, resource constraints, and human caring.

What would be different? We can imagine that there might be less burnout, fewer errors, more collaboration, excellent teamwork, and higher patient satisfaction. Clinicians would be able to know themselves intimately, practice in ways that uphold their vows and codes of ethics, be buoyant amid ethical challenges, be confident and capable in recognizing and addressing ethical problems and demonstrate their commitment to self-stewardship in their day-to-day choices and actions. Healthcare organizations would become sanctuaries of health and healing; clinicians and leaders would respectfully co-create and design solutions; leaders would align their essential values with strategic priorities and budget allocations. Ethics infrastructure, including ongoing surveillance, assessment,

Cynda Hylton Rushton, *Afterword* In: *Moral Resilience*. Second Edition. Edited by: Cynda Hylton Rushton, Oxford University Press. © Oxford University Press 2024. DOI: 10.1093/oso/9780197667149.003.0013

feedback loops, robust ethics consultation, and education, policies, and processes to address and resolve ethical concerns, would be part of day-to-day operations. The healthcare industry would take seriously and commit to systemic changes to create cultures that support ethical practice and address the factors that produce moral suffering and burnout. Adequate human and material resources would enable safe, quality care for all. Incentives within the system would be oriented toward essential values and commitments and would disable those that undermine integrity. A new dashboard of tools would measure the impact of initiatives to address the multi-faceted dimensions of moral adversity. Institutions responsible for training clinicians would reform their curricula to integrate ethics and moral resilience into the fabric of their programs and would work with accrediting bodies to align their focus with licensure examinations. New programs of research would be launched with the support of funding collaboratives. Societal expectations regarding health and healthcare would be clarified through authentic dialogue and actionable design. The societal contract between nurses, doctors, and others would be re-imagined through a bidirectional social covenant that upholds relational integrity for everyone.[1] Patients, families, and communities would become learning partners with clinicians, healthcare organizations, and community institutions. Education about health and personal responsibility would be a thread woven through all levels of preparation beginning with K–12. Beyond these, there are vast possibilities for individuals to leverage and strengthen their innate and learned abilities to address moral adversity and to collaborate with leaders to reform systems to create a sustainable culture of ethical practice.

We are not naïve, nor are we denying the severity of moral suffering in healthcare. Moral suffering in healthcare is not going to go away; the likelihood is that it will continue and will even intensify as national and global realities unfold. As evidenced by the COVID-19 pandemic, current models are insufficient to meet future demands. We must unlock the potential of a new paradigm by opening our hearts and minds to new understandings and possibilities that we have heretofore not seen or understood. We need supportive and collaborative spaces to allow our minds to rest enough to shift from our entrenched ways of being and thinking to discover what is indeed attainable and necessary. We need new skills to allow ourselves to recognize when we are stuck in a repeating narrative of disempowerment and despair and to be able to let go of what no longer serves and embrace a vision for our desired future. When we mindfully come together and a critical mass arises, real change is possible.

Beginning the process starts with believing that change is possible and working together to launch a vision of possibility and hope. We must take the long view of culture change to begin intentionally and incrementally to shift the patterns that undermine personal and professional integrity and ethical practice by grounding our efforts in our essential values. As outlined in this book, we must invest in supporting clinicians to leverage and strengthen their innate and learned abilities to address moral adversity and eliminate the root causes of moral adversity for individual strategies to be sustainable and ethical practice environments to flourish. Solutions must align the dynamic interplay among individuals, teams, organizations, and the broader society. We need to find solutions at the local level, to build infrastructure to monitor and respond to ethical challenges and moral adversity, and to co-create mechanisms to address the root causes of threats to integrity and to modify the sources of moral adversity.

Much more work is needed—more empirical research, better measurement tools, more transdisciplinary forums, more groundbreaking reports from our professional associations and healthcare advocacy groups. There is an urgent need to refine, study, and systematically address some of the systemic factors that contribute to moral suffering and to devise innovative, effective, sustainable, and scalable methods for addressing them. What we offer in this book is only the beginning of large-scale innovation and culture change in healthcare that leverages the excellent scholarship of pioneers in transdisciplinary initiatives aimed at documenting the sources, consequences, and possible solutions for addressing moral adversity in healthcare. Multi-faceted approaches must harness the commitment and moral fortitude for system change that take into account the need for mindfulness, resilience, and joy.[2,3] Along with leading healthcare organizations, we embrace a "both/and" vision of what is needed to make meaningful and sustainable change in our healthcare ecosystem that includes both individual and systemic strategies and a robust research agenda.[4,5,6,7,8,9,10] Everyone must come together in a spirit of shared commitment to create the conditions for meaningful and sustainable change. Real change comes from the inside out. Clinicians and leaders must bridge the apparent gaps between their values and worldviews to co-create new patterns and paradigms that truly serve everyone. We are all fellow travelers on the journey to wholeness.

There is urgency for everyone—patients, families, clinicians, leaders, organizations, and communities—to come together in new ways. We invite others to add to the repertoire of promising practices and initiatives and to refine the concepts outlined in this book[11]. The time is now for releasing the residue of the past and focusing on the potential within the present to create a future that reflects who we really are, our commitments to the people we serve, and our dedication to bring integrity, compassion, and equity into our moment-to-moment experience.

In closing, we leave you with the wisdom of elders of the Hopi Nation:[12]

> There is a river flowing now very fast.
> It is so great and swift, that there are those who will be afraid.
> They will try to hold on to the shore.
> They will feel they are being torn apart and will suffer greatly.
> Know the river has its destination.
> The elders say we must let go of the shore,
> push off into the middle of the river, keep our eyes open,
> and our heads above the water.
> And I say, see who is in there with you and celebrate.
>
> At this time in history, we are to take nothing personally.
> Least of all, ourselves.
> For the moment that we do, our
> spiritual growth and journey comes to a halt.
>
> The time of the lone wolf is over. Gather yourselves!
>
> Banish the word *struggle* from your attitude and your vocabulary.
> All that we do now must be done in a sacred manner and in
> celebration.
>
> WE ARE THE ONES WE'VE BEEN WAITING FOR.

References

1. Fry-Bowers E, Rushton C. Reimagining nursing's social contract with the public. American Nurse Journal.18(9).ahead of print.
2. Sinsky CA. What if joy in practice were a metric? In Physician burnout: the root of the problem and the path to solutions. Waltham, MA: NEJM Catalyst; 2017: 41–42. http://join.catalyst.nejm.org/download/physician-burnout-collection.

3. Joseph R. Performance training and public health for physician burnout. In Physician burnout: the root of the problem and the path to solutions. Waltham, MA: NEJM Catalyst; 2017:43–46. http://join.catalyst.nejm.org/download/physician-burnout-collection.
4. Rushton CH, Schoonover-Shoffner K, Kennedy MS. A collaborative state of the science initiative: transforming moral distress into moral resilience in nursing. Am J Nurs. 2017;117(2):S2–S6.
5. American Nurses Association Professional Issues Panel on Moral Resilience. Exploring moral resilience toward a culture of ethical practice. Silver Spring, MD: American Nurses Association; 2017. http://nursingworld.org/ExploringMoralResilience.
6. Perlo J, Balik B, Swensen S, Kabcenell A, Landsman J, Feeley D. IHI framework for improving joy in work. Cambridge, MA: Institute for Healthcare Improvement; 2017. http://www.ihi.org/resources/Pages/IHIWhitePapers/Framework-Improving-Joy-in-Work.aspx.
7. Johnson Foundation. A gold bond to restore joy to nursing: a collaborative exchange of ideas to address burnout. Racine, WI: Johnson Foundation; 2017. http://www.qpatientinsight.com/uploads/2/0/7/1/20710150/nurses_at_wingspread__final.022217.pdf.
8. Johnson Foundation. Physician burnout in America: a roadmap for restoring joy and purpose in medicine. Racine, WI: Johnson Foundation; 2016. http://www.qpatientinsight.com/uploads/2/0/7/1/20710150/healingbringsmejoy_final_print.pdf.
9. US Department of Health and Human Services. Addressing health worker burnout: The U.S. Surgeon General's advisory on building a thriving health workforce. Published 2022. Accessed February 24, 2023. https://www.hhs.gov/surgeongeneral/priorities/health-worker-burnout/index.html.
10. US Department of Health and Human Services. Current priorities of the U.S. Surgeon General. Published 2022. Accessed March 7, 2023. https://www.hhs.gov/sites/default/files/workplace-mental-health-well-being.pdf.
11. Rushton, C. Transforming moral suffering by cultivating moral resilience and ethical practice. Amer J of Crit Care.2023, 32 (4): 238–248.
12. Anonymous. Untitled poem [We are the ones we've been waiting for]. Inauguration Ceremony of Arnold Schwarzenegger [Program]. Sacramento, CA: State of California, 2007.

Index

For the benefit of digital users, indexed terms that span two pages (e.g., 52–53) may, on occasion, appear on only one of those pages.

Tables and figures are indicated by an italic t and f following the page/paragraph number.

act/acting. *see* CFSR approach; inner sphere
acting (inner sphere), 289–90, 298–301
Action Collaborative on Clinician Well-Being and Resilience, 148–49
acupuncture, 180
adaptation/adaptability
  buoyancy and, 170
  neurobiological resilience, 135–37
adversity. *see also* moral adversity
  buoyancy and, 169–71
  psychological resilience and, 137–41
  resilience and (*see* resilience)
affective empathy, 208–9
Albaqawi, H., 263
allostasis, 136–37
Alrashidi, M. S., 263
American Hospital Association, 323–24
American Journal of Nursing, 49, 324–25
American Medical Association, 102–3, 117*t*
American Nurses Association, 117*t*, 324–25, 342–43
American Nurses Association Code of Ethics for Nurses, 175–76
American Organization of Nurse Leaders, 323
American Society for Bioethics and Humanities, 341–42
amygdala, 136–37
anger
  moral distress and, 30–31, 37–39
  moral outrage and, 65*f*, 82–89
  moral potential of, 39
  respect and respond to, 199–200
  voicelessness and, 39–40
antecedent-focused emotion regulation strategies, 179–80
Antonsdottir, I., 260–61
anxiety
  anticipatory, 30–31, 71–72
  buoyancy, 169–71
  COVID-19 effects, 262–63
  crescendo effect, 45–46
  decision-making and, 178–79, 197–98
  imperiled integrity and, 69–70
  mindfulness and, 202

anxiety (*cont.*)
  moral adversity and, 68
  moral distress and, 30–31, 45–47, 68, 75–77, 80, 275–76
  moral sensitivity and, 213
  moral suffering and, 13, 20, 243–45
  physiologic/somatic responses to stressors, 198
  powerlessness and, 108–9
  self-stewardship and, 175–76, 217–20
  solutions to relieve, 285
appreciative inquiry, 289

Bandura, A., 85–87
Bartky, Sandra, 44
Beil, Mary Ann, 320
being (outer sphere), 287–88, 291–93
Being With Dying program, 3–4, 250–51
Berman Institute of Bioethics, 324–25
Beryl Institute, 175–76
bioethics performance improvement, 320
biofeedback, 203
Buddhism, 3
buoyancy
  adaptation/adaptability and, 170
  adversity and, 169–71
  anxiety and, 169–71
  capacities for moral resilience, 169–71
  flexibility and, 170
  hope and, 170
  moral adversity and, 169–71
  positive (supportive) relationships and, 169–71
  RMRS conceptual domain, 259*t*
burnout syndrome, 146–47, 148–49, 316–17

call of conscience, 49, 112–14, 123–24, 228–31, 238
Call to Action, 324–25
capacities for moral resilience. *see also* integrity
  buoyancy, 169–71
  in clinicians, 68, 72–73, 144–47
  competing moral/ethical claims, 213–15
  concept development, 5–6
  conscience, 49, 109–14, 238
  defined, 89–90
  determining action to take, 216–17
  expressive repair, 245–46
  fostering, 48–49, 135
  general discussion, 193–94
  individual level, 266
  inner sphere, 289–90, 298–301
  integrity
    heeding call of conscience, 112–14, 123–24, 228–31, 238
    Integrity begins with "I" statements, 103*t*
    meaning and purpose, 240–43
    moral adversity, 106
    moral agency, 69–70, 72–73, 75–76, 123–24
    moral courage, 237–39
    moral repair, 66, 90–93, 166–86, 243–52
    organizational integrity, 124–25, 126, 272–73, 279, 286, 290–91, 310
    personal integrity, 123–26, 168–69, 290
    potential responses to threats to, 250*t*
    response and repair strategies, 236–40
  limitations, acknowledging, 239–40
  listening skills, 207
  meditations, 140–41
  mindfulness and self-attunement, 194–95, 196–203
    acknowledging what our bodies tell us, 197–98
    mindfulness practices, 202–3

monitoring thought patterns, 200–2
mindfulness self-care program studies, 263–64
moral agency, 215–16
moral attunement, 211–12
moral compromise, 231–36
moral efficacy, 209–17
moral/ethical analysis, 210, 212–13
moral sensitivity, 210–11
open mindset, 204–6
overview, 7–8
pausing, 206–7, 206*t*
peer support systems, 208–9
practicing empathy, 208–9
protective factors, 8, 263
reflection and insight, 203–9
respecting and responding to emotions, 199–200
self-stewardship, 217–20
standing for what matters most, 195–96, 196*t*
transformational learning, 220–21, 311–15
values, 194–96

Carse, Alisa, 4
CFSR approach, 279–87. *see also* system design strategies
applying, 286–87, 310*f*, 310, 344–45
cognitive capacities bias in, 285
development of, 5
information flow, 281–82, 320–21
inner sphere, 282–83
interventions for individuals, 287–90
inner sphere, 289–90
middle sphere, 288–89
outer sphere, 287–88
interventions for teams and organizations, 290–301
inner sphere, 298–301
middle sphere, 293–98
outer sphere, 291–93
leveraging, 323–24
Nurse Residency Collaborative, 314–15
outer sphere, 283
overview, 8, 279–83
TCEP model, 5, 331–32
Toward a Culture of Ethical Practice (TCEP), 331–32
transparency, 320–21
universal values in, 283–84
change-makers, supporting, 281–82, 310, 325–28
chaplains, 21, 30, 33, 92–93, 258
clinicians
acknowledging what our bodies tell us, 197–98
advocacy by, 323–24
burnout syndrome, 146–47, 148–49, 316–17
call of conscience, 228–31
capacities for moral resilience in, 68, 72–73, 144–47
dedication to integrity, 100–1, 102
dissonance among, 14–15, 17–19, 100–1, 337
peer support systems, 208–9
personal transformational learning, 220–21, 311–15
resilience in, 144–47
respecting and responding to emotions, 199–200
RMRS moral injury scores/themes, 261–62
self-stewardship, 217–20
supporting/CFSR approach, 300
values in integrity, 101–4, 114–15, 119
voice, finding, 233–36
Codes of Ethics for Medicine and Nursing, 116–19, 117*t*
cognitive capacities, bias towards, 285. *see also* mindfulness
cognitive control, 201–2
cognitive dissonance. *see* dissonance
cognitive empathy (perspective-taking), 105, 208–9

cognitive residue, 45–46, 75–76, 126–27
Communities of Practice, 49
Compassionate Care Initiative, 5, 290
compassion fatigue, 179
Compassion in Action Review, 317
competitive culture, 339
compromise, 231–36
Connor-Davidson Resilience Scale (CD-RISC), 147–48, 256–57
conscience
  call of conscience, 49, 112–14, 123–24, 228–31, 238
  claims of, 126–29
  defined, 109–10
  dissonance and, 110–13, 126–27
  memory and, 229
  moral agency and, 105
  moral distress and, 32
  moral injury and, 77
  observing actions of others, 15, 126
  relational and socially mediated nature of, 111–12
  threats to, 126–29
  voicing moral adversity, 236, 246
Conscious Full Spectrum approach. *see* CFSR approach
consequent-focused emotion regulation strategies
  discernment, 71–72
  emotional suppression, 179–80
  reflection and insight, 203–9
conspiracy of silence, 14
control, sense of, 13–14
courage (moral courage), 237–39
COVID-19 pandemic
  as cause of burnout syndrome, 148–49
  cumulative risk of negative outcomes, 142–43
  mindfulness self-care program studies, 263–64
  moral apathy and, 81–82, 333
  moral distress and, 29–30, 34
  moral suffering and, 6, 17–19, 266
  narratives, reframing, 251–52
  opportunities arising from, 344
  oppressive narratives of nurses, 248
  RMRS moral distress measures, 262–64
  social fragmentation due to, 120–21, 341
  threats to integrity, 21, 311–12
creative mind, 283
crescendo effect, 45–46, 47
Cribb, A., 19, 71
critical reflection, 203–9
critical resilience, 184–85
culpability, 20, 71–72, 92–93
culture. *see also* ethical practice; resilience
  competitive, 339
  ethical culture, 273–75
  of self-stewardship, 23–24
cumulative risk (social ecological resilience), 142–43

Dalai Lama, 3
Daniels, N., 232
debriefings, 241–42
decision-making
  accountability in, 338–39
  anxiety and, 178–79, 197–98
  CFSR approach to, 296
  disempowering patterns of teams and organizations, 182, 331*t*, 337–41
  end-of-life decisions, 299
  information flow, 281–82, 320–21
  large-scale change and, 310
  mindfulness interventions and, 200–2
  system design strategies, 315–25
  transparency and, 320–21
decompensation, 293–94

denial, 19, 24, 43, 46, 75, 81, 218, 234–35, 244, 249–50
depersonalizing patients, 47–48
despair. *see also* moral suffering
buoyancy and, 169
changing narrative of, 240–41, 341–42, 357–58
contagious nature of, 18–19
isolation and, 44
language of, 234
mindfulness practices, 208–9
moral adversity and, 68–69, 169
moral agency and, 181–82
moral disengagement and, 85–86
moral distress and, 29–30, 36–37, 100–1
moral resilience and, 89–90, 184–85
moral suffering and, 13–14, 64, 133
powerlessness and, 38–39, 174, 183–84
transformation of, 7, 250–51, 295–96
voiceless suffering, 243–45
Didion, Joan, 238
diminished moral responsiveness, 41–43
Dinndorf-Hogenson, G. A., 238–39
disappointment, 13, 18–19, 20, 85–86, 302
discernment. *see also* CFSR approach
conscience and, 49, 113
integrity and, 66, 91–92, 93, 103–6, 116, 123–24
limitations, acknowledging, 239–40
moral agency, 215–16
moral efficacy and, 209–17
moral/ethical analysis, 212–13
pausing, 206–7, 206*t*
reflection and insight, 203–9
standing for what matters most, 195–96
when engaging in moral repair process, 167, 243–52
disciplinary mind, 283
disempowering patterns, 331*t*, 337–41
disillusionment, 41–43
dissonance, 17–19
among clinicians, 14–15, 17–19, 100–1, 337
conscience and, 110–13, 126–27
monitoring thought patterns, 200–2
moral adversity and, 163
moral apathy and, 244
moral injury and, 79
moral sensitivity development, 210–11
moral stress and, 71–72
moral suffering and, 74–75, 107–8, 120
powerlessness and, 229–30
reconciliation of, 92–93, 195–96, 212, 214–16, 242, 275–76, 285–86, 320–21
relational integrity and, 122
trust and, 274
doctrine of double effect, 18–19
do no harm commitment, 197–98, 299–300
double effect doctrine, 18–19

Eisenberg, Nancy, 198
either/or thinking, 83–84, 204, 338–39
electronic medical record, 184, 318–19, 334–35
embodying values, 64*f*, 119, 167, 171, 194, 208–9, 216–17, 281, 290, 331–32
emotional inhibition, 173–74
emotional residue, 30–31, 75–76, 126–27
emotional suppression, 179–80
emotion regulation. *see* self-regulation
emotions, respecting and responding to. *see* respecting and responding to emotions
empathic arousal
modulating, 236–37
neuroscience, 178–80
somatic remembering and, 198

empathic concern, 179
empathic distress, 178–80
empathic over-arousal, 42–43, 179–80, 208–9, 236–37, 244
empathy
affective, 208–9
cognitive, 105, 208–9
empathy fatigue, 179
listening skills, 177–78
monitoring thought patterns, 200–2
practicing, 208–9
end-of-life decisions, 299
ethical arrogance, 19
ethical competence, 4, 172, 173–74, 201–2, 205–6, 283, 345–46
ethical conflicts, 282–83, 299
ethical culture, 273–75
ethical laziness, 19
ethical practice
acknowledging what our bodies tell us, 197–98
approach for sustainable results, 279–83, 282*t*
CFSR approach, 283–87
applying, 286–87
interventions for individuals, 287–90
interventions for teams and organizations, 290–301
creating new narrative, 246–47, 272
cultivating culture of, 272, 301–2, 303*t*
ethical conflicts, 282–83, 299, 324
ethical culture, 273–75, 340
future of, 356–59
guidelines, development of, 3, 272
integrity, 271–72, 299 (*see also* integrity)
moral adversity in healthcare, 271–73
moral distress and, 34–36, 38, 45–46
moral residue and, 80–82
moral resilience and ethical practice template, 280*f*
moral weakness, 40–41
partial responses to moral adversity and suffering, 275–79, 276*f*
limitations of partial responses, 279
overview, 275–79
personal development only, 276*f*, 278*f*, 278–79
policy and patterns only, 276*f*, 277*f*, 277–78
tactics only, 276*f*, 276–77
personal transformational learning, 220–21, 311–15
social contract/covenant, 120–21
system design strategies
avoiding quick fixes, 285–86
creating new narrative, 296, 341–46, 342*t*
decision-making, 296
developing new patterns and rules, 295–97, 331–32, 335–37
embodying values, 274–75, 281–82, 332–35
enabling work environment, 293–98, 299–300, 337–41
external factors impacts, 297–98
general discussion, 310*f*, 310–28
pattern identification, 296–97
personal transformational learning, 220–21, 311–15
supporting change-makers/risk-takers, 281–82, 310, 325–28
transcending disempowering patterns, 296
transformational design for sustainable results, 298–301, 328–46, 331*t*
treatment access/payment, 298
typology, 64*f*, 64, 67*f*, 180–86, 181*f*
weigh competing moral/ethical claims, 213–15
ethics consultation, 2, 233, 277, 294–95, 300, 320–22, 324, 327–28, 334–35

eustress, 71–72, 73–74
experiential, council process, 250–52
expressive repair, 245–46
expressive suffering, 245–47
expressive writing/journaling, 247
external threats (neurobiological resilience), 135–37

fear
conscience and, 49
integrity and, 106
role stress response, 136–37, 199–200
fight, flight, or freeze response, 136–37, 197–98, 199–200
five minds, 283
flexibility, buoyancy and, 170
Framework for Workplace Mental Health & Well-Being, 329–30
Frankl, Victor, 203–4
frustration
moral distress, 83, 84–87
moral outrage, 65*f*, 83, 234

gag clauses, 333
Gillespie, B. M., 145
G.R.A.C.E. process, 119, 289, 335
gratitude
embodying, 102
gratitude circle, 313–14
of patient/family, 240–42
self-regulation and, 139–41, 173–75
in teams and organizations, 294–95, 313–14
value of expressing, 140, 145
conscience and, 112–14
growth orientation, 170–71
guilt. *see also* moral suffering
accepting feelings of, 88–89, 230, 238, 242–43
conscience and, 109–14
crescendo effect, 45–46, 47
disengagement and, 88–89
moral courage and, 238
moral distress and, 20, 30–31, 45–46
moral injury and, 78–79
moral outrage and, 229–30, 234
moral residue and, 80–81, 230
powerlessness and, 37–38

Halifax, Joan, 4, 102
HALT tool, 219–20
Healer's Art program, 3
Healing Healthcare Initiative, 322–23
healthcare system
as brittle organization, 6, 293–94
clinicians as moral anchor in, 37–38, 293–94, 301
clinicians' frustration with, 29–30, 344
ethical conduct within, 273–75
future vision of, 79, 332–35, 336, 356–59
moral adversity in, 89, 271–73
organizational integrity, 124–25, 126, 272–73, 279, 286, 290–91, 310
Health Decisions Act (Maryland), 324
Hippocratic Oath, 116–19
Holtz, H. K., 263
homeostasis
negativity bias, 137
neuroscience, 135–37, 178–80
Nightingale Pledge, 116–19
honesty and truthfulness. *see also* integrity
conscience and, 101–2, 110–11
moral repair and, 91–92
personal integrity, 119, 167
resilience and, 145
hope. *see also* resilience
buoyancy and, 170
eustress, 73
moral repair and, 243
resilience and, 140, 145, 309
Hopi Nation, 359

Hospital Consumer Assessment of Healthcare Providers and Systems survey, 315–16
humility
  acknowledging limitations, 232
  integrity and, 102
  moral resilience and, 174–75, 177
  self-regulation and, 206–7

IEWeb database, 321–22
imagination, 209–10
imperiled integrity, 107–9, 110*t*
indicators, 315–25
individual interventions (CFSR approach)
  inner sphere, 289–90, 298–301
  middle sphere, 288–89
  outer sphere, 287–88
infants of substance abusing mothers (ISAM), 85–87
informed consent, 35, 111, 295–97
initial moral distress, 47
inner sphere, 276, 281–83, 287, 289–90, 298–301
insight, reflection and, 203–9
insight practices, 203
Institute for Healthcare Improvement, 294, 315–17, 323–24
integrity. *see also* capacities for moral resilience
  claims of conscience, 126–29
  clinicians' dedication to, 100–1, 102
  clinicians' values in, 101–4, 114–15, 119
  conscience, 109–14
  defined, 166–69
  environment factors in, 5, 24
  ethical laziness/arrogance, 19
  ethical practice/moral resilience typology, 63–64, 64*f*, 67*f*
  heeding call of conscience, 112–14, 123–24, 228–31, 238
  limitations, acknowledging, 239–40
  moral agency, 104–6, 215–16
  organizational integrity, 124–25, 126, 272–73, 279, 286, 290–91, 310
  overview, 7
  personal integrity, 123–26, 290
  personal/professional, 101–4, 103*t*, 116, 167
  potential responses to threats to, 250*t*
  powerlessness and, 17–19
  preserving, 228
    Integrity begins with "I" statements, 103*t*
    integrity-preserving actions, 180–86, 181*f*
    meaning and purpose, 240–43
    moral courage, 237–39
    moral repair, 166–86
    moral sensitivity, 210–11
    relational integrity, 114–21, 167
    response and repair strategies, 70–71, 73–74, 76–77, 236–40, 245–46
    shared responsibility, 108, 122–23, 207, 252, 325–26
    sustaining, 102–4, 105–6, 119, 123–26, 168–69
  relational integrity, 90–91, 167, 168–69
  restored integrity (*see* restored integrity)
  self-stewardship, 175–76
  shifting patterns that undermine, 70
  threats to, 16–17, 20–22, 30–31, 69–71, 74–75, 88–89, 106–9, 110*t*
  values and, 194–96
internal threats (neurobiological resilience), self-stewardship and, 175–76
interventions, CFSR approach. *see* CFSR approach
isolation
  ethical practice impacts, 274, 277
  moral distress and, 39–41, 44, 92, 235–36

narrative impacts on, 247
negative emotions and, 199–200
self-regulation and, 36–37
self-stewardship and, 141–42, 219
social resilience and, 92, 141–42
voicelessness and, 16, 36–37, 39–41

Jameton, A., 30–31, 47, 63
job gratification, 145–46
Johns Hopkins Hospital Ethics Committee and Consultation Service, 3
Johns Hopkins University School of Nursing, 324–25
Joint Commission, 323–24
Journal of Christian Nursing, 324–25

Kazniack, Al, 4
Kornfeld Fellowship, 3
Kovanci, M. S., 264

Lamott, Anne, 238
language
in expressive repair, 245–46
of moral adversity, 233–35
of moral compromise, 231–36
of moral distress, 36–37, 86–87
in response/recognition, 22–23
of self-attunement, 203
large-scale change, 184–85. *see also* CFSR approach
enabling work environment, 283–84
personal transformational learning, 220–21, 311–15
in relational integrity, 114–21
supporting change-makers/risk-takers, 310
leadership. *see also* ethical practice
accountability to, 321, 338–39
change-makers, supporting, 281–82, 310, 325–28
culture change implementation role, 19, 184, 272–74, 290, 300–2, 303*t*, 322–23, 331–35, 342–43
ethics consultation process, 2, 233, 277, 294–95, 300, 320–22, 324, 327–28, 334–35
moral injury by, 77–78
personal transformational learning, 220–21, 311–15
professional integrity in, 116
in relational integrity, 252
3-factor model of, 147–48
learning in action communities, 302
LGBTQIA+ community, 319
limitations, acknowledging, 239–40
listening skills, 177–78, 207

Maslach Burnout Inventory (MBI), 148–49
Maslow's theory, 218
McCammon, Susan, 37–38, 39–40
McCullough, L. B., 285–86
Mead, Margaret, 290
meaninglessness, 242–43
measurement tools, 315–25
meditation, 140–41, 196–97, 203
Memorial Health, 320
memory
conscience and, 229
embodied, moral distress and, 46–47
moral distress and, 46–47
negative memory activation, 46
projecting past experiences onto current reality, 198, 288–89
somatic remembering, 198
working memory, 194–95
mentors, 299–300
MEPRA. *see* Mindful Ethical Practice and Resilience Academy (MEPRA)
Miller, S., 243–44

Mindful Ethical Practice and Resilience Academy (MEPRA), 4, 265, 313–15, 323, 337
mindfulness
acknowledging what our bodies tell us, 197–98
conscience and, 113
meditation training, 196–97
mindfulness practices, 202–3
monitoring thought patterns, 200–2
narratives and, 246–47
practices, 202–3
qualities and skills to support, 177–80
resilience and, 146–47
respecting and responding to emotions, 199–200
alternative orientation, 63–64, 64*f*
courage to maintain integrity, 119
imperiled integrity, 107–9, 110*t*
mindset, 204–6
moral agency, 104–6, 215–16
moral apathy, 65*f*, 81–82
moral compromise, 231–36
moral decline, 65*f*, 80–81
moral disengagement, 65*f*, 84–89, 126–27, 244
moral efficacy, 209–17
moral injury, 77–82
moral outrage, 65*f*, 82–89
moral repair, 66, 90–93, 243–52
moral resilience, 89–90
moral stress, 71–74
restored integrity, 75, 93–94
response and repair strategies, 236–40
self-care, 175–76, 263–64, 323
self-care program studies, 263–64
sensing into the body practice, 202
Mindfulness-Based Stress Reduction (MBSR), 3, 203, 289
mindsets, 4, 8–9, 68–69, 169, 200, 204–6, 302, 314–17, 319–20
mirror neurons, 179, 281–82
moral adversity
alternative meanings, 240–43
apathy, 65*f*, 81–82
buoyancy and, 169–71
claims of conscience, 126–29
defined, 68–69
disengagement, 65*f*, 84–89, 126–27, 244
integrity and, 106
integrity-preserving actions, 180–86, 181*f*
language of, 233–35
open mindset, 204–6
overview, 6–7, 8–9
resilience and, 135
responses to, 65*f*, 65–68, 67*f*, 138–39, 169, 244–45
self-regulation, 173–75
transformation of, 22–23, 73–74
voice, finding, 233–36
moral agency
courage and, 104–6
defined, 104–5
integrity and, 69–70, 72–73, 75–76, 123–24
narratives and, 247
respecting and responding to emotions, 104–6
responses to adversity, 138–41
social network and, 92–93
understanding boundaries of, 82, 101, 104–5, 108
upholding commitments in face of moral adversity, 89–90
moral attunement, 72, 93, 211–12
moral blindness, 72
moral compass
ethical practice culture creation, 301–2
fundamental values and, 100–1, 167, 194–96, 281
moral adversity and, 68, 271
moral injury and, 77–78

relational integrity interface with, 123, 291
self-stewardship, 175
standing for what matters most, 114–15, 195–96, 228, 314–17
moral compromise, 231–36
moral courage, 119
moral distress, 7. *see also* moral suffering
anger, 30–31, 37–39, 82–89
cognitive residue, 45–46, 75–76, 126–27
concept of, 30–32
contours/costs of, 36–43
cumulative dynamic of, 45*f*, 45–48, 65*f*
differing characterizations of, 232, 327
diminished moral responsiveness, 41–43
disempowerment, 39–40, 44
disillusionment, 41–43
emotional residue, 30–31, 75–76, 126–27
frustration, 30–31, 37–39
general discussion, 29–30
gradual onset of, 48, 50
initial *vs.* reactive, 47
isolation, 39–41, 44, 92
language of, 36–37, 86–87
mitigation of, 48–49
moral adversity and, 75–77
moral outrage and, 82–83
moral residue, 230
moral toll of, 36–43
opportunities created by, 48–49, 65*f*, 66, 73
personal narratives of, 35–40, 42–43, 45–46
physical residue, 44–47, 65*f*, 75–76, 80–82, 126–27
powerlessness, 37–39, 86–87, 293
selected individual-level responses to, 43
shame, 41–44
sources of, 33–36
unresolved, 43, 45–48
variations in frequency/intensity, 75–76, 135–36, 138
voicelessness, 39–41, 44, 172
moral efficacy, 171–72
capacities for moral resilience, 209–17
competing moral/ethical claims, 126–29
conflict of conscience and, 110–11, 238
courage and, 119
determining action to take, 216–17
moral agency, 104–6, 215–16
moral attunement, 211–12
moral/ethical analysis, 210, 212–13
moral outrage, 65*f*, 82–89
moral repair, 66, 90–93, 166–86, 243–52
moral sensitivity, 210–11
response and repair strategies, 236–40
responses to adversity, 138–39
RMRS conceptual domain, 259*t*
self-regulation, 173–75
self-stewardship, 175–76, 217–20
weigh competing moral/ethical claims, 213–15
moral harmony, 232
moral imagination, 177–78, 209–10, 238
moral injury
conscience and, 77
defined, 77–82
dissonance and, 79
guilt and, 78–79
military context, 77–78, 312
moral outrage and, 82–83
moral resilience and, 66
of physicians, 78
protective factors, 261, 263
RMRS scores/themes, 261–62
traumatic manifestations of, 78–79

moral nerve, 238
moral outrage, 65*f*, 82–89
moral repair, 66, 90–93, 243–52
moral residue, 80–82
moral resilience. *see* resilience
moral sensitivity, 210–11
moral stress. *see also* moral distress
  defined, 71–74
  integrity and, 70–71
  outrage, 65*f*, 82–89
  overview, 7
moral suffering. *see also* guilt
  adjusting view of, 22–24
  compassion in response to, 15–16
  defined, 2
  disengagement, 65*f*, 84–89, 126–27, 244
  feelings associated with, 15–16, 20
  future changes in, 22–24
  integrity-preserving actions, 180–86, 181*f*
  life-affirming view of, 75
  moral adversity and, 15, 18–19, 22–23, 74–75
  moral dimensions of suffering, 15–22
  moral dissonance in, 17–19, 71–72
  overview, 7
  phases of, 243–52
  reality of clinical practice, 12–14
  responses to, 65*f*, 67*f*
  Rushton's background, 1–6
  soul pain, 16–17, 74–75
  threats triggering, 20–22
moral weakness, 40–41
Morley, G., 184–85
movement practices, 203
mute suffering, 243–45

narratives
  alternative meanings, 240–43
  creating new narrative, 246–47, 296, 341–46, 342*t*, 357–58
  effects of, 205–6
  narrative repair, 247–49
  patterns of protest, 233–35
  power of, 246–47
National Academy of Medicine, 49, 148–49
National Center for Ethics in Health Care (NCEHC), 321–22
negative feelings/emotions
  dissonance, 46–47
  moral repair and, 66, 90–93, 243–52
  self-regulation and, 139–40
  SNS activation and, 197–98, 199–200
negativity bias, 137
Nelson, H. L., 248, 261
neonatal and pediatric settings, 35–36
neurobiological resilience, 135–37
Nightingale Pledge, 116–19
Nurse *Antigone,* The, 251–52
Nurse Residency Collaborative, 314–15

ombudsman, 277*f*, 277
open mindset, 204–6
organizational ethics
  organizational integrity, 120, 124–25
  for teams and organizations, 125–26
organizational integrity, 124–25, 126, 272–73, 279, 286, 290–91, 310
organizations. *see* teams and organizations

Palmer, Parker, 175–76
parasympathetic nervous system (PNS), 197, 200
partial responses to moral adversity in healthcare, 275–79, 276*f*
  limitations of, 279
  limitations of partial responses, 279
  overview, 275–79
  personal development only, 276*f*, 278*f*, 278–79
  policy and patterns only, 276*f*, 277*f*, 277–78
  tactics only, 276*f*, 276–77
patterns
  of decision-making, 182, 331*t*, 337–41

disempowering, 331*t*, 337–41
middle sphere, CFSR approach, 288–89, 293–98
monitoring thought patterns, 200–2
shifting patterns that undermine integrity, 70
tend and befriend, 197–98
transformational design for sustainable results, 298–301
pausing, 206–7, 206*t*, *see also* mindfulness
Pavlish, C., 345–46
peer coaches, 299–300
peer support systems, 208–9
personal agency, 138–40, 204
personal integrity, 123–26
in CFSR approach, 290
conceptualization, 167
interface between relational integrity and, 123–26
as precondition for relational integrity, 114–21, 167
RMRS conceptual domain, 259*t*
perspective-taking (cognitive empathy), 105, 208–9
phases of moral suffering
experiential, council process, 250–52
expressive repair, 245–46
understanding/engagement, 243–52
voiceless suffering, 243–45
physical residue, 44–47, 65*f*, 75–76, 80–82, 126–27
physicians. *see also* clinicians; moral distress
call of conscience, 107, 112–14, 123, 228–31
ethics consultation process, 327–28
moral injury, 78
powerlessness and, 80–81, 86–87, 107
Pike, A. W., 82–83
PNS (parasympathetic nervous system), 197, 200
policy and patterns only response to moral adversity, 276*f*, 277*f*, 277–78
positive emotionality
gratitude (*see* gratitude)
hope (*see* hope)
PNS activation, 197, 200
psychological resilience, 137–41
positive (supportive) relationships
buoyancy and, 169–71
listening skills, 207
moral outrage, 65*f*, 82–89
open mindset, 204–6
pausing, 206–7, 206*t*
practicing empathy, 208–9
psychological context (self-regulation), 139–41
psychological resilience, 137–41
reflection and insight, 203–9
resilience and, 145
self-regulation and, 139–41, 173–75
social ecological resilience, 141–44, 144*f*
positivity resonance, 200
post-traumatic growth, 180–86, 181*f*
powerlessness
anxiety and, 108–9
despair and, 38–39, 174, 183–84
dissonance and, 229–30
guilt and, 37–38
integrity and, 17–19
moral distress, 37–39, 86–87, 293
physicians and, 80–81, 86–87, 107
power on culture, 1
productivity-focused metrics, 339
Providence/St. Joseph Health, 311–12
psychological integrity, 20–21
psychological resilience, 137–41

quick fixes, avoiding, 285–86
Quigg, Laura, 263–64

reactive moral distress, 47
redemptive value of suffering, 13–14

Reich, Warren T., 2, 4, 17, 243, 244, 249–51
Reina Trust and Betrayal Model©™, 261
reintegration of self (psychological resilience), 137–41
relational context (social ecological resilience), 141–44, 144f
relational integrity, 114–21
  in clinical practice, 122–26, 167
  dissonance and, 122
  heeding call of conscience, 112–14, 123–24, 228–31
  leadership in, 252
  limitations, acknowledging, 239–40
  moral compromise, 231–36
  moral courage, 237–39
  moral repair and, 66, 90–93, 243–52
  personal integrity and, 123–26, 168–69
  RMRS conceptual domain, 259t
  solidarity of purpose, 116
resilience
  in clinicians, 144–47
  defined, 163, 256
  gender differences in, 263
  general discussion, 134–44
  integrity-preserving action, 180–86
  measurement of, 147–48, 256–57
  measurement tools, 315–25
  meditations and, 140–41
  mindfulness self-care program studies, 263–64
  moral complexity and, 257
  neurobiological resilience, 135–37
  neuroscience, 178–80
  outcome variables, 148–49
  predictors of, 146
  psychological resilience, 137–41
  qualities and skills to support, 177–80
  research directions, 147–48
  scholarship on, 162–66, 164t
  self-stewardship, 175–76
  social ecological resilience, 141–44, 144f
  typology, 180–86, 181f
Resilience in Stressful Events (RISE), 300
resource allocation, 22, 184, 285–86, 296, 332–33, 336–37
respectful mind, 283
respecting and responding to emotions, 199–200
  alternative orientation, 63–64, 64f
  courage to maintain integrity, 119
  imperiled integrity, 107–9, 110t
  mindset, 204–6
  moral agency, 104–6, 215–16
  moral apathy, 65f, 81–82
  moral compromise, 231–36
  moral decline, 65f, 80–81
  moral disengagement, 65f, 84–89, 126–27, 244
  moral efficacy, 209–17
  moral injury, 77–82
  moral outrage, 65f, 82–89
  moral repair, 66, 90–93, 243–52
  moral resilience, 89–90
  moral stress, 71–74
  restored integrity, 75, 93–94
  self-attunement and, 199–200
response and repair strategies (integrity), 236–40
responsibility
  alternative meanings, 240–43
  displacing onto others, 87–88
  open mindset, 204–6
  shared responsibility, 92–93, 108, 122–23, 207, 252, 325–26
  social contract/covenant, 120–21
  transparency and, 207, 273, 288, 296–97, 320–21
  understanding boundaries of, 23–24, 35, 73–75, 82, 101, 104–6, 108

restitution, 92–93
restored integrity, 228
  alternative meanings, 240–43
  general discussion, 75
  limitations, acknowledging, 239–40
  meaning and purpose, 240–43
  moral courage, 237–39
  moral efficacy and, 209–17
  moral resilience and, 93–94
  response and repair strategies, 236–40
  self-regulation, 139–41, 173–75
  self-stewardship, 7–8, 23–24, 73, 163, 175–76, 259*t*, 312–15, 356–57
  shared responsibility, 252
  voice, finding, 233–36
RISE (Resilience in Stressful Events), 300
risk-takers, supporting, 281–82
RMRS. *see* Rushton Moral Resilience Scale (RMRS)
R^3 (Renewal, Resilience & Retention) program, 314–15
Rushton, C. H., 256, 261–62, 264–65
Rushton Moral Resilience Scale (RMRS)
  applying, 318, 329–30
  conceptual domains, 259*t*
  cross-sectional analyses, 262, 263, 264–65
  cross-sectional online surveys, 261, 262–63
  development process, 258–60
  future directions of, 265–66
  mindfulness self-care program studies, 263–64
  mixed-methods analysis, 261, 263
  moral distress measures, 262–64
  overview, 8
  qualitative analysis, 263
  research studies, 260–64
  revised, 264–65
  secondary analysis, 261–62
  testing/validation of, 260, 264
  themes, 261–62, 265
  Turkish translation of, 264

Sabin, J. E., 232
sadness, 1, 13, 36–37, 199, 202, 244. *see also* moral suffering
scarcity paradigm, 336–37
scarcity thinking, 204
Schwartz Center for Compassionate Care, 322–23
secondary trauma, 42–43
self-attunement, 113
  acknowledging what our bodies tell us, 197–98
  general discussion, 196–203
  language of, 203
  mindfulness practices, 202–3
  monitoring thought patterns, 200–2
  respecting and responding to emotions, 199–200
  response and repair strategies, 236–40
self-awareness
  integrity and, 167
  moral disengagement and, 85–86, 244
  moral resilience and, 177–78
  neuroscience, 178
  outer sphere, CFSR approach, 278, 281–83, 287–88
  standing for what matters most, 195–96
self-betrayal, 75–76, 100–1, 103–4, 232
self-care, 175–76, 263–64, 323. *see also* self-stewardship
self-centered psychological functioning, 179
self-efficacy, 139
self-expression, 288–89

self-harm, 78–79, 238
self-regulation, 139–41
  creating culture of, 23–24
  isolation, 36–37
  middle sphere, CFSR approach, 277–83, 288–89
  mindfulness and self-attunement, 196–203
  moral efficacy and, 173–75
  response and repair strategies, 236–40
  RMRS conceptual domain, 259*t*
  self-stewardship, 175–76
  sensing into the body practice, 202
  shame, 41–43
self-related distress, 41
self-stewardship, 175–76, 217–20
  cultivation of, 313
  culture of, 23–24
  moral compass in, 175
  RMRS conceptual domain, 259*t*
Selye, H., 71
Serenity Prayer, 174–75
shame, 30–31, 36–37, 41–43. *see also* moral distress
shared responsibility, 92–93, 108, 122–23, 207, 252, 325–26
Sharma, Monica, 5, 283–84
Sherman, N., 77
Siegel, Dan, 203
silence
  conspiracy of silence, 14
  marginalization, 205
  reflection and insight, 7–8, 183, 199, 203–9
  as response to suffering, 244
  voicelessness, 39–41, 44, 172
SMART goals, 329
SNS (sympathetic nervous system), 197–98, 199–200
social ecological resilience, 141–44, 144*f*
  community response to adversity, 143
  cultivating positive relationships, 142
  cumulative risk, 142–43
  interdependence of individuals/ecosystems, 143
  interplay between personal/moral agency, 142–44
  overview, 141
  relational context, 141–42
  social ecological interdependence, 141–42
  social resilience, 141–42, 143
  social support, 142
social justice, 323–24, 336–37
social neuroscience, 178–80
social workers, 21, 30, 33, 258
Soelle, D., 75
solitude, value of, 203
somatic attunement, 202
somatic remembering, 198
soul pain, 16–17, 74–75
spaciousness, 203–9
Spilg, E., 262–63
Standards for Establishing and Sustaining Healthy Work Environments
  applying, 322–23
  experiential, council process, 250–52
  expressive repair, 245–46
  narrative, 246–47
  narrative repair, 247–49
  transformation, 249–50, 250*t*
  voiceless suffering, 243–45
storytelling, 205–6
stress contagion effect, 199–200, 281–82
stress response, 136–37
supportive (positive) relationships. *see* positive (supportive) relationships
Swavely, D., 263
SWOT (Strengths, Weaknesses, Opportunities, Threats) analyses, 329

sympathetic nervous system (SNS), 197–98, 199–200
Symposium on Transforming Moral Distress to Moral Resilience, 324–25
synergistic operational strategies, 310*f*
synthesizing mind, 283
system design strategies
  avoiding quick fixes, 285–86
  creating new narrative, 246–47, 296, 341–46, 342*t*
  decision-making, 296, 315–25
  developing new patterns and rules, 295–97, 331–32, 335–37
  embodying values, 274–75, 281–82, 332–35
  enabling work environment, 293–98, 299–300, 337–41
  external factors impacts, 297–98
  general discussion, 310*f*, 310–28
  integrity-preserving actions, 180–86, 181*f*
  pattern identification, 296–97
  personal transformational learning, 220–21, 311–15
  supporting change-makers/risk-takers, 281–82, 310, 325–28
  transcending disempowering patterns, 296
  transformational design for sustainable results, 298–301, 328–46, 331*t*
  treatment access/payment, 298
systems transformation/leadership, 5

tactics only responses to moral adversity, 276*f*, 276–77
tai chi, 203
Taking Action Against Clinician Burnout: A Systems Approach to Professional Wellbeing, 6
Tanahashi, Kazuaki, 126
TCEP (Toward a Culture of Ethical Practice), 5, 331–32
teams and organizations
  CFSR interventions for, 290–301
  competitive culture, 339
  disempowering patterns, 182, 331*t*, 337–41
  gratitude in, 294–95, 313–14
  measurement tools, 315–25
  shared decision-making, 338–39
tend and befriend pattern, 197–98
Theater of War: Frontline, 251–52
Thich Nhat Hanh, 63–64
Thomas, T. A., 262, 285–86
thought patterns, monitoring, 200–2
Toward a Culture of Ethical Practice (TCEP), 5, 331–32
toxic stress, 137
transformational design for sustainable results
  creating new narrative, 246–47
  developing new patterns and rules, 295–97
  system design strategies, 298–301
  transformational power, 249–50, 250*t*
  voice, finding, 233–36
transformational learning, 220–21, 311–15
transparency
  in CFSR approach, 320–21
  decision-making and, 320–21
  responsibility and, 207, 273, 288, 296–97, 320–21

understanding (middle sphere), 288–89, 293–98
universal values, 283–84
University of Virginia's Compassionate Care Initiative, 5, 290
unsettledness, 13
Upaya Institute, 250–51

us *vs.* them attitude, 311

Veterans Health Administration (VHA), 321–22
visualization, 203
voice, finding, 233–36
voicelessness, 39–41, 44, 172
  anger and, 39–40
voiceless suffering, 243–45

Walker, Margaret, 209–10, 252
walking wounded, 44
wandering mind, 201–2
West, C. P., 146–47
Wexton, P., 84–89
Winslow, B. J., 232
Winslow, G. R., 232
work-life climate measurement, 316–17
Wright, M. O., 139

yoga, 203